Clinical Anatomy of the Nose,
Nasal Cavity and Paranasal Sinuses

Clinical Anatomy of the Nose,
Nasal Cavity and Paranasal Sinuses

This book is to be returned on or before the last date stamped below.

PERMANENT LOAN TO E.N.T. OFFICE
I.A.K. ROOM

Clinical Anatomy of the Nose, Nasal Cavity and Paranasal Sinuses

Johannes Lang

Translated by P. M. Stell
Foreword by B. Proctor

183 Illustrations, most in color
14 Tables

1989
Georg Thieme Verlag
Stuttgart · New York

Thieme Medical Publishers, Inc.
New York

Prof. Dr. J. Lang
Vorstand des Anatomischen Instituts
der Universität Würzburg
Koellikerstr. 6
8700 Würzburg
FRG

Translator:
Prof. P. M. Stell, Ch. M., F.R.C.S.
University of Liverpool
Royal Liverpool Hospital
Prescot St.
P.O. Box 147
Liverpool L69 3BX
UK

Cover drawing by Renate Stockinger

Library of Congress Cataloging-in-Publication Data

Lang, Johannes.
  [Klinische Anatomie der Nase, Nasenhöhle, und Nebenhöhlen.
English]
  Clinical anatomy of the nose, nasal cavity, and paranasal sinuses
/ Johannes Lang ; translated by P. M. Stell ; foreword by B. Proctor.
  Translation of: Klinische Anatomie der Nase, Nasenhöhle, und
Nebenhöhlen.
  Includes bibliographies references.
  1. Nose--Atlases. 2. Nasal fossa--Atlases. 3. Paranasal sinuses-
-Atlases. I. Title.
  [DNLM: 1. Nasal Cavity--anatomy & histology. 2. Nose--anatomy &
histology. 3. Paranasal Sinuses--anatomy & histology. WV 300
L269k]QM505.L3613 1989 611'.86--dc20

© 1989 Georg Thieme Verlag, Rüdigerstrasse 14, D-7000 Stuttgart 30,
Germany
Thieme Medical Publishers, Inc., 381 Park Avenue South,
New York, N.Y. 10016

Typesetting by Druckhaus Götz KG, D-7140 Ludwigsburg
(System 5 [202] Linotype)
Printed in West-Germany by Druckhaus Götz KG,
D-7140 Ludwigsburg

ISBN 3-13-7384-01 (Georg Thieme Verlag, Stuttgart)
ISBN 0-86577-330-0 (Thieme Medical Publishers, Inc., New York)

1 2 3 4 5 6

Foreword

An important timely review of the clinical anatomy of the nose, nasal cavity, and paranasal sinuses, is presented by Professor Lang. He has intensively researched the anatomy of these structures for a quarter of a century, with emphasis on exact measurements of these vital structures as they relate to surgical intervention.

The history of the various surgical operations in this area is reviewed carefully and brought up to date. Structures of the nasal septum are given in detail. Septal deviations are described with causes. Vestibular cysts (nasoalveolar), hematomas, abscess and polyps of the septum are discussed.

The nasal cavity, its conchae, meatuses, orifices of the osteums of the paranasal sinuses etc. are described. Precautions during surgery are indicated. Particular attention is given to the variations in the osteums of the paranasal sinuses.

The size of the various paranasal sinuses and their relation to adjacent structures are detailed. Important surgical landmarks are pointed out and most important – their measured distance from vital structures are included.

The frontal sinus with its nasofrontal duct are discussed. The variations of its size and extent noted. Meningoencephalocele, mucocele, empyema of the frontal sinus and trauma are discussed.

A careful presentation of the maxillary sinus includes important measurements, its growth, the various recesses, septa and mucosal folds. A good discussion on "blowout" fractures, maxillary sinusitis, and pneumosinus dilatans follows.

Significant anatomy of the ethmoid cells is stressed. A detailed description and measurements of the sphenoid sinus follows. Important relations with the internal carotid artery, optic and other cranial nerves – lying in the adjacent cavernous sinus – are indicated.

Of clinical importance is the lacrymal duct and its nasal osteum which is carefully described and measured from important landmarks.

Measurements of the choana are shown. We then see the vessels of the nose, septum, and paranasal sinuses demonstrated, followed by a good description of the innervation of the nasal cavity.

The variable mucosa of the nasal cavity and paranasal sinuses are presented with a discussion of ciliary beat and mucus transport. Finally we have an exciting description of the optic canal and the medial approach for relief of optic compression.

In summary, Prof. Lang's book – The Clinical Anatomy of the Nose, Nasal Cavity, and Paranasal Sinuses – is of particular importance for the large number of measurements between specific landmarks (averaged and with upper and lower limits) – to help guide a nasal surgery of this difficult operation area. We thus avoid injury to important structures – while at the same time diseased tissue is removed – to effect a satisfactory cure.

This book is valuable information for the rhinologist's library as an important reference, and should also be available in operating rooms for immediate reference, should the need arise.

Bruce Proctor,
M.D., F.A.C.S.,
Clinical Professor of Otolaryngology; and Research Associate – Kresge Hearing Institute,
Ann Arbor, Michigan

Preface

This book is the distillate of many papers and courses for otorhinolaryngologists, neurosurgeons, neuroradiologists, oral and maxillofacial surgeons, neurologists, anatomists and physiologists. Its aim is to provide them all with their basic need for illustrations of nasal anatomy.

Anatomy is the oldest medical science. Therefore, I have taken great care to name the author who gave the original description of each structure. Ever since I started teaching anatomy, I have devoted my time to clinical anatomy and to contacts with clinicians, particularly those working on the head and neck. I am very grateful to the following Professors (in alphabetical order), and many other otorhinolaryngologists, neurosurgeons, neuroradiologists and neurologists, who have provided me with numerous ideas for research, and who have also provided illustrations:

Dr. Bumm, Chefarzt der HNO-Klinik Augsburg,
Dr. Denecke, HNO-Klinik, Heidelberg,
Dr. Draf, Chefarzt HNO-Klinik Fulda,
Dr. Helms, Direktor der Univ. HNO-Klinik, Würzburg,
Dr. Kley, em. Direktor der Univ. HNO-Klinik, Würzburg,
Dr. Wigand, Direktor der Univ. HNO-Klinik, Erlangen.

I am particularly grateful to Professor Dr. Naumann of Munich for extensive discussions about the choice of topics.

The statistical basis of measurements, counts, etc. could not have been achieved without the help of my current and former assistants, and numerous doctoral candidates. I would like to record my gratitude to them all.

All the diagrams have been prepared from photographs of my own sections of the nose and related structures. The measurements have been added by Mr. Cristof. I wish also to record my particular thanks to my secretary of many years standing, Mrs. K. Maak, to my technicians, Mrs. E. Engel and Mrs. I. Schatz, and to my photographer Mrs. E. Nenninger.

Also I wish to thank the Georg Thieme Verlag, particularly Dr. med. h. c. Günther Hauff and his colleagues, for their high technical standards and their cooperation in the preparation of this book.

I hope that this volume will contribute to surer diagnosis and safer surgery.

Würzburg, July 21, 1989   Johannes Lang

Recording of the data

Measurements throughout the book are shown by the mean (in millimeters) followed by the range, given in brackets. Angles are similarly shown as the mean (in degrees) with the range in brackets.

Contents

Prenatal Development of the Nose

Normal Development and Developmental Disturbances

(Figs. **1** and **2**)

The nasal cavity begins to develop in the 5 mm (32 day) embryo with a thickening of the ectoderm of the frontal process, termed the olfactory placode (Fig. **1**). The nasal placode sinks rapidly to form the nasal fovea and then the nasal sac; then it splits off a medial and a lateral nasal process from the frontonasal process. For a short period the stomatodeum and the nasal cavity are separated by the oronasal membrane. The latter ruptures at the 15 mm stage; the nasal cavity and the primitive choanae are then formed. The part of the roof of the mouth in front of the choana is the premaxilla (primitive palate). The nasal sac initially has epithelial connections with the ectoderm which are penetrated by mesenchyme and then disintegrate. Retention of this epithelial connection leads to clefts and anomalies of the skin of this region, termed *cheiloschisis*. However, Otto and Opitz (1987) state that the epithelial partition is formed by the two epithelial layers, and does not disintegrate. The secondary nasal cavity arises by incor-

poration of part of the stomatodeum (primitive oral cavity) to form the nasal cavity.

The thick nasal septum, its precartilage and cartilage grow downwards in the 19 mm embryo. At the same time the maxillary processes develop medially and inferiorly on each side from the alveolar process (Fig. **2**). Initially, in the 18–20 mm stage, the tongue lies between these palatine processes. Later, at the 26 mm stage, the tongue sinks downwards as the mandible and tongue develop; the palatine processes expand in a horizontal plane at the 30–32 mm stage. In the 35 mm embryo the palatine processes fuse anteriorly with the primitive palate and posteriorly with each other: fusion proceeds in a posterior direction (Peter, 1913; Diewert, 1983). Initially epithelial cords arise in the fusion zone between the two alveolar processes and the inferior edge of the nasal septum. Later they usually disappear completely. The dorsal part of the stomatodeum does not divide into two compartments, but persists as the pharynx. A part of the stomatodeum is included in the nasal cavity by growth and elevation of the alveolar processes and by their fusion with each other and with the nasal septum.

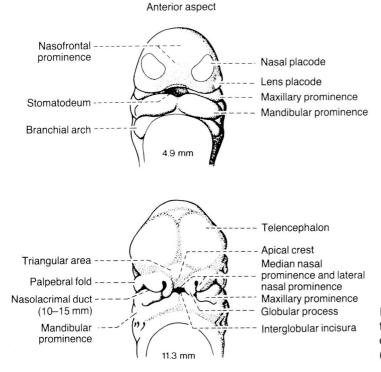

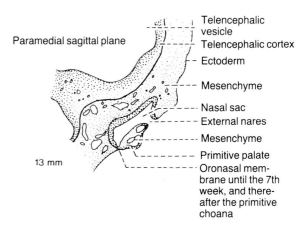

Fig. **1** Development of the olfactory placode and definition of the external nostril and the oronasal membrane. The primitive choana appears after dissolution of the oronasal membrane (Fischel, 1929)

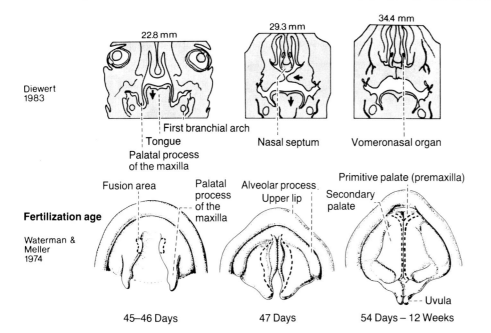

Fig. **2**   Development of the secondary palate, in frontal section viewed from below (adapted from various authors)

Anomalies

The processes fuse from the front backwards: thus, the most minor anomaly of fusion of the two palatine processes is the bifid uvula. Non-fusion of the two palatine processes causes a cleft of the secondary palate (palatoschisis) which is often combined with a cleft lip (cheiloschisis) and/or a cleft of the primary palate (gnathoschisis). Cleft lip and palate occur in 0,82% of neonates. The cleft may be total, and lie on either the left or right side. If the alveolar processes are very underdeveloped the nasal septum can be seen from below through the mouth, a condition termed uranoschisis. It is curious that almost all investigators have found more palatal clefts on the left side than on the right (Koelliker, 1882). A gnathoschisis can run through the canine tooth dividing it into a pre-canine and a canine tooth. Underdevelopment of the middle part of the middle nasofrontal process produces the bifid nose which is often combined with other anomalies. Atresia of the nose, partial or complete obstruction of the nasal cavity, choanal atresia and narrowing of the pharynx by posterior displacement of the maxilla also occur (Lang, 1985).

Development of the Nasal Cavity

(Fig. **3**)

The cartilaginous anlage of the external nose and nasal cavity develops in 7–8 week embryos, initially in the region of the nasal septum and later in the lateral wall of the nose. Further centers follow: for the inferior concha in the 8th week, the middle concha in the 9th week and the superior concha in the 12th week. The paraseptal cartilages (Jacobson's cartilage) rapidly develop anteroinferiorly on the septal cartilage.

The nasal capsules form at the end of the 3rd month of embryonal life, connecting posteriorly with the cartilaginous anlage of the body of the sphenoid bone and the lesser wing of the sphenoid. Wide foramina are present for the olfactory filaments, the vomeronasal nerve (Jacobson's nerve), the ethmoidal nerves, the nervus terminalis and the nasal branches of the ethmoidal arteries (Fig. **4**). These large openings divide up later into smaller and more numerous foramina.

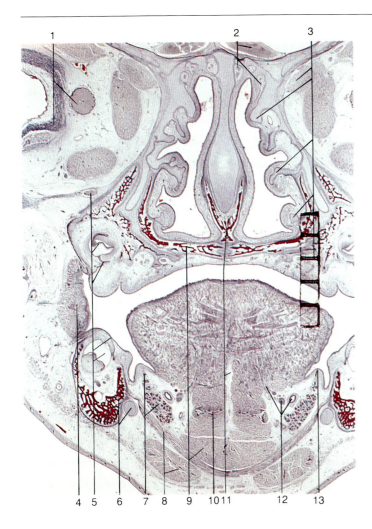

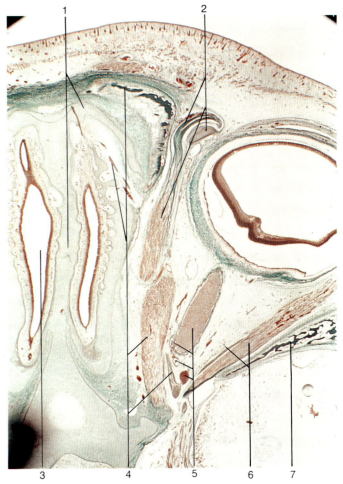

Fig. **3** Frontal section of an 18-cm-long fetus at the level of the posterior part of the ocular bulb
 1 Sclera and optic nerve
 2 Olfactory bulb and filaments
 3 Superior, middle and inferior nasal conchae, and superior oblique and medial rectus muscles with a millimeter strip
 4 Buccinator muscle
 5 Infraorbital nerve and tooth buds with dental anlage
 6 Mandible and Meckel's cartilage
 7 Plica and sublingual gland
 8 Mylohyoid muscle and anterior belly of the digastric muscle
 9 Palatine process of the maxilla, and the geniohyoid muscle
10 Genioglossus muscle
11 Vomer and lingual septum
12 Lingual nerve and submandibular duct
13 Sublingual ductule

Fig. **4** Transverse section through the roof of the nasal cavity and orbit in a 14-cm-long fetus
 1 Nasal septum
 2 Cartilaginous trochlea and tendon of superior oblique muscle
 3 Superior segment of the nasal cavity
 4 Frontal bone, medial rectus muscle with the muscular ramus of the third cranial nerve, and the anterior ethmoidal nerve
 5 Optic nerve, ophthalmic artery and ciliary ganglion
 6 Lateral rectus muscle and the abducens nerve
 7 The greater wing of the sphenoid bone

Development of the External Nasal Skeleton

(Fig. 5)

The cartilaginous segments involute but contribute to the shape of the skeleton of the external nose. The greater alar cartilages appear in the sixth fetal month. A section of a 35 cm fetus illustrates this stage of nasal development (Fig. 6). Excessive resorption of the cartilage leads to floppiness of the nasal ala which then prolapse against the septum during inspiration, causing nasal obstruction (Broman, 1911).

The nasal bone arises by desmal ossification during the tenth and eleventh week. Its lower edge forms the upper boundary of the piriform aperture. The lateral wall and floor of the piriform aperture are formed by the maxilla. The first ossification centers for the maxilla appear in the sixth to eighth embryonal weeks. The maxilla arises during the sixth and seventh weeks from five small desmal ossification centers lateral and inferior to the cartilaginous nasal capsule (Gilbert et al., 1958). In the fourth fetal month the centers fuse to form the alveolar and palatine processes, the floor of the orbit, the zygomatic process and the frontal process of the maxilla. Between the eighth and ninth weeks an area of ossification appears in the medial part of the floor of the piriform aperture called the *premaxilla*. The superior incisor teeth develop in this area. The premaxillary wings develop early on the nasal surface, and then push obliquely upwards and laterally to fuse with the posterior part of the anterior nasal spine (Fig. 7). The premaxillary wings fuse with the septal cartilage above, and the vomeronasal cartilage laterally. The premaxilla arises from two ossification centers. The vomer is embedded in the posterior part of the premaxillary wings (Klaff, 1956). Anteriorly the premaxilla forms the anterior nasal spine. Posteriorly it borders the anterior and lateral wall of the incisive foramen and canal. We have observed a process of the premaxilla which was under the frontal process of the maxilla.

Rosenmueller (1804) gave the first description of the suture between the premaxilla and the maxilla on the facial surface, and called it the facial incisive suture.

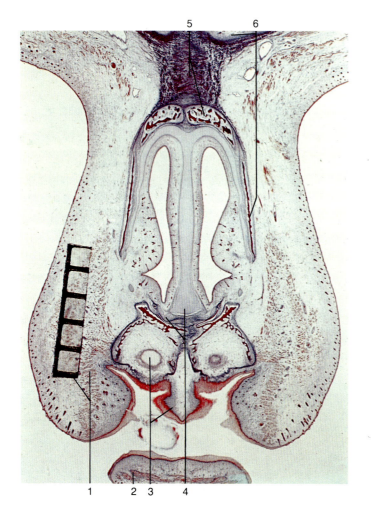

Fig. 5   Frontal section through the nose at the level of the first incisor tooth in an 18-cm-long fetus
1 Orbicularis oris muscle within the upper lip
2 Lower lip
3 First incisor tooth, anlage and incisive papilla
4 Nasal septum and vomeronasal cartilage
5 Nasal bone and transverse connective tissue fibers
6 Frontal bone and premaxilla

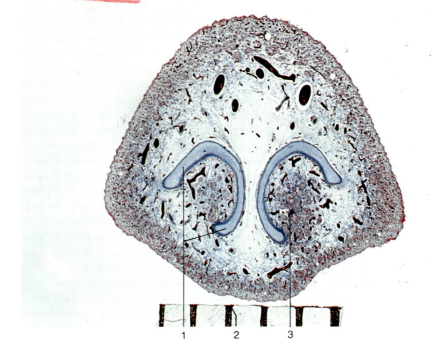

Fig. **6** Frontal section through the nose: the greater alar cartilage is complete (35 cm fetus)
1 Horseshoe-shaped greater alar cartilage
2 Millimeter strip
3 Glands of the nasal vestibulum in horizontal section

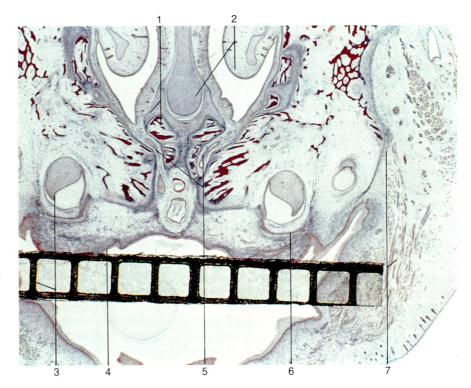

Fig. **7** Incisive duct in frontal section (18 cm fetus)
1 Vomeronasal cartilage and premaxillary wing
2 Nasal septum and inferior concha
3 Anlage of the canine tooth, and a millimeter strip
4 Palatal mucosa
5 Right and left nasopalatine duct in the incisive canal
6 Dental rim
7 Buccinator muscle

External Nose

Skeleton

Nasal Bones

(Fig. **8**)

The nasal bones unite above with the frontal bone at the nasofrontal suture, and laterally with the frontal process of the maxilla at the nasomaxillary suture. Within the nasal cavity a thick spur, *the nasal spine of the frontal bone,* projects inferiorly and anteriorly. It supports the nasal bones which lie upon it; they receive further support in the midline from the *perpendicular plate* of the ethmoidal bone (Fig. **9**).

The normal nasal bone resembles a long irregular rectangle, narrower above and wider below, and shorter laterally than medially. The narrowing of the upper third was termed the isthmus by Hovorka (1893) (Fig. **10**). If the isthmus of both sides lies at the same level then the nose is usually straight; if not the nose is scoliotic. The nasal bone is usually convex and smooth externally, but concave and rough internally. It carries a median groove for the perpendicular plate, and for the nasal spine of the frontal bone. Foramina for vessels and nerves are often found in the lower third of the nasal bone. The postnatal growth of the length and breadth of the nasal bone in our material is given in Fig. **11.** The different shapes of the nasal bone are shown in Fig. **10** (Lang and Baumeister, 1982). Zuckerkandl (1893) reported the following variations:

1) nasal bones which were too small, often triangular in shape and which did not articulate with the frontal bone;
2) rudimentary nasal bones connected with the frontal bone;
3) nasal bones of unequal width;
4) absent nasal bones;
5) extremely broad nasal bones, in which case the frontal process of the maxilla was narrow.
   Further details are given in Fig. **12.**

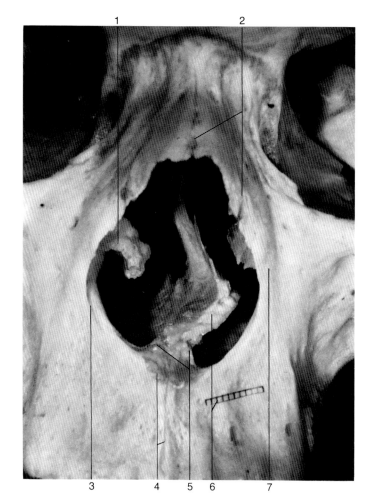

Fig. **8** Asymmetrical piriform aperture and premaxilla; septal deviation
1 Inferior nasal concha
2 Internasal and nasomaxillary sutures with the left nasal bone between them
3 Lateral edge of the piriform sinus
4 Anterior nasal spine and intermaxillary suture
5 Premaxillary alae
6 Septal deviation of the vomer, with a millimeter strip
7 Frontal process of the maxilla

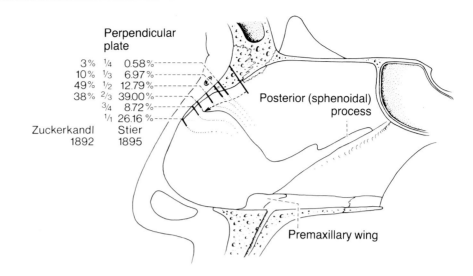

Fig. 9 Boundary zone of the perpendicular plate and nasal bone (adapted from Stier, 1895 and Zuckerkandl, 1892)

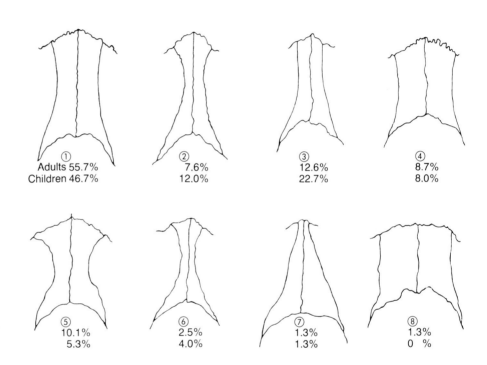

Fig. 10 Shapes of nasal bone found in our material (Lang and Baumeister, 1982)

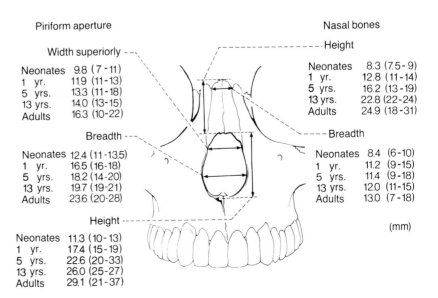

Fig. 11 Length and breadth of the nasal bone and size of the piriform aperture (Lang and Baumeister, 1982)

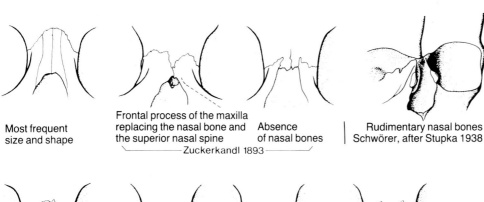

Most frequent
size and shape

Frontal process of the maxilla
replacing the nasal bone and
the superior nasal spine

Absence
of nasal bones

⎣————— Zuckerkandl 1893 —————⎦

Rudimentary nasal bones
Schwörer, after Stupka 1938

Perpendicular plate
of the ethmoid bone

Nasal bone absent
on the left side

Synostosis of the
nasal bones

small nasal bones with no
suture with the frontal bone

⎣————————— van der Hoeven 1860 —————————⎦

Fig. **12** Normal appearance and rare variants of the nasal bone, for example the two frontal processes of the maxilla may abut (upper row) or the nasal bone may be completely or partially absent (adapted from various authors)

Nasal Fistulae

(Figs. **13** and **14**)

Streit (1911) showed that middle clefts of the nose are exceedingly uncommon. He reported a dermoid with a fistula in the midline of the nose in an 18-year-old boy who was known to have had a small swelling of the dorsum of the nose in the neonatal period. Later the swelling grew to the size of a cherry. He removed the tumor. Dermoids of the nose constitute about 1% of congenital dermoids of the entire body (Bruck and Kittinger, 1963). They present as small pits or openings in the glabella or the dorsum of the nose, and are easily confused with comedones, sebaceous cysts, etc. The cyst originally lies between the two halves of the septum and grows slowly due to desquamation: then it penetrates the dorsum of the nose between the frontal bone and the nasal bones, or between the nasal bones and the septal cartilage, or it may penetrate the nasal bone itself (Pfeifer, 1986)

Fracture of the Nasal Bones

Fractures of the nasal bones are by far the most common injury of the facial skeleton, causing scoliosis or prolapse of the nose, nasal obstruction, anosmia and, occasionally, crepitation (Guelzow, 1979). Of 1037 patients undergoing a nasal operation in a 15-year period, 403 (39%) had a history of previous trauma (Helms, 1973).

The nasal bones are anchored to the neighboring bones by rigid syndesmoses. In simple fractures the break usually does not lie at the sutures but in the frontal process of the maxilla (Naumann, 1966). The pyramid of the dorsum of the nose is indeed often depressed or dislocated, but only rarely is its outline completely disorganized. The ethmoidal cells or the floor of the frontal sinus can extend into the nasal bone, so that the nasal sinuses too, can be injured. The terminal branch of the anterior ethmoidal nerve and its accompanying blood vessels run on the inner surface of the nasal bone, and they, too, are at risk of injury.

Piriform Aperture

(Figs. **8** and **11**)

The piriform aperture is bounded below and laterally by the maxilla, and above by the nasal bones. The medial part of its lower border may be sharp or rounded. This part arises from the premaxillary bone; it ends anteromedially in the anterior nasal spine. A little lateral to it lies the sharp edge of the piriform aperture. This edge is single in 57% of cases, and is then described as an anthropine type. An infantile form with an incomplete edge between the medial and lateral parts of the lower boundary of the piriform aperture is found in 22% of cases (Hovorka, 1893). Finally, a pre-nasal fossa is found in 12% of cases. In these cases a shallow depression extending to the alveolar arch of the incisor teeth lies on the inferior sharp border of the piriform aperture on both sides. Medially, the anterior and posterior edges merge into the anterior nasal spine.

Leicher (1928) stated that a pre-nasal fossa is inherited as a recessive trait, as is the short anterior nasal spine, whereas a protruding anterior nasal spine is a dominant inherited factor.

The lateral part of the inferior edge of the piriform aperture merges roundly into its lateral wall formed by the frontal process of the maxilla. It tapers superiorly, and inclines medially and posteriorly. It is bounded superiorly by the nasal part of the frontal bone, and superomedially by the lateral edge of the nasal bone. The inferior edge swings externally in a slightly curved arch to provide the piriform aperture with fairly sharp edges. Hovorka (1893) pointed out that, in a narrow nose, the border between the segment without a suture (the aperture) and the segment with a suture, is characterized by a marked kink.

The instrument used for a reduction osteotomy should be placed on the outermost angle of the piriform aperture (Naumann, 1966). The upper border of the piriform aperture is formed by the free ends of the nasal bones. Its edge is curved concave downwards. Less commonly it is straight or angled, and occasionally jagged or

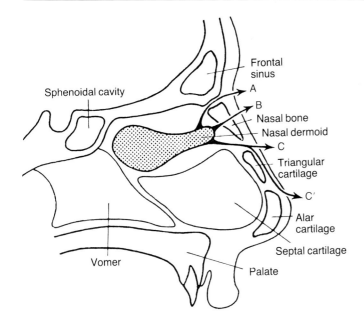

Fig. **13** Pathways of penetration of dermoid fistulae through the nose. A = superior fistula, B = penetration through the nasal bone, C and C' = inferior fistula (Bruck and Kittinger, 1963)

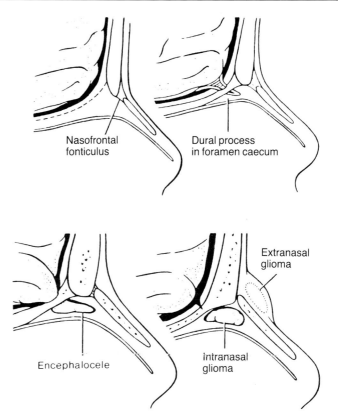

Fig. **14** Encephaloceles resembling nasal gliomas area (Whitaker et al., 1981)

notched, or even doubly notched. Thus the aperture may have a double or single convexity pointing upwards. The internasal suture seldom lies exactly in the midline. Hovorka (1893) found that it was straight in only 4.5%, irregular in about 2.5% and in 93% it was curved. A total synostosis of the internasal suture is uncommon, but partial synostosis is found in 1.3% of young subjects.

Variations
(see Fig. **12**)

The upper border of the piriform aperture is defective in hypoplasia of the nasal bones, if the nasal bones are free and do not synostose in the upper part of the piriform aperture, and in aplasia of the nasal bones. Zuckerkandl (1892) reported small, round or polygonal small bones up to the size of a hemp seed on the inner surface of the nasal bone. They may fuse either with the nasal bone or with the perpendicular plate (Hovorka, 1893). Values for the height and width of the aperture during post-natal development in our material are shown in Fig. **11** (Lang and Baumeister, 1982). Welcker (1882) investigated 666 adult skulls, and found 37 (5.5%) with oblique nasal bones or an inequality of the lower part of the piriform aperture.

The nasal bones lie straight in about 89% of cases, and in the remainder are more often orientated towards the right than the left (Stier, 1895). Straight nasal bones are more common in brachycephalic than in mesocephalic skulls. The superolateral angle of the nasal bone (the lateral process of the orbital sulcus) projects between the frontal bone and the frontal process of the maxilla (Perna, 1906). It is usually about 3–4 mm long, but occasionally as much as 12 mm. In the latter case the frontal process of the maxilla does not reach the frontal bone. In 20% these lateral processes are absent, but in 10% they are well developed. Hoeven (1860) described a part of the perpendicular plate projecting between the nasal bones in a Portuguese subject.

Anterior Nasal Spine

The anterior nasal spine is said to correlate with the shape of the soft tissues of the nose and the position of the alveolus. It is 2.1 (0–3) mm long in neonates, 3.2 (2–4.5) mm in two-year-olds, and 4.1 (0–9) mm in adults (Lang and Baumeister, 1982).

In cadavers the spine is up to 15 mm in length (Lang and Sakals, 1982) (Fig. **11**). The anterior nasal spine is related superiorly to the anteroinferior, free, end of the septal cartilage from which it is separated by perichondrium, periosteum and an intervening mobile layer. Behind it two flat processes, the alae of the pre-maxilla, project superiorly and laterally.

Cartilage of the External Nose

(Figs. **15–18**)

The nasal cartilages consist of hyaline cartilage which may occasionally be ossified. The 1983 edition of the Nomina Anatomica describes a lateral nasal cartilage, a greater alar cartilage with a medial and a lateral crus, minor alar cartilages and accessory nasal cartilages. It has been known for a long time that the upper part of the septal cartilage merges directly into the lateral cartilage. Therefore it was described in the Nomina Anatomica of 1935 as the septodorsal cartilage. Distally there is no immediate connection between the lateral nasal cartilages and the septal cartilage. Most authors state that the minor alar cartilage lies at the posteroinferior edge of the lateral crus of the greater alar cartilage. Accessory nasal cartilages are also reported lying at the upper edge of the lateral crus of the greater alar cartilage, or at the lower edge of the lateral

nasal cartilage as well as in the posterior part. The individual cartilages are united relatively rigidly to the neighboring skeleton at the piriform aperture, but are joined loosely by connective tissue towards the nasal tip. The lateral nasal cartilage in our material was 23.6 (18–31) mm long (Fig. **19**). In the midline the lateral cartilage was overlapped by the nasal bones for a distance of 6.8 (3–15) mm. The lateral crus of the greater alar cartilage overlapped the lateral cartilage over a distance of 2.9 (1–4) mm provided that there are no separate cartilaginous fragments in this area. The maximal width of the lateral cartilage measured from the lateral side was 14.4 (11–21) mm (Lang and Mundorff-Vetter, 1986). The maximal length of the lateral crus of the greater alar cartilage measured from the nasal tip in a superolateral direction was 23.1 (18–27) mm, and its greatest width 12.8 (10–15) mm (Fig. **20**). The distance of the posterior end of the lateral crus from the base of the nose was 13.8 (9–18) mm. The longitudinal axis through the lateral crus forms an angle with the base of the

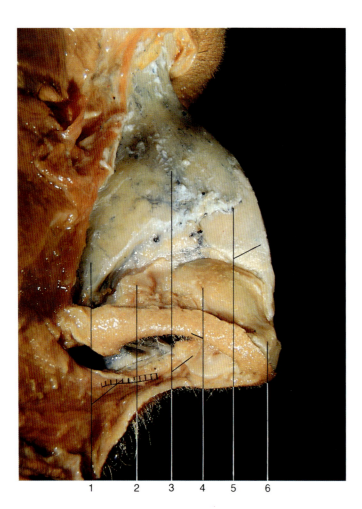

Fig. **15**   Lateral view of the cartilage of the external nose
1 Frontal process of the maxilla and depressor muscle of the septum (millimeter strip)
2 Accessory cartilage
3 Nasomaxillary suture and medial crus of the greater alar cartilage
4 Lateral crus of the greater alar cartilage and nares
5 Distal edge of the nasal bone and lateral nasal cartilage
6 Point of union of the medial and lateral crura of the greater alar cartilage

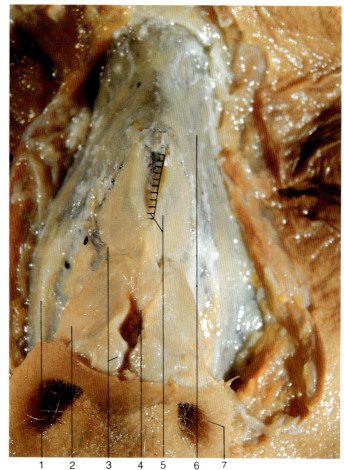

Fig. **16**   View of the nasal cartilage from in front
1 Piriform aperture (frontal process of the maxilla)
2 Lateral crus of the greater alar cartilage
3 Accessory alar cartilage at a rare site, and the junction of the medial and lateral crura of the greater alar cartilage
4 Lower edge of the septal cartilage (septal angle and weak triangle)
5 Lateral nasal cartilage, with a millimeter strip
6 Left nasal bone
7 Nares

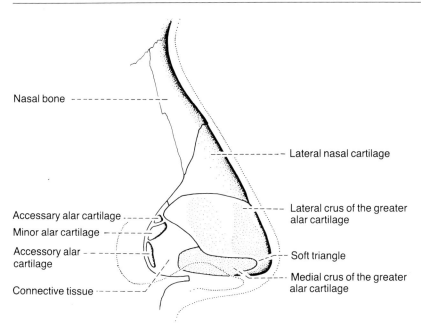

Nasal bone

Lateral nasal cartilage

Lateral crus of the greater alar cartilage

Accessary alar cartilage

Minor alar cartilage

Accessory alar cartilage

Soft triangle

Medial crus of the greater alar cartilage

Connective tissue

Fig. **17**   Diagram of the nasal cartilage showing the most common arrangement in our material (Lang and Mundorff-Vetter, 1986)

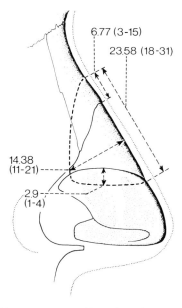

6.77 (3-15)

23.58 (18-31)

14.38 (11-21)

2.9 (1-4)

Fig. **19**   Measurements of length and overlapping zone of the lateral nasal cartilage. Overlapping by the nasal bone and by the lateral crus of the greater alar cartilage. Breadth of the lateral cartilage is also given (Lang and Mundorff-Vetter, 1986)

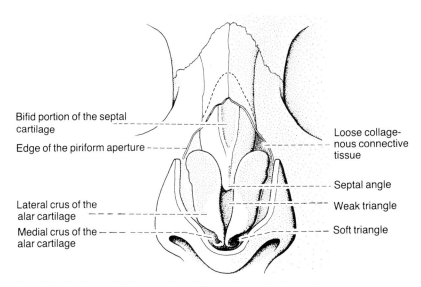

Bifid portion of the septal cartilage

Edge of the piriform aperture

Loose collagenous connective tissue

Septal angle

Weak triangle

Lateral crus of the alar cartilage

Medial crus of the alar cartilage

Soft triangle

Fig. **18**   A view of the nasal cartilages from in front. Loose connective tissue lies between the lateral nasal cartilage and the piriform aperture

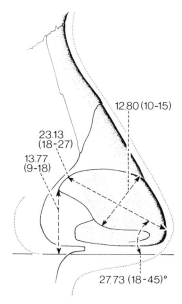

12.80 (10-15)

23.13 (18-27)

13.77 (9-18)

27.73 (18-45)°

Fig. **20**   Length of the lateral crus of the greater alar cartilage, width and angle with the base of the nose, and distance of its posterior end from the plane of the base of the nose (Lang and Mundorff-Vetter, 1986)

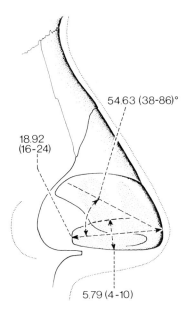

54.63 (38-86)°

18.92
(16-24)

5.79 (4-10)

Fig. 21 Length and breadth of the medial crus of the greater alar cartilage, and the angle between the middle zone of the lateral and medial crura (Lang and Mundorff-Vetter, 1986)

nose of 27.7° (18°–45°). The medial crus of the greater alar cartilage was 18.9 (16–24) mm long and 5.8 (4–10) mm wide (Fig. **21**). The angle between the medial and lateral crura of the greater alar cartilage was 54.6° (38°–86°). (The upper value is a rare, extreme, variant). The lengths of the nasal cartilages were measured both in projection and on the curve (Tables **1–7**).

On average 2.3 (1–4) minor and accessory nasal cartilages were found in our material. The nasal cartilage has been investigated by Zuckerkandl (1893), Ilberg (1935), Straatsma and Straatsma (1951), Gunter (1969), Seifert (1969), Krmpotic-Nemanic, Draf and Helms (1985) and many others. The medial crus is usually convex towards the septum. In our material other curves of the medial crus were also found, as previously described by Natvig et al. (1971). If the medial crus is convex medially its posterior tip can push the nasal columella forwards (see Figs. **22** and **23**).

Particularly detailed investigations of the skeleton of the external nose have been carried out from a clinical viewpoint by Converse (1955), Cottle (1955) and Masing (1964). They described the *keystone area* where the lateral nasal cartilages clearly separate from the septal cartilage (Cottle, 1955). The distal point of attachment of the lateral nasal cartilage is particularly important for the stability of the dorsum of the nose (Masing, 1964). Converse (1955) termed this area the weak triangle (Fig. **18**). If the superior parts of the lateral crura of the greater alar cartilages do not overlap the lateral nasal cartilage in the midline the edge of the septum lies free in the midline. Septal resection in these cases leads to a depression of this soft triangular area.

The *soft triangle* lies at the junction of the medial and lateral crura of the greater alar cartilage. This area is

Table 1 Lateral nasal cartilage

Length

a) Length in projection

	n	x̄	s	max.	min.
Total	30	23.58	3.46	31	18
Right	12	21.88	3.02	28	18
Left	18	24.72	3.40	31	20

b) Length on the curve

	n	x̄	s	max.	min.
Total	30	25.95	3.83	34	19.5
Right	12	23.50	2.37	30	19.5
Left	18	27.60	3.76	34	21

The mean difference between the length measured in projection and on the curve was 2.23 mm (0–5 mm)

Width

a) Measured in projection

	n	x̄	s	max.	min.
Total	30	14.38	2.82	21	11
Right	12	15.08	2.97	21	12
Left	18	13.92	2.70	20	11

b) Measured on the curve

	n	x̄	s	max.	min.
Total	30	16.30	3.08	23	12
Right	12	16.58	3.12	23	13
Left	18	16.11	3.14	22	12

The mean difference between the width measured in projection and on the curve was 1.88 mm (1–4 mm)

Table 2 Size of the overlapping zone at the nasal bone and at the lateral crus

a) Nasal bone

	n	x̄	s	max.	min.
Total	30	6.77	2.91	15	3
Right	12	6.92	3.37	15	3
Left	18	6.56	2.81	11	4

b) Lateral crus

	n	x̄	s	max.	min.
Total	30	2.90	0.75	4	1
Right	12	2.58	0.76	4	1
Left	18	3.11	0.67	4	2

Table **3**   Lateral crus of the greater alar cartilage

Length

a) Measured in projection

	n	x̄	s	max.	min.
Total	30	23.13	2.58	27	18
Right	12	23.33	2.96	27	18
Left	18	23.00	2.40	27	19

b) Measured on the curve

	n	x̄	s	max.	min.
Total	30	27.87	3.06	32	23
Right	12	28.41	3.53	32	23
Left	18	27.50	2.75	32	23

The mean difference between the length measured in projection and on the curve was 4.73 mm (1−9 mm)

Width

a) Measured in projection

	n	x̄	s	max.	min.
Total	30	12.80	1.56	15	10
Right	12	12.67	1.50	15	10
Left	18	12.83	1.62	15	10

b) Measured on the curve

	n	x̄	s	max.	min.
Total	30	14.37	1.82	17	10
Right	12	13.92	1.93	16	10
Left	18	14.67	1.75	17	10

The mean difference between the width measured in projection and on the curve was 1.57 mm (0−4 mm)

Table **4**

a) Angle between the axis and the edge of the nasal ala

	n	x̄	s	max.	min. (x°)
Total	30	27.73	6.51	45	18
Right	12	25.83	5.94	40	20
Left	18	29.06	6.70	45	18

b) Distance from the lateral end to the edge of the nasal ala

	n	x̄	s	max.	min.
Total	30	13.77	2.19	18	9
Right	12	13.33	2.23	18	9
Left	18	14.06	2.18	18	11

Table **5**   Medial crus of the greater alar cartilage

Length

a) Measured in projection

	n	x̄	s	max.	min.
Total	24	18.92	2.04	24	16
Right	9	18.78	2.33	24	17
Left	15	19.00	1.93	23	16

b) Measured on the curve

	n	x̄	s	max.	min.
Total	24	22.50	1.69	27	20
Right	9	22.11	2.03	27	21
Left	15	22.73	1.49	26	20

The mean difference between the length measured in projection and on the curve was 3.6 mm (1−7 mm)

Width

a) Measured in projection

	n	x̄	s	max.	min.
Total	24	5.79	1.22	10	4
Right	9	6.33	1.58	10	5
Left	15	5.47	0.83	7	4

b) Measured on the curve

	n	x̄	s	max.	min.
Total	24	7.25	0.90	10	6
Right	9	7.67	1.00	10	7
Left	15	7.00	0.76	8	6

The mean difference between the width measured in projection and on the curve was 1.5 mm (1−3 mm)

Shape

No.	Shape
11	Convex towards the septum
5	Asymmetrical S-shape
5	Symmetrical S-shape
3	Concave towards the septum

Table **6**   Angle between the lateral and medial crura

	n	x̄	s	max.	min. (x°)
Total	24	54.63	12.67	86	38
Right	9	53.11	11.85	75	40
Left	15	55.53	13.45	86	38

Table **7**   Greater alar cartilage

Correlations	Correlation coefficient	Significance level (%)
Length of the lateral nasal cartilage measured in projection: overlapping by the nasal bone	0.40	90
Nasal cheek depth: lateral crus (width measured in projection)	0.42	90
Length of the lateral crus of the greater alar cartilage measured in projection: nasobuccal depth	0.57	99
Isthmus of the lateral end of the lateral crus to the edge of the nasal ala: angle between the lower axis of the lateral crus and the edge of the nasal ala	0.44	90
Lateral nasal cartilage (length measured in projection): lateral nasal cartilage (length measured on the curve)	0.91	99.9
Lateral nasal cartilage (breadth measured in projection): lateral nasal cartilage (breadth measured on the curve)	0.95	99.9
Lateral crus (length measured in projection): lateral crus (measured on the curve)	0.69	99
Lateral crus (breadth measured in projection): lateral crus (breadth measured on the curve)	0.78	99.9
Medial crus (length measured in projection): medial crus (length measured on the curve)	0.82	99.9
Medial crus (breadth measured in projection): medial crus (breadth measured on the curve)	0.75	99.9

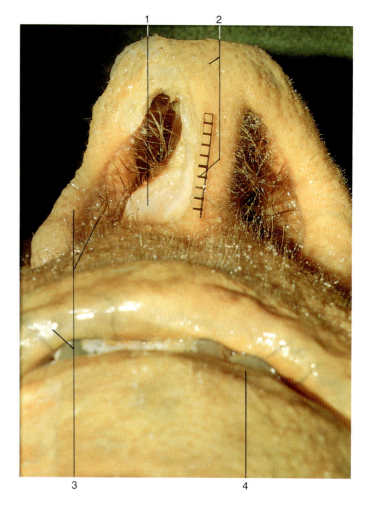

Fig. **22**   Columella (mobile part of the nasal septum) and medial crus of the greater alar cartilage)
1 Medial crus of the greater alar cartilage dissected and showing a medial convexity
2 Tip of the nose, columella and a millimeter strip
3 Lower edge of the nasal ala, vibrissae and the upper lip
4 Lower lip

separated from the free edge of the nares by a triangle consisting of two layers of skin, the external skin and the skin of the nasal vestibule with the intervening connective tissue. The transition between the medial and lateral crus is termed the dome (Fig. **23**). Incision of this zone from within the nasal cavity should be avoided to ensure that the soft triangle is not divided.

The *perichondrium* is divided into a fibrous and a chondral layer. The former consists mainly of collagen fibers running in a anterosuperior-posteroinferior direction in the lateral view. The cartilage of the external nose and the chondral layer possess different cleavage lines. In the greater alar cartilage they mainly run transverse to the longest extent of its limb (Ilberg, 1935) (Figs. **9** and **10**). The cleavage lines of the central part of the lateral nasal cartilage run towards the piriform aperture, in the upper part they run parallel to the nasal bone whereas below they merge in the cleavage lines of the lateral crus of the greater alar cartilage. The external perichondrium also serves to

unite the nasal cartilages to each other and with the periosteum of the facial skeleton.

A few fibers are found lying parallel to the edge only in the dome of the greater alar cartilage, but in other parts in flat noses (Ilberg, 1935).

Columella: Mobile Part of the Nasal Septum

The part of the septum running between the tip of the nose and the philtrum is termed the columella; it bounds the nares medially. The posterior part is thicker than the anterior because the medial crura of the greater alar cartilage are embedded in this area: they diverge slightly to grasp the inferior end of the septal cartilage. The contour of the columella depends on the shape and course of the medial crura. A relatively short columella may be due to the alar region being long, or it may be due to congenital lesions, trauma, inflammation of the cartilage or over-

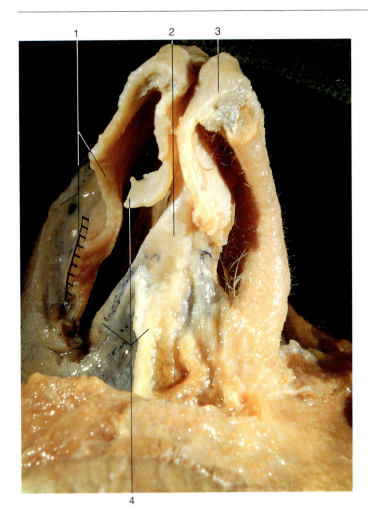

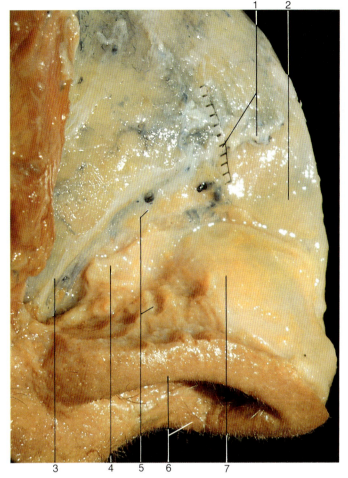

Fig. 23   Nasal cartilage exposed from below
1 Piriform aperture, lateral crus of the greater alar cartilage and a millimeter strip
2 Lower edge of the septal cartilage
3 Nasal dome
4 Medial crus of the greater alar cartilage and a well developed vomeronasal cartilage with the anterior nasal spine in between

Fig. 24   Lateral view of the skeletal part of the nose
1 Inferior edge of the nasal bone and a millimeter strip
2 Lateral nasal cartilage
3 Piriform aperture with a small periosteal edge
4 Accessory alar cartilage
5 Connective tissue (the suspensory ligament of the tip of the nose) (Converse, 1955)
6 Nares
7 The lateral crus of the greater alar cartilage

generous submucosal resection of cartilage. Syphilis can cause the columella to disappear. Surgical management of the columella is described by Millard (1963), and by Denecke and Meyer (1964).

Ligaments of the Nose

(Fig. 24)

Fig. 19 demonstrates the overlapping of the lateral nasal cartilage by the nasal bones. The overlapping zone in the midline is termed the keystone area. Firm connective tissue anchors the lateral cartilage to the nasal bones. Parkes and Kanodia (1981) gave a thorough description of tearing of this ligamentous apparatus, and the treatment of the resulting deformity of the nose and nasal obstruction. Converse (1955) termed the aponeurotic tissue between the

lateral cartilage and the lateral crus of the greater alar cartilage (including its perichondrium) the suspensory ligament of the apex of the nose. The connective tissue is also fixed to the septal angle. The tip of the nose prolapses if the support of the septal cartilage is lost due to trauma or surgery. However, in our material the external nose was surprisingly little deformed in the presence of almost complete loss of the nasal septum (see Figs. 2 and 3 in Lang and Kley [1981]).

The lateral crus of the greater alar cartilage overlaps the lateral nasal cartilage in 72% of cases. Both cartilaginous edges interdigitate with each other in 52% cases, whereas they overlap in 20% of cases, an end-to-end abutment is found in 17% of cases, and reverse overlap, that is the lateral nasal cartilage overlaps the greater alar cartilage, is found in 11% (Dion et al., 1979).

Muscles of the External Nose

Depressor Muscle of the Septum

(Fig. 25)

This muscle arises from the alveolus of the incisor tooth, and runs medially and superiorly to reach the medial crus of the greater alar cartilage; its fibers spread out in the perichondrium of the latter structure. Loose connective tissue can be found between the medial crus of the alar cartilage and the septal cartilage. The muscle fibers are difficult to demonstrate since they pass through, or are incorporated in, the fibers of the orbicularis oris muscle.

The muscle depresses the septum and the nasal tip slightly, and expands the nares during deep inspiration. Its nerve supply arises from the superior buccal branches of the facial nerve.

Nasal Muscle

(Fig. 26)

According to the Nomina Anatomica the nasal muscle has a transverse and an alar part. The transverse part arises immediately lateral to the piriform aperture, and its fibers pass superiorly and medially. In the dorsum of the nose they often merge into a thin aponeurosis which is attached

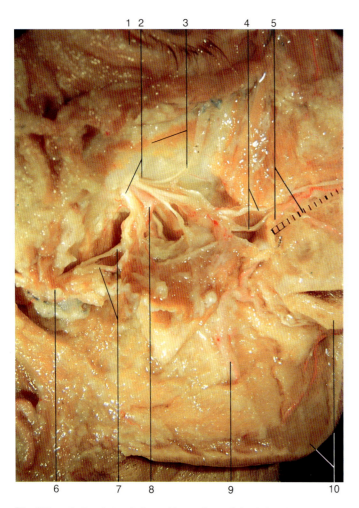

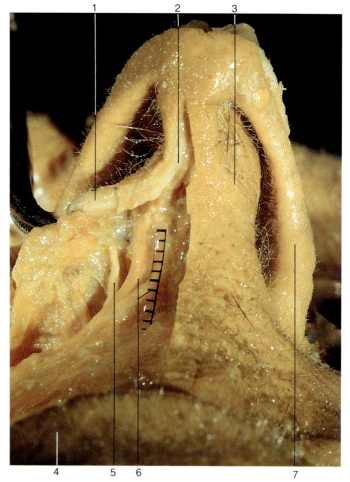

Fig. **25a**   Anterolateral view of branches of the infraorbital nerve
1 Palpebral cleft
2 Branches of the infraorbital nerve at the infraorbital foramen
3 Inferior palpebral ramus and cut edge of the levator labii superioris alaequae nasi muscle
4 Lateral nasal rami
5 Superior alar rami with a millimeter strip
6 Zygomaticus major muscle displaced laterally
7 Superior buccal rami of the facial nerve (lesser pes anserinus)
8 Infraorbital artery and levator muscle of the upper lip displaced inferiorly
9 Facial artery
10 Columella and upper lip

Fig. **25b**   Depressor muscle of the septum seen from below
1 Cutis of the columella dissected and retracted laterally
2 Anterior edge of the medial crus of the greater alar cartilage
3 Cutis of a thick columella
4 Upper lip
5 Branch of the infraorbital nerve
6 Depressor muscle of the septum with millimeter strip
7 Ala nasi at the nares

to the corresponding muscle of the opposite side. Fibers of the procerus muscle also run into this aponeurotic area.

The alar part (termed the alar muscle by Eisler in 1912) arises beneath the nasomaxillary suture and above the connective tissue layer of the nasal alae at the piriform aperture, as well as from the minor alar cartilages. The muscle is 15–18 mm long. It runs inferiorly, laterally and anteriorly and is attached by a short thin tendon to the skin of the nasal ala anterior to the alar groove as far as the middle of the nostril. The muscle can be as much as 2 mm thick, but its development varies with that of the transverse part of the nasal muscle (Eisler, 1912). It runs below the skin of the dorsum of the nose, but is elsewhere covered by the levator muscle of the upper lip, the orbicularis oculi and the incisive muscle of the upper lip. The alar part of the muscle draws the nasal alae inferiorly and laterally, thus expanding the nares. Fomon et al. (1950) and Fomon (1960) termed this part of the muscle the posterior dilator of the nose. Also, they described an additional anterior nasal dilator that grasps the superior part of the lateral crus in the tip area (Fig. 4 in Fomon et al., 1950). Therefore the muscle is termed the apical nasal muscle.

Muscle of the Nasal Tip

(see Fig. 26)

This muscle was first described by Luschka (1853, 1867). It arises from the posteroinferior angle of the lateral cartilage, displaces the alar part of the nasal muscle anteriorly and runs forward under it immediately above the lower edge of the greater alar cartilage and then under the skin. Then it runs via the apical area of the alar cartilage. It can be as long as 18 mm. The muscle inserts into the junction of the medial and lateral crura of the greater alar cartilage. The muscle dilates the anterior segment of the nares, but it can narrow the nasal aperture anteriorly and expand it posteriorly if the greater alar cartilage is thin.

The transverse part of the nasal muscle can narrow the nasal cavity at the junction of the vestibule and the nasal cavity, and is therefore known as the compressor muscle. The transverse part of the nasal muscle, its alar part and the depressor muscle of the septum pull the dorsum of the nose downwards and elongate it.

Procerus Muscle

(see Fig. 27)

Muscle fibers arise from the medial segment of the frontal belly of the occipitofrontalis muscle, swing inferiorly and blend into the aponeurosis on the nasal dorsum. This aponeurosis lies over the lower part of the nasal bones and the upper part of the lateral nasal cartilage. Some fibers run to the skin between the eyebrows. Virchow (1912) suggested that the procerus muscle should be called the depressor of the glabella because it was responsible for facial movement in the hirsute area between the eyebrows. Its attachment to the bone or to the aponeurosis of the nasal dorsum seldom extends inferiorly beyond the midzone of the nose, but occasionally it reaches as far as the nasal tip or the nasal ala. The muscle then spreads out superiorly and laterally to meet the superciliary depressor muscle which is also fanning out. Behind the lateral edge of the muscle lies the root of the nose. This gap is filled with fatty tissue between the corrugator and procerus muscles. If the fat pad is fairly well developed a modest deepening of the surface at this point conveys a fine modelled appearance to the root of the nose. The muscle partially bridges the region of the paranasion and determines its skin relief. It pulls the medial segment of the eyebrow inferiorly, and produces transverse folds in the region of the root of the nose.

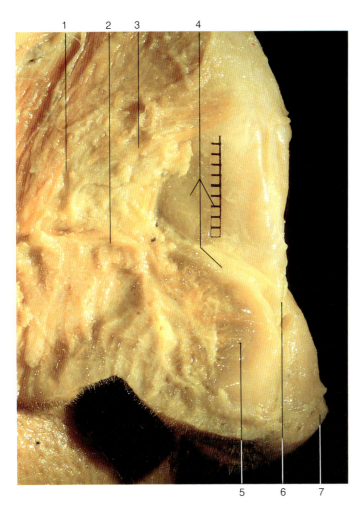

Fig. 26 Poorly developed nasal muscle seen from the side
1 Levator labii superioris alaequae nasi muscle
2 Fibers of the muscle of the nasal tip
3 Transverse part of the nasal muscle
4 Lateral nasal cartilage and superior edge of the lateral crus with a millimeter strip
5 Apical nasal muscle
6 Septal angle
7 Tip of the nose

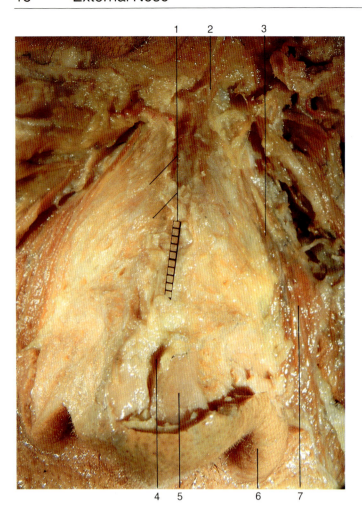

Fig. 27   Nasal muscles from the front
1 Transverse part of the nasal muscle with a millimeter strip
2 Procerus muscle
3 Levator alae nasi muscle
4 Weak triangle
5 Dome of the greater alar cartilage
6 Inferior edge of the nasal ala
7 Levator labii superioris alaequae nasi muscle

Levator Labii Superioris Alaequae Nasi Muscle

The part of this muscle belonging to the nose was previously known as the angular head. It arises from the frontal process of the maxilla and blends into the perichondrium of the lateral crus of the greater alar cartilage. It can pull the lateral crus superiorly, and is therefore termed the dilator of the nares. The other part of the muscle elevates the upper lip. Its nerve supply comes from the zygomatic and superior buccal branches of the facial nerve (Quiring and Warfel, 1969).

Electromyography shows that the nasal dilators are respiratory muscles whose function correlates directly with the ventilatory resistance (Sasaki et al., 1976). The afferent limb of the reflex arc runs in the thoracic segment of the vagus nerve carrying impulses from the mechanoreceptors and the lungs to the inspiratory centre of the medulla oblongata: the efferent fibers run in the facial nerve.

Vessels

Arteries

(Fig. 28)

The outer part of the nose receives its blood supply from branches of the external carotid, ophthalmic and infraorbital arteries. The number and origin of the branches of the facial artery vary widely, and they anastomose with the infraorbital, transverse facial ("buccinator") arteries. An angular artery may arise from the transverse facial artery; the facial artery then ends as the inferior labial artery (Hyrtl 1885). The superior artery of the nasal ala and the end branch of the anterior ethmoidal artery may anastomose (Denecke and Meyer, 1964). The facial artery ends as the angular artery in 58% of cases, as the superior labial artery in 20% and the inferior labial artery in 22%. The arteries of the right and left sides anastamose (Kozielic and Jozwa, 1977). Hovorka (1893) gave a particularly thorough description of the nasal arteries. He demonstrated that two branches arise from the superior labial artery; one runs downwards to the upper lip and the other upwards to the nasal septum. The angular artery usually runs close to the anterior edge of the levator labii superioris alaeque nasi, lying partly under and partly over it. From this point arises an inferior alar branch to the inferior edge of the nasal ala, and a larger superior alar branch for the superior edge of the lateral crus of the greater alar cartilage. He termed the larger branch to the lateral part of the nose the nasal dorsal artery, and the nasal end branch of the ophthalmic artery as the external nasal artery. The latter arises at the medial angle of the orbit and divides into two branches. The smaller medial branch supplies the root of the nose and the procerus muscle; a larger lateral branch runs on the levator labii superioris alaeque nasi inferiorly, and anastamoses with the dorsal artery arising from the facial artery. Fine branches from this vessel penetrate the nutrient foramina of the nasal bones. Four types of nasal artery were represented in our material, in addition to a group of six rarer variations. If the facial artery was developed normally it ran superomedially and anteriorly on the anterior edge of the masseter muscle. One or more small arterial branches arose close to the mandible and ran upwards, anterior or posterior to the facial nerve. These are called the premasseteric branches. Another branch penetrates the muscle. Next, the vessel runs into the area where the fibers of the zygomaticus major muscle irradiate, embedded in the fatty tissue lying under the muscle. Occasionally it also ran through the deep fibers of this muscle. Next, it runs under the lateral part of the levator muscle of the upper lip, penetrates the deep layer of the medial part of the muscle and curves around its medial border in a superior direction. Its further course is then either within the superficial fibers of the levator muscle of the upper lip and nasal wing or deep to it. In our material the deeper vessels ran in a relatively straight line, the vascular segments lying between individual muscles were curved with deviations of 10 mm or more. The largest curves were found superior and inferior to the zygomaticus major muscle in the fatty tissue. Within this muscle the direction of the vessels usually changed, in a more medial and superior direction, and then superiorly

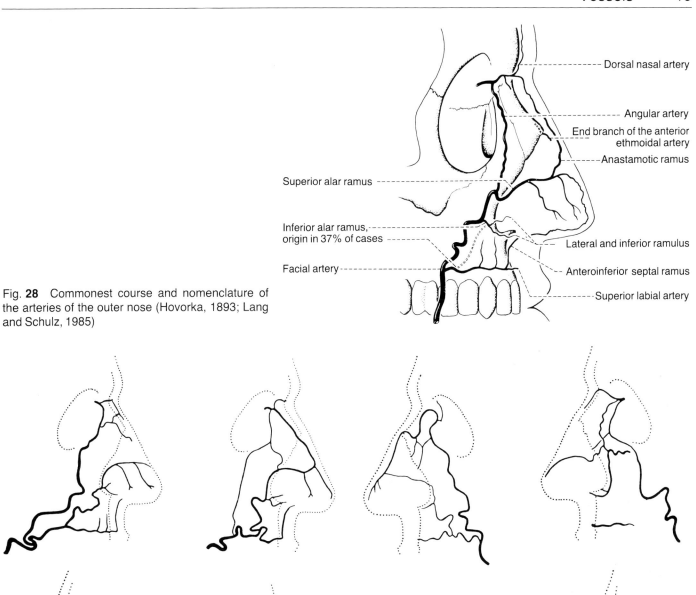

Dorsal nasal artery

Angular artery

End branch of the anterior ethmoidal artery

Anastamotic ramus

Superior alar ramus

Inferior alar ramus, origin in 37% of cases

Facial artery

Lateral and inferior ramulus

Anteroinferior septal ramus

Superior labial artery

Fig. **28** Commonest course and nomenclature of the arteries of the outer nose (Hovorka, 1893; Lang and Schulz, 1985)

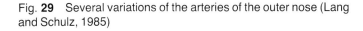

Fig. **29** Several variations of the arteries of the outer nose (Lang and Schulz, 1985)

Fig. **30** Rarer variations of the arteries of the outer nose (Lang and Schulz, 1985)

again in the area of the levator muscle of the upper lip. Fig. **28** shows the course of the nasal vessels which we found in 27.4% of our material, and in Fig. **29** the course and types of branching which were found in 17.5%. Fig. **30** shows the less common variants. The latter included a more dorsal course of the facial artery, a retrograde supply from the facial artery via the inner canthus, replacement of the

superior facial area by a vessel from the opposite side via the superior alar branches and the lateral nasal branches from the angular artery, supply of the inferior nasal area from the infraorbital artery, replacement of the facial artery by the transverse facial artery which supplied the inferior part of the nose, and replacement of the facial artery by the ophthalmic artery. In the latter case the left superior labial artery was fed from the artery of the same name on the right side. We also measured the external diameter of the vessels (Table **8** and **9**). There was no significant difference between the right and left sides, either of the stem of the facial artery at the angle of the mouth, or of the angular artery. The superior nasal alar branch was significantly wider on the left side than on the right.

Group ≙ 27.5%	n	$\bar{x}$	s	$s_{\bar{x}}$	x_{sup}	x_{inf}	$\sum x$
Facial artery	18	1.56	0.42	0.10	2.50	0.80	28.10
Superior labial artery	7	1.21	0.44	0.17	2.00	0.80	8.50
Inferior alar ramus	11	0.83	0.33	0.10	1.40	0.50	9.10
Superior alar ramus	17	0.97	0.38	0.09	2.00	0.50	16.50
Branches of the superior alar ramus	9	0.31	0.11	0.04	0.50	0.20	2.80
Angular artery	15	0.77	0.35	0.09	1.40	0.20	11.50
Lateral nasal rami	12	0.37	0.21	0.06	0.80	0.10	4.40

Table **8** External diameter of the branches of the facial artery (Lang and Schulz, 1985)

	n	$\bar{x}$	s	$s_{\bar{x}}$	x_{sup}	x_{inf}	$\sum x$
Facial artery	45	1.64	0.46	0.07	2.5	0.7	73.60
Superior labial artery	20	1.11	0.35	0.08	2.0	0.5	22.20
Inferior alar ramus	31	0.57	0.32	0.06	1.4	0.2	17.60
Superior alar ramus	64	0.92	0.39	0.05	2.0	0.2	58.80
Nerves of the superior alar ramus	28	0.54	0.29	0.05	1.2	0.2	15.10
Angular artery	62	0.61	0.38	0.05	1.9	0.1	37.90
Lateral nasal rami	24	0.35	0.20	0.04	0.8	0.1	8.30

Table **9** Average values of the external vascular diameter (Groups I–IV) (Lang and Schulz, 1985)

Veins

The venous networks arise in the post-capillary veins of the nasal tip and the nasal ala (Krmpotic-Nemanic, 1978). Their drainage does not run parallel to the arteries, but corresponds to territories termed arteriovenous units (Lassau et al.; quoted by Krmpotic-Nemanic, 1978). The frontomedian region of the face belongs to the region of the facial vein, and the orbitopalpebral area to the region of the ophthalmic veins. The upper lip drains by an ascending venous trunk into the facial vein (Ricbourg et al., 1976). The connections of the veins of the nose, upper lip and cheek with the drainage area of the ophthalmic vein are of clinical significance in inflammatory lesions of this area, such as orbital phlegmon and cavernous sinus thrombosis. Connections to the anterior ethmoidal vein also occur. The facial vein arises by the union of the supratrochlear and supraorbital veins in the inner canthus; it is termed the angular vein in its superior part. In its further course inferiorly it runs increasingly posterior to the facial artery, and is covered by the facial muscles inferiorly. Usually a transverse venous anastamosis, termed the nasal venous arch, lies between the supratrochlear veins in the root of the nose. Small veins from the root and the dorsum of the nose run into this area. Occasionally a supratrochlear vein arises in the frontal area, splits at the root of the nose, and opens into the first part of the facial (angular) veins.

Lymphatics

(Fig. **31**)

Lymph drainage from the external nose runs along with that of the cheek, the upper lip and the lateral part of the lower lip to the submandibular group of nodes. Buccal lymph nodes lying close to the facial vein may form an intermediate station. There are further connections with the parotid lymph nodes which also receive direct drainage of lymph from the root of the nose and the forehead.

Nerves

(Figs. **32** and **33**)

The skin of the outer part of the nose is supplied by branches of the trigeminal nerve, that of its root and dorsum by the ophthalmic division, and that over the nasal alae by the maxillary division. The anterior ethmoidal artery and nerve run through the canal of the same name to the anterior segment of the olfactory fossa. The nerve then runs anteriorly and medially in the ethmoidal sulcus (which is about 8 mm long) to the cribro-ethmoidal foramen, giving off branches to the dura mater of the anterior cranial fossa and the falx cerebri. Then it pierces the cribro-ethmoi-

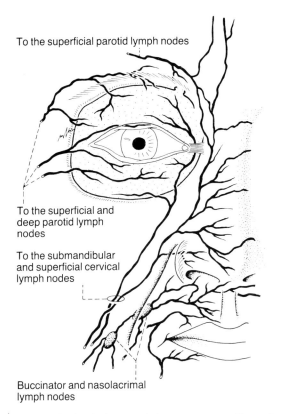

Fig. **31** Lymphatic drainage of the outer nose (from the nasal vestibule) and the orbital area

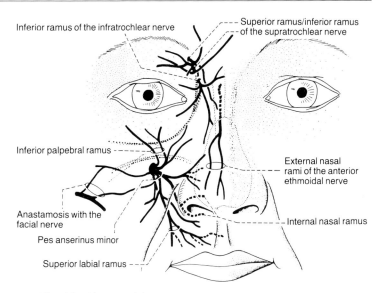

Fig. **32** Nerves of the outer nose

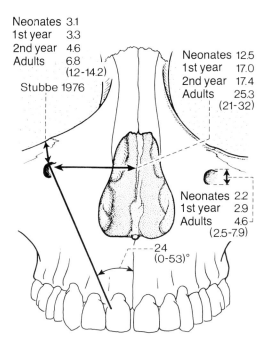

Fig. **33** Position of the infraorbital foramen, its postnatal change in position and growth (adapted from Stubbe, 1976), and the angle of the most anterior segment of the infraorbital canal in adults (Hassmann, 1975)

dal foramen to reach the nasal cavity, where it supplies the lateral and anteromedial segments of the nasal cavity via its lateral and medial nasal branches. The external nasal branch runs downwards on the inner surface of the nasal bone, often in a groove, and then usually between the lateral nasal cartilage and the nasal bone to reach the skin of the dorsum of the nose which it supplies as far as the tip of the nose. The lateral surface of the root of the nose receives fine twigs from the inferior branch of the infra-trochlear nerve. The nerve supplies the inner canthus, and the lacrimal caruncle and sac.

The infraorbital nerve is the sensory end-branch of the maxillary nerve. Usually it divides into external and internal nasal branches with is the last part of its canal. The infraorbital nerve also gives off inferior palpebral and superior labial branches. In the loose connective tissue of the canine fossa the branches are covered by the levator labii superioris alaeque nasi; they anastamose with superior buccal branches of the facial nerve to form the *pes anserinus minor*. The external nasal branches reach the nasal alae, and the internal nasal branches pass to the skin of the nasal vestibule.

A further branch of the infraorbital nerve runs 2–3 mm behind the piriform aperture: this is the nasodental ramus of the anterior superior alveolar branch (Knox 1853). The nasodental ramus arises 15 mm behind the infraorbital foramen, runs firstly in the floor of the orbit

8–10 mm anterolateral to the infraorbital foramen, and then turns downwards towards the anterior wall of the maxillary sinus lying about 6 mm below the orbital rim and 10 mm lateral to the infraorbital foramen. Then, the nerve runs 3–4 mm downwards and finally turns medially and upwards again to reach the piriform aperture. Its course is about 22 mm long lying with in the anterior wall of the maxillary sinus (Fig. **34**) (Wood-Jones, 1939). In the region of attachment of the inferior nasal concha it gives off branches to the inferior nasal concha, to the inferior nasal meatus, to the nasolacrimal duct and also to the region

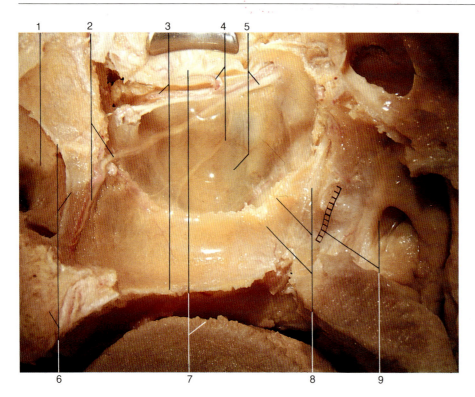

Fig. **34** Nasodental nerve arising from the superior medial alveolar nerve, seen from the medial side
1 Nasal vestibule
2 Nasodental nerve and its accompanying artery exposed
3 Infraorbital artery and hard palate
4 Branch of the infraorbital artery to the orbital cavity, and the posterior alveolar nerve
5 Infraorbital nerve and the lateral wall of the maxillary sinus
6 Piriform aperture and alveolar process of the maxilla
7 Orbital contents retracted superiorly, and the tongue
8 Greater palatine nerve, the lateral wall of the nasal cavity and the area of section of the bone
9 Anterior edge of the ostium of the pharyngotympanic tube with a millimeter strip

around the piriform aperture (Lang and Papke, 1984). The course of these nerves is of clinical significance in local anesthesia for rhinoplasty and operations on the upper jaw. Denecke and Meyer (1964) summarize the various methods of local anesthesia of the external nose (see their Figs. 33–38).

Skin of the External Nose

The soft tissues at the paranasion are between 2 and 5 mm thick, in the center of the nasal bone 3.2 mm thick and at the tip of the nasal bone 2–2.2 mm thick. The skin of the dorsum of the nose and the nasal alae is usually thin, and fixed by loose connective tissue to the nasal aponeurosis and to the muscle fibers fanning out within it. Over the tip and the ala it is thicker, anchored more securely, and contains numerous large sebaceous glands. In our material the skin was about 7 mm thick in the alar region and 5 mm thick at the nasal tip. Elastic fibers run from the corium of the skin through the subcutis to the thin corial layer of the nasal vestibule.

The elasticity and mobility of the skin depend on the texture of its collagen fibers and on their anchorage to the underlying layer. On the dorsum of the nose the skin can only be displaced by 2–4 mm compared with 2–6 mm over the forehead and 4–6 mm in the philtrum of the upper lip (Friederich and Moerike, 1962).

Shape and Growth

Parts of the Nose

(Fig. **35**)

The current Nomina Anatomica defines the root, dorsum and tip of the nose, and the nasal alae. A zone of particularly thin skin lies at the root of the nose, where the forehead meets the nose. The nasal alae merge laterally into the skin of the cheek, and below and medially into the upper lip. Inferolaterally lies the nasolabial sulcus. The alae, the floor of the nasal cavity and the columella of the nasal septum define the nares.

The *root of the nose* may be narrow, medium or broad. From the lateral aspect it may appear high, moderate or deeply depressed. Its position relative to the eyeball varies widely. The depression between the nose and the forehead is termed the *sella nasi*. Usually this region is gently curved in children, is more marked in women, and it is most pronounced in men. (See also the paranasion in Figs. 35 and 43.)

The *dorsum of the nose* has two parts: the upper is supported by the nasal bones of varying width and curvature: the lower part, towards the tip, is supported only by cartilage. The lower part can be broader or narrower than, or of similar width to, the upper part.

The nasal alae may be narrow or flared. Their lower border may hang low, be normally placed or lie superiorly.

They are bounded above by a flat, or a curved *nasal-alar furrow,* or may be divided by a dimple from the remaining segment of the nasal alae. The shape of the nose provides one of the most obvious human characteristics (hereditary and further details, and a review of the literature are provided by Ziegelmayer, 1969). A nasal tip shaped in the literal meaning of the word is very unusual. The shape of the *nasal tip* depends on the shape and on the connections of the greater alar cartilages with each other and with the neighboring cartilages. The nasal tip can be broad or narrow, blunt or pointed, angular or globular. If the medial parts of the greater alar cartilages diverge from each other the nasal tip appears to be cleft or hooked downwards. A pointed nose is termed a nasus avicularis.

Nasal Folds

The *nasal alae* (pinnulae nasi) begin above at the alar *sulcus* and then continue inferiorly as the *nasal lobules.* The depth of the alar sulcus determines whether the nasal alae are clearly demarcated from the lateral part of the dorsum of the nose. Medially and anteriorly the alae merge smoothly into the tip of the nose. The nasal lobules may be oval, round or pointed in shape. Deeply arched lobules, curves interrupted in the middle as well as lobules without any curves can also occur. They possess neither a bony nor a cartilaginous support.

The alar sulcus is a groove in the skin which bounds the nasal alae above and joins the nasolabial sulcus. Below it runs in a curve towards the nasal tip but does not reach it. In the absence of the furrow, particularly during childhood, the lateral part of the nose merges smoothly into the nasal ala. If the furrow is particularly well developed an alar fossa is found.

Nares and Alar Lobules

(Fig. 36)

The region of the *nares* is also termed the base of the nose. If the nose is regarded as the surface of an upright pyramid, the nasal aperture forms the base, its tip points towards the nasal apex and its base joints the upper lip.

The alar *lobules* may be high-standing so that the nasal septum is visible from the side. Conversely, if the lobules hang low they conceal the nasal septum in the lateral view. Occasionally the base of the nose may slope downwards towards the tip of the nose in Europeans during puberty (Keiter, 1933), but this shape is relatively unusual in adults. The shape of the nares when observed from below varies widely. Usually the medial part of the nares, that is the columella, runs towards the tip in the shape of a bridge. Therefore this area is also termed the ponticulus or nasal bridge. Usually the ponticulus possesses an hour-glass shape, and its basal part is bigger and wider than its apex.

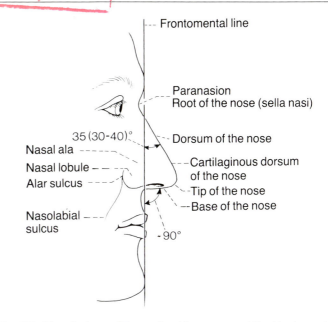

Fig. **35**   Terminology of the parts of the nose and the ideal nasal angle. The nasofacial angle should be 30–35° (Joseph, 1931)

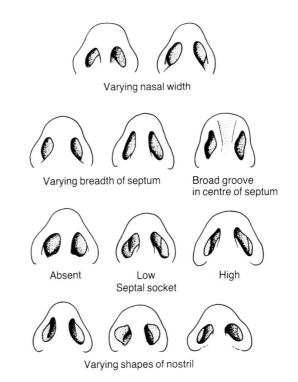

Fig. **36**   Nares and base of the nose showing various different shapes (Ziegelmayer, 1969)

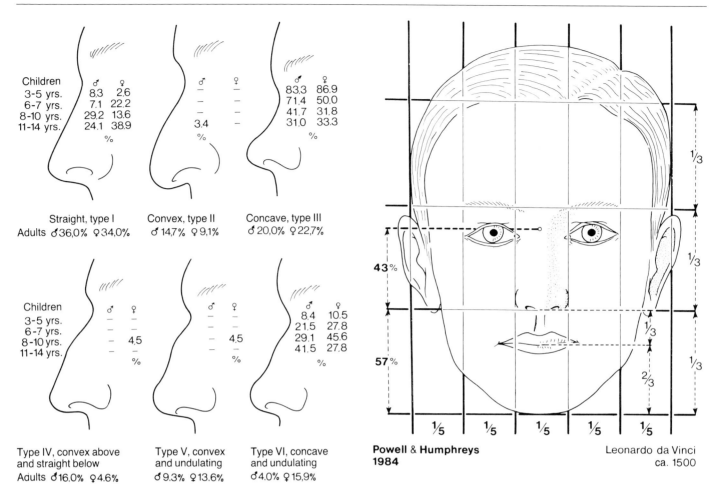

Children	♂	♀		♂	♀		♂	♀
3-5 yrs.	8,3	2.6		—	—		83,3	86.9
6-7 yrs.	7,1	22.2		—	—		71,4	50.0
8-10 yrs.	29.2	13.6		3.4	—		41,7	31.8
11-14 yrs.	24.1	38.9		—	—		31,0	33.3
		%			%			%

	Straight, type I	Convex, type II	Concave, type III
Adults	♂36,0% ♀34,0%	♂14,7% ♀9,1%	♂20,0% ♀22,7%

Children	♂	♀		♂	♀		♂	♀
3-5 yrs.	—	—		—	—		8,4	10.5
6-7 yrs.	—	—		—	—		21,5	27.8
8-10 yrs.	—	4.5		—	4.5		29,1	45.6
11-14 yrs.	—	—		—	—		41,5	27.8
		%			%			%

Type IV, convex above and straight below	Type V, convex and undulating	Type VI, concave and undulating
Adults ♂16.0% ♀4.6%	♂9.3% ♀13.6%	♂4.0% ♀15,9%

Fig. 37 Types of nasal profile in adolescents and adults (Würzburg material, Lang et al., 1987)

Powell & Humphreys 1984   Leonardo da Vinci ca. 1500

Fig. 38 Facial proportions from in front, divided into thirds as described by Leonardo da Vinci; other lines and measurements made by Powell and Humphreys (1984) are also given

Nasal Profile, Height and Depth

Broca (1872) carried out thorough measurements of the nasal skeleton on the skull. Collignon (1883) and Topinard (1888) later applied this method to the nasal soft tissues. Hovorka (1893) described five types of nasal shape. We used six types of nasal profile as described by Ziegelmayer (1969) for an investigation of 201 children between the ages of 3 and 14 years and 119 students. Fig. **37** shows the frequencies of the various types of nasal profile.

Basler (1931) investigated the nasal shape of 73 of his students in China: 42.5% had a straight nasal dorsum, 28.5% were very convex, 15.0% were slightly convex, 6.8% were concave-convex, 5.5% were slightly concave and 1.4% had a markedly concave nose. Altogether 28.8% has a curved nasal dorsum, and 2.8% had a Roman nose.

Proportions of the Nose and Face from in Front

(Fig. **38**)

Leonardo da Vinci (1452–1519) divided the face into three equal segments: the forehead reaches from the hairline to the medial insertion of the eyebrow, the central part from here to the base of the nose, and the lower segment runs from the base of the nose to the point of the chin (without the soft parts). More recent authors describe roughly the same thirds of the face as Leonardo da Vinci (Fig. **38**).

The esthetic face and the "ideal" nasal shape are an important working basis for plastic surgeons. The proportions of the face were therefore analyzed again by Powell and Humphreys (1984). They state that the upper third of the face extends from the hairline to the glabella, the middle third runs between the glabella and the subnasale, and the lower third between the subnasale and the chin. These authors also include the upper and lower lips in their scheme. The upper lip between the subnasal area and the orifice of the mouth thus constitutes one third of the lower third of the face, the lower lip together with the chin constitutes two thirds. Measurement of the distance from the paranasion to the chin allows two segments to be distinguished. The upper part, constituting 43% of this length in the ideal case, extends from the paranasion to the subnasale, and the lower part, constituting 57%, extends from the subnasale to the chin. Vertical lines through the angle of the mouth in directly forward gaze should run approximately through the medial edge of the iris, whereas a vertical line through the external boundary of the nasal alae should roughly coincide with the inner canthus (Naumann, 1966). If the nasal alae extend beyond a verti-

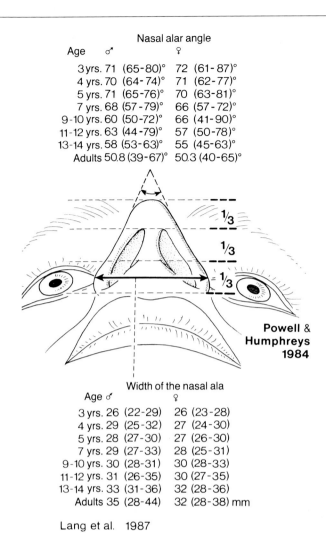

Nasal alar angle

Age	♂	♀
3 yrs.	71 (65-80)°	72 (61-87)°
4 yrs.	70 (64-74)°	71 (62-77)°
5 yrs.	71 (65-76)°	70 (63-81)°
7 yrs.	68 (57-79)°	66 (57-72)°
9-10 yrs.	60 (50-72)°	66 (41-90)°
11-12 yrs.	63 (44-79)°	57 (50-78)°
13-14 yrs.	58 (53-63)°	55 (45-63)°
Adults	50.8 (39-67)°	50.3 (40-65)°

Powell &
Humphreys
1984

Width of the nasal ala

Age	♂	♀
3 yrs.	26 (22-29)	26 (23-28)
4 yrs.	29 (25-32)	27 (24-30)
5 yrs.	28 (27-30)	27 (26-30)
7 yrs.	29 (27-33)	28 (25-31)
9-10 yrs.	30 (28-31)	30 (28-33)
11-12 yrs.	31 (26-35)	30 (27-35)
13-14 yrs.	33 (31-36)	32 (28-36)
Adults	35 (28-44)	32 (28-38) mm

Lang et al. 1987

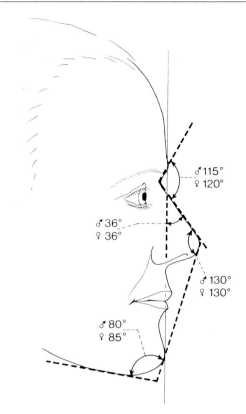

Fig. 40 Nasal, nasofacial, nose-chin, nasomental and other angles (Powell and Humphreys, 1984)

◀ Fig. 39 Angles and breadth of the nasal ala (Lang et al., 1987; Powell and Humphreys, 1984)

cal line through the inner canthus the nose then appears too broad, whereas conversely it appears too narrow (Fig. **39**).

A further useful line runs horizontally through both points of insertion of the nasal alae to the upper lip. The tip of the nose should lie only slightly below this horizontal plane. If the nose lies lower, then it appears to be too long, whereas if it lies above this horizontal plane it appears to be too short. The shortest distance between the inner canthus and the nasal dorsum should be not less than 1.5 cm.

The rhinoplastic surgeon should be aware not only of the ideal facial form and the current concepts of beauty, but also of the entire harmony of the face, taking account of the patient's personality and racial characteristics (Becker, 1961). The harmony of the face should never be sacrificed solely to preserve a beautiful nose (Daley, 1945). The face must be regarded as a unit, and the nose should have a good structural relationship with the balance of the face (Naumann, 1966). Photographs of the left and right sides often reveal entirely different facial expressions (Lang, 1937).

Profile View

(Figs. **37** and **40**)

Apart from the varying shapes of the nose, the profile of the face is influenced considerably by the teeth. Ideally the occlusion should be Class I. In Class II the mandible lies too far posteriorly, and in Class III too far anteriorly. Further details of orthognathia, retrognathia and prognathia of various types are described in the section on the maxillary skeleton. The shape of the forehead is also important for the facial profile; it may be convex, flat or even concave. Powell and Humphreys (1984) also demonstrated the projection of the nasal tip, and the increase or decrease of the length of the alar-lobular nasal complex. The nasal base may appear short or long in the lateral view.

Nasofacial Angle

(Fig. **40**)

A tangent to the nasal dorsum should form an angle between 30° and 35° with a line between the glabella and the chin (Joseph, 1931). This is the esthetic profile angle. Powell and Humphreys (1984) state that well-proportioned noses should have a naso-facial angle between 36° and 40°.

The tangent should not run through the protuberant zone but rather between the paranasion and the nasal tip if the nose is humped.

Baum (1982) described a vertical line between the paranasion and the subnasale, and another between this line and the nasal tip; the ideal ratio between the length of these two is 2 : 1. In the Goode method a vertical line is drawn between the paranasion and the alar sulcus and a horizontal line is drawn from this line to the nasal tip. The ratio between the length of the line from the ala nasi to the nasal tip and that between the paranasion and the point of intersection of the above two lines should lie between 0.55 and 0.6 (Powell and Humphreys, 1984). The columella should extend at most 3–5 mm below the nares. A tangent to the nasal base should divide the fronto-mental tangent at an angle of about 90° in a well-proportioned nose, and the tangent to the nasal dorsum should form an angle of about 60° with the tangent to the nasal base (Martin-Saller, 1957; Sercer, 1962; Denecke and Meyer, 1964).

The angle between the edge of the mandible and the subnasale should be about 100°. The angle between a line from the glabella to the pogonion and the edge of the mandible should be about 85°.

The authors also describe a nasofrontal angle: one tangent runs along the dorsum of the nose as far as the paranasion, and the other runs from the paranasion to the glabella. This nasofrontal angle should be 120° (115°–130°). The nasomental angle lies between a tangent to the dorsum of the nose extending as far as the tip, and a line from the nasal tip to the pogonion; it should measure 130° (120°–132°) (Fig. 40). Finally the angle between a vertical line from the glabella and the pogonion, and the lower edge of the mandible (the mentocervical angle) should be 85° (80°–95°) (Powell and Humphreys, 1984).

Arc Segments

(Fig. 42)

Baud (1982) drew an arc based on the mid-point of the external auditory meatus with its radius extending to the nasal tip (Fig. 41). In the ideal case the arc includes the frontal hairline and the point of the chin. For the average Frenchman he calculated an angle of 29° for the upper segment between the frontal hairline and the medial segment of the eyebrow, an angle of 23° for the middle segment between the frontal hairline and the nasal tip, and 30° for the lower angle between the nasal tip and the chin.

We measured the *height of the nose* between the paranasion (that is the deepest point of the saddle overlying the nasion) and the subnasale (the soft tissue area overlying the subspinale, see Fig. 42). In 3-year-old subjects we found values of 34 mm in boys, and 35 mm in girls. In girls there was a growth spurt between 3 and 4 years of age which produced an average growth of 4 mm, with further spurts between the ages of 11 and 12 and between 13 and 14. The average values in adult women were only 1 mm greater than those for 13–14 year-old girls. In males there were growth spurts between the ages of 3 and 4, 8 and 11, 11 and 12, and 13 and 14 years of age. After puberty the male nose grew on average by 6 mm.

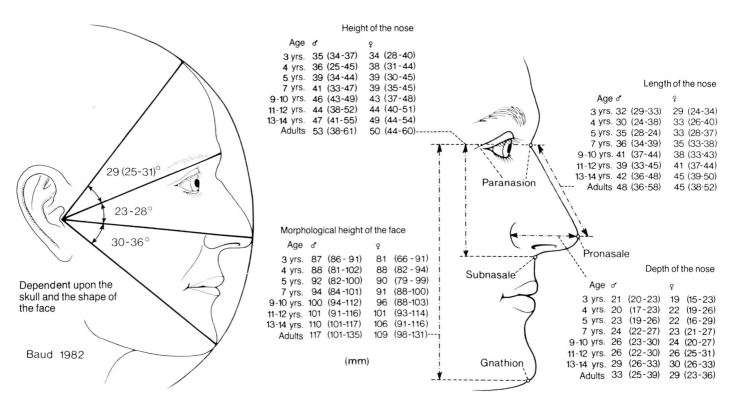

Fig. 41 "Crossbow" segments measured on the facial profile showing the relation to the shape of the skull and face (Baud, 1982)

Fig. 42 Postnatal growth of the nose after the third year of life (Lang et al., 1987)

Height of the nose

Age	♂	♀
3 yrs.	35 (34-37)	34 (28-40)
4 yrs.	36 (25-45)	38 (31-44)
5 yrs.	39 (34-44)	39 (30-45)
7 yrs.	41 (33-47)	39 (35-45)
9-10 yrs.	46 (43-49)	43 (37-48)
11-12 yrs.	44 (38-52)	44 (40-51)
13-14 yrs.	47 (41-55)	49 (44-54)
Adults	53 (38-61)	50 (44-60)

Length of the nose

Age	♂	♀
3 yrs.	32 (29-33)	29 (24-34)
4 yrs.	30 (24-38)	33 (26-40)
5 yrs.	35 (28-24)	33 (28-37)
7 yrs.	36 (34-39)	35 (33-38)
9-10 yrs.	41 (37-44)	38 (33-43)
11-12 yrs.	39 (33-45)	41 (37-44)
13-14 yrs.	42 (36-48)	45 (39-50)
Adults	48 (36-58)	45 (38-52)

Morphological height of the face

Age	♂	♀
3 yrs.	87 (86-91)	81 (66-91)
4 yrs.	88 (81-102)	88 (82-94)
5 yrs.	92 (82-100)	90 (79-99)
7 yrs.	94 (84-101)	91 (88-100)
9-10 yrs.	100 (94-112)	96 (88-103)
11-12 yrs.	101 (91-116)	101 (93-114)
13-14 yrs.	110 (101-117)	106 (91-116)
Adults	117 (101-135)	109 (98-131)

(mm)

Depth of the nose

Age	♂	♀
3 yrs.	21 (20-23)	19 (15-23)
4 yrs.	20 (17-23)	22 (19-26)
5 yrs.	23 (19-26)	22 (16-29)
7 yrs.	24 (22-27)	23 (21-27)
9-10 yrs.	26 (23-30)	24 (20-27)
11-12 yrs.	26 (22-30)	26 (25-31)
13-14 yrs.	29 (26-33)	30 (26-33)
Adults	33 (25-39)	29 (23-36)

29 (25-31)°

23-28°

30-36°

Dependent upon the skull and the shape of the face

Baud 1982

Paranasion

Pronasale

Subnasale

Gnathion

We measured the *depth of the nose* in projection between the apex of the nose (pronasale) and the most posterior insertion of the nasal ala. Fig. **42** shows the growth of the depth of the nose between the third year of life and adulthood. The length of the dorsum of the nose is the distance in a straight line between the paranasion and the pronasale. The growth in length of the nasal dorsum is shown in Fig. **42**.

Breadth of the Root of the Nose, Width of the Alae, the Nasal-Alar Angles and Nasal Indices

In anthropological terms the *width of the root of the nose* is defined as the length of a straight line between the two inner canthi with the eyelids open (medial intercanthal distance). The values are shown in Fig. **43**. Our results for 3- and 12-year-old children were on average 0.5–1.5 mm less than that those of Feingold (1974), whereas after the age of 12 our values were about 1 mm greater. Our findings were similar to those of Dekaban (1977). In his subjects values greater by about 1 mm were found in a few age groups.

The *breadth of the nasal alae* is the distance in a straight line between both alae. Our results can be seen in Fig. **43**. Between the age of 3 and 14 we found rather higher values than Houze (1891) and Hoyer (1895). The differences were usually less than 1 mm. Davenport (1939) observed relatively wide nasal alae in 3-year-old girls,

followed by suspension of growth between the ages of 4 and 7. The values at the age of 8 were the same in his subjects and ours (Lang et al. 1987).

The *alar angle* (inferior nasal angle) (Fig. **39**) depends especially on the width of the nasal ala and the depth of the nose. The angle becomes smaller from the age of 3 onwards, and this reduction is rouhgly continuous. After puberty the angle in the female is reduced to 50.3° (40°–65°) and in males to 50.8° (39°–67°). The shape of the nose and the alar angle show very marked racial differences.

The *nasal index* is calculated from the following formula:

Breadth of the nasal ala × 100 / Height of the nose.

A high index shows a broad nose, and a low index a narrow nose. Table **10** shows that in the male sex there are initially more mesorrhine noses with average values above 75; the mean nasal index then becomes discontinuously smaller. The external nose becomes relatively narrower during maturation.

The *elevation index* of the nose is calculated from the formula:

Lateral depth of the nose × 100 / Breadth of the nasal alae.

The index provides information about the steepness of the alae: low values indicate flat alae, whereas high values define steeper alae. Table **11** shows that the alae become continuously steeper during maturation. In young adults therefore the nasal alae in our material are on average steeper than in small children. Girls reach a high elevation index rather earlier than boys.

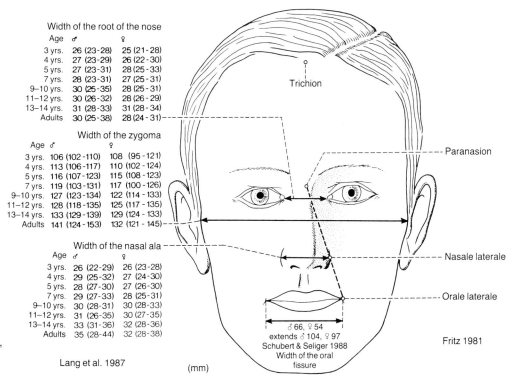

Width of the root of the nose

Age	♂	♀
3 yrs.	26 (23-28)	25 (21-28)
4 yrs.	27 (23-29)	26 (22-30)
5 yrs.	27 (23-31)	28 (25-33)
7 yrs.	28 (23-31)	27 (25-31)
9–10 yrs.	30 (25-35)	28 (25-31)
11–12 yrs.	30 (26-32)	28 (26-29)
13–14 yrs.	31 (28-33)	31 (28-34)
Adults	30 (25-38)	28 (24-31)

Width of the zygoma

Age	♂	♀
3 yrs.	106 (102-110)	108 (95-121)
4 yrs.	113 (106-117)	110 (102-124)
5 yrs.	116 (107-123)	115 (108-123)
7 yrs.	119 (103-131)	117 (100-126)
9–10 yrs.	127 (123-134)	122 (114-133)
11–12 yrs.	128 (118-135)	125 (117-135)
13–14 yrs.	133 (129-139)	129 (124-133)
Adults	141 (124-153)	132 (121-145)

Width of the nasal ala

Age	♂	♀
3 yrs.	26 (22-29)	26 (23-28)
4 yrs.	29 (25-32)	27 (24-30)
5 yrs.	28 (27-30)	27 (26-30)
7 yrs.	29 (27-33)	28 (25-31)
9–10 yrs.	30 (28-31)	30 (28-33)
11–12 yrs.	31 (26-35)	30 (27-35)
13–14 yrs.	33 (31-36)	32 (28-36)
Adults	35 (28-44)	32 (28-38)

Lang et al. 1987

Trichion

Paranasion

Nasale laterale

Orale laterale

♂ 66, ♀ 54
extends ♂ 104, ♀ 97
Schubert & Seliger 1988
Width of the oral fissure

Fritz 1981

(mm)

Fig. 43 Breadth of the root of the nose (medial intercanthal distance), of the zygoma and of the nasal ala (Lang et al., 1987)

Hyperleptorrhine	x−54.9			
Leptorrhine	55.0−69.9			
Mesorrhine	70.0−84.9			
Chamaerrhine	85.0−99.9			
Hyperchamaerrhine	100.0−x			

Table **10**   Nasal indices (Lang, Bachmann and Raabe, 1987)

Age		$\bar{x}$	s	$s_{\bar{x}}$	n	$x_{min.}$	$x_{max.}$
3 years	f	75.5	9.5	2.9	11	62.2	92.9
	m	75.2	10.3	6.0	3	64.7	85.3
4 years	f	71.3	8.8	2.6	11	61.4	90.3
	m	73.7	10.8	4.1	6	65.8	83.8
5 years	f	69.8	7.0	1.8	15	59.1	80.6
	m	72.6	7.7	2.4	10	64.3	88.2
6 years	f	68.3	3.2	1.1	8	64.4	74.4
	m	74.2	4.8	1.5	11	62.5	81.1
7 years	f	70.2	5.7	2.0	8	63.6	81.6
	m	72.9	10.4	3.0	12	61.4	100.0
8 years	f	71.9	3.7	1.5	6	68.2	77.5
	m	71.1	4.3	1.2	13	65.1	78.6
9/10 years	f	69.4	7.1	2.0	13	54.2	82.1
	m	65.6	4.1	1.3	10	59.2	72.1
11/12 years	f	68.7	6.3	2.0	10	57.5	80.0
	m	70.3	7.7	1.8	19	52.9	81.4
13/14 years	f	67.4	7.0	2.6	7	59.3	76.1
	m	69.3	7.6	2.7	8	58.5	78.3
Adults	f	63.3	6.2	9.9	44	53.3	82.2
	m	66.1	7.9	9.2	73	52.6	92.9

Distribution of individual values for the nasal index (%)

Girls	3−5 years	6−7 years	8−10 years	11−14 years	**Women**
Hyperleptorrhine	−	−	5.3	−	4.5
Leptorrhine	51.4	62.5	42.1	52.9	79.5
Mesorrhine	43.2	37.4	52.6	47.1	15.9
Chamaerrhine	5.4	−	−	−	−
Boys					**Men**
Hyperleptorrhine	−	−	−	3,7	4.1
Leptorrhine	42.1	26.1	56.5	44.4	68.54
Mesorrhine	47.4	69.6	43.5	51.9	24.7
Chamaerrhine	10.5	4.3	−	−	2.7
Hyperchamaerrhine	−	−	−	−	−

The sagittal (nasofacial index) is calculated from the following formula:

Nasal height × 100 / Morphological height of the face (see Table **12**)

The *morphological height of the face* is the distance in a straight line between the paranasion and the gnathion. Fig. **42** shows the increase of this distance from the third year onwards. The sagittal nasofacial index defines relatively short and relatively long noses. In girls the sagittal nasofacial index increases between 3 and 14 years of age, from 42.2 to 45.6. Similar values are observed in young women. In the male, values of 38.8 are found in the third year of life, and 41.2 at the age of 4. Thereafter the sagittal nasofacial index increases to a value of 45.5 (33.6−54.6) in young adult men, with spurts between 7 and 11 years of age.

The *interalar-jugular* index relates the width of the nasal alae to the width of the zygomatic arch. It defines nasal alae which appear narrow or broad. It is also termed the transverse nasofacial index. The development of the width of the zygomatic arch after the age of 13 can be seen in Fig. **43.** The index is calculated as follows:

Width of the nasal ala × 100 / Width of the zygomatic arch.

During adolescence the index in our subjects lay between 23.4 and 25.6. The interalar-jugular index increases in both sexes during development, but more obviously in girls than in boys. Nasal alae which appear broad are somewhat commoner in girls than in boys. We found values 1−2 mm higher for the length of the nasal dorsum than Hoyer (1895). Bach (1925, 1926) found an average height of 169.2 cm in young men compared with

Table **11**   Elevation index of the nose

Age		x̄	s	s_x̄	n	x_min.	x_max.
3 years	f	73.4	12.0	3.8	10	51.0	88.0
	m	81.5	9.2	4.6	4	69.0	90.9
4 years	f	80.3	9.2	3.1	9	67.9	92.0
	m	73.0	10.2	3.4	9	61.3	88.5
5 years	f	80.1	10.6	2.7	16	61.5	96.7
	m	77.2	2.4	2.3	8	67.9	83.3
6 years	f	83.0	6.2	2.5	6	75.0	92.9
	m	76.7	9.3	2.3	16	58.6	93.3
7 years	f	82.4	4.9	1.6	9	73.3	88.9
	m	80.3	7.6	2.3	11	66.7	93.1
8 years	f	81.2	4.4	1.8	6	76.7	86.7
	m	78.1	5.3	1.6	11	69.0	86.2
9/10 years	f	81.5	8.3	2.3	13	68.8	96.4
	m	82.9	4.9	1.7	8	77.4	93.5
11/12 years	f	87.1	5.1	1.6	10	81.3	96.4
	m	83.9	6.7	1.6	18	74.3	96.4
13/14 years	f	94.0	8.7	3.3	7	81.3	106.5
	m	87.5	8.3	2.8	9	75.0	100.0
Adults	f	92.9	9.4	1.4	44	74.2	109.4
	m	95.7	10.4	1.2	75	72.9	118.7

Table **12**   Sagittal nasofacial index

Age		x̄	s	s_x̄	n	x_min.	x_max.
3 years	f	42.2	3.2	1.0	11	38.0	48.2
	m	38.8	4.7	2.7	3	33.7	43.0
4 years	f	42.9	4.0	1.2	11	35.6	47.8
	m	40.2	3.9	1.3	9	33.7	44.3
5 years	f	43.4	4.4	1.1	16	36.4	51.1
	m	42.3	2.3	0.8	9	38.9	46.3
6 years	f	44.7	2.1	0.8	8	42.1	48.5
	m	42.0	4.4	1.1	16	34.0	52.0
7 years	f	45.6	2.0	0.7	8	43.2	48.9
	m	44.0	4.4	1.3	12	34.4	50.6
8 years	f	45.0	2.5	0.9	7	41.2	48.4
	m	41.9	1.9	0.5	13	38.9	44.6
9/10 years	f	45.0	3.3	0.9	15	39.8	50.5
	m	45.4	2.7	0.9	10	41.1	49.0
11/12 years	f	44.1	3.6	1.1	10	37.0	50.0
	m	43.6	2.6	0.6	20	39.0	49.1
13/14 years	f	45.6	6.3	2.2	8	33.3	52.3
	m	43.1	3.2	1.1	9	39.8	47.8
Adults	f	45.5	–	–	–	33.6	54.6
	m	45.5	–	–	–	33.6	54.6

Distribution of individual values for the sagittal nasofacial index (%)

					Women
Girls	3–5 years	6–7 years	8–10 years	11–14 years	18–32 years
x–39.9	23.7	–	4.6	11.1	4.5
40.0–47.9	65.8	87.5	81.8	61.1	65.6
48.0–x	10.5	12.5	13.6	27.8	29.7
Boys					**Men**
x–39.9	28.6	25.0	4.3	10.3	5.4
40.0–47.9	71.4	60.7	82.6	86.2	75.8
48.0–x	–	14.3	13.1	3.5	18.9

181.1 cm in our material, and 158 cm for women compared with 167 cm for our subjects. Thus the micro-evolution has had only a trivial effect on the nasal dorsum.

Keiter measured the angle between the Frankfurt horizontal and the nasal dorsum. This appeared to be smaller in children because of the lesser nasal depth. However, the dorsum of the nose is usually relatively short due to the inclination of the base of the nose. Overall, the child's nose is as prominent as that of the adult (Keiter, 1933).

Elongation of the nasal dorsum during ageing has been studied particularly by Pellnitz (1962) and Krmpotic-Nemanic et al. (1971). Krmpotic-Nemanic et al. think that sinking of the nasal tip during ageing is due to fracture of the lateral cartilage and of the lateral crus of the alar cartilage; this had already been described as early as 1912 by Virchow. Dion et al. (1978) on the other hand have emphasized that fragmentation only occurs at the zone connecting the individual cartilages of the nose, and not elsewhere.

The *nasal index* reflects the height to breadth ratio of the nose. A broad nose has a high index, and a narrow nose a low index. Table **11** shows the various nasal indices in mature adults and adolescents in our subjects. Blind (1890) showed that 75% of Bavarian neonates are hyper-platyrhine, 21% are platyrhine and 4%, mesorrhine. He could find no examples of leptorrhine nasal types. The mothers noses were usually mesorrhine.

Nasal Cavity

Nasal Septum

In this section the nasal septum, the narrow nasal roof, the broad nasal floor, the lateral wall of the nose and the choanae will be discussed in turn. The nasal cavity is the space between the nasal vestibule and the choanae, and is bounded by the ethmoidal labyrinth, the ethmoidal conchae, the lacrimal bone, the maxilla and the inferior concha, and the septum medially. Vertically the nasal cavity extends from the palate to the inferior surface of the cribriform plate. The nasal cavity can be divided into an introitus (the internal nostril), a main part encompasing the nasal cavity itself and an outlet at the choanae. The nasal septum divides the upper airway into two nasal cavities extending from the nares to the choanae.

Development

(Fig. **44**)

The nasal septum has a membranous part in front at the columella, a cartilaginous part overlying the septal cartilage and a bony part formed by the perpendicular plate of the ethmoid bone and the vomer.

The cartilage of the nasal septum begins to develop in the 7th to 8th week of embryonal life (Broman, 1911). At the end of the 2nd embryonal month the nasal capsule is uniformly chondrified. The vomer develops in the 3rd embryonal month by desmal ossification in two bony laminae which unite below. Above, the lamellae diverge from each other in a V shape. The lower edge of the cartilaginous nasal septum is grasped by the anterior part of

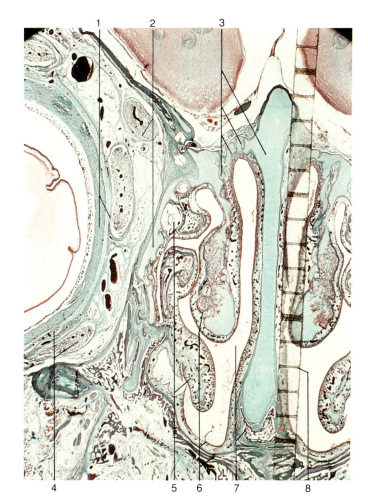

Fig. **44** Nasal cavity and nasal septum. Frontal section of a 35 cm fetus. The vessels are injected in black. The nasal crest of the maxilla has not yet developed
1 Sclera and medial rectus muscle
2 Superior oblique muscle and cartilaginous medial wall of the orbit
3 Olfactory filaments and septal cartilage
4 Inferior rectus and inferior oblique muscles
5 Developing ethmoidal cells, and the inferior concha
6 Middle concha and floor of the nasal cavity (maxilla)
7 The common nasal meatus and vomer
8 Millimeter strip

this groove. Posteriorly the two lamellae form the ala of the vomer which grasps the sphenoid rostrum. Later the lower part of the vomer elongates, so that in a frontal section the vomer is V-shaped anteriorly, and Y-shaped posteriorly. Chondral ossification of the perpendicular plate begins in the 6th month in the crista galli, and extends superiorly and inferiorly (Zuckerkandl, 1892; Schultz-Coulon and Eckermeyer, 1976). The nasal septum is of fundamental significance for the growth of the nose (Scott, 1953): it constitutes an epiphyseal plate for the entire skeleton of the upper face. Ossification of the perpendicular plate has reached the vomer in the third year of life. A bony canal is found between the two structures in which the posterior (sphenoidal) process of the septal cartilage extends backwards as far as the body of the sphenoid bone. This can be ossified laterally and appear distended (see also page 32).

Perpendicular Plate and Nasal Bones

(see Fig. **9**)

The nasal spine of the frontal bone forms the most anterosuperior segment of the roof of the nasal cavity in the septal area. Below it lies the perpendicular plate extending anteriorly for a varying distance on the posterior surface of the nasal bone. In 0.6% of specimens the perpendicular plate lay only along one-quarter of the length of the nasal bone, in 7% it covered one-third, in 13% half of the nasal bone, in 39% two-thirds of its length and in 9% three-quarters of its length. In 26% the perpendicular plate abutted the nasal bone in its entire length (Stier, 1895).

The anterior edge of the perpendicular plate extends to the middle of the nasal bones in 49% of cases, in 38% to the junction between the middle and inferior thirds of the nasal bone (Zuckerkandl, 1892). In 10% the contact between the perpendicular plate and nasal bones lies at the junction between the upper and middle thirds. In 3% of cases there is no connection between these two parts of the skeleton, and the perpendicular plate supports only the nasal spine of the frontal bone.

Premaxilla and Nasal Septum

(Figs. **8, 9** and **45**)

Koelliker showed in the last century that the premaxilla possesses its own bony center. Klaff (1956) found two bony centers within the later premaxilla which fuse to a large extent with the upper jaw of the same side before birth.

Fawcett (1911) showed that the vomer develops from one or two connective tissue bone centers. Two ossification centers were found in his material, one in the lower part of the nasal septum, slightly posterior and medial to the paraseptal cartilage. This ossification center appeared in the 45 mm embryo. In the 50–60 mm embryo both anlages unite at their lower edges, the vomer then appears U-shaped in frontal section, and later at the 100 mm stage as Y-shaped. The vomer therefore arises mainly by membranous ossification, but a small part arises from chondral ossification. The two bony plates of the vomer unite from

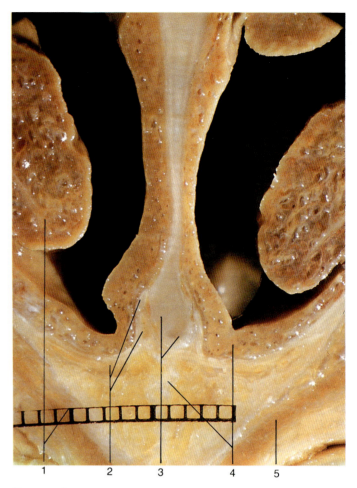

Fig. **45** Septal cartilage and septal groove in frontal section from behind
1 Inferior nasal concha with a millimeter strip
2 Paraseptal cartilage (Jacobson's cartilage) and ala of the premaxilla
3 Lower edge of the septal cartilage (footplate)
4 Floor of the nasal cavity and interincisive suture
5 Area of origin of the incisive muscle

behind forwards during the 3rd to the 15th year of life (Gilbert et al., 1958).

The anterior nasal spine projects downwards from the anterior surface of the premaxilla. Klaff (1956) thought that the maxilla also took part in its development. Before birth the premaxillary wings grow upwards from the posterior two-thirds of the superior surface of the premaxilla on both sides. The upper edges of the alae can be curved laterally. Therefore in frontal section the alar region can arise from a median ridge. The alae grow very little from birth to the 6th year of life, but then grow rapidly (Fig. **45**). In adults each ala measures about 12 mm along its upper edge but only 6 mm along its lower edge. This pedicle of the alar region lies immediately anterior to the incisive canal. In the 15th year of life the apex of the vomer unites with the alar region (Mosher, 1907). This area of union was previously known also as the subvomeral bone. Mosher was the first to show that it forms part of the premaxilla.

Incisive suture. The premaxilla synostoses in the first year of life with the maxilla, initially on the nasal surface. In our material the incisive suture persisted on the palatine surface up to the sixth year of life, but occasionally later.

Perpendicular Plate of the Ethmoid Bone

The anterior edge of the thin perpendicular plate of the ethmoid bone runs downwards and backwards from the anterior middle third of the nasal bone to reach the upper edge of the vomer immediately behind the ala of the premaxilla. The anterior edge may lie almost vertical or almost horizontal. In the latter case the lower segment of the septal cartilage is prolonged. Rarely the upper part of the perpendicular plate is pneumatized from the frontal sinus (see Fig. **96,** page 68).

Nasal Crest of the Maxilla

After birth the nasal crest of the maxilla projects beneath the vomer (see Fig. **61**) and enfolds its inferior edge. The vault of the maxilla begins behind the incisive canal. In our material the distance between the subspinale (the bony point inferior to the anterior nasal spine) and the anterior edge of the incisive foramen was 7.5 mm in the newborn, 9 mm in the second year of life, and 11.6 (8–18) mm in adults (Lang and Baumeister, 1982).

Palatine Bone and Nasal Crest

The most posterior part of the floor of the nasal cavity is formed by the horizontal plate of the palatine bone which runs on both sides immediately lateral to the midline into the posterior nasal spine. In the newborn its mean length is 0.9 (0–1.5) mm, in the two-year-old 1.6 (0.5–3.0) mm and in adults 3.9 (0–7.0) mm. In the midline the nasal crest of the palatine bone projects superiorly from the palatine bone. Its height was 1.6 (1–2) mm in the newborn, 2.0 (1–4) mm at the age of 2 and 5.6 (3–10) mm in the adult (Lang and Baumeister, 1982).

Figs. **70** and **71** illustrate the postnatal increase of the height of the nasal cavity, and the migration of the nasal conchae.

Vomer

The vomer forms the posterior and inferior part of the nasal septum. The alae of the vomer rest upon the sphenoidal rostrum. Rarely a recess of the sphenoidal sinus extends into the vomer (see also pages 41 and 90).

Septal Cartilage

(Fig. **46**)

The septal cartilage is 3–4 mm thick: parallel cartilaginous surfaces are present over wide areas (Cottle et al., 1957). The anteroinferior part of the septal cartilage expands into an area 4–8 mm wide, termed the *footplate*. Zuckerkandl (1896) described this thickening and called it the lateral anterior process. Similar expansions of the cartilage are present at the junction with the lateral nasal cartilage, termed the lateral posterior process (Cottle, 1957). It is firmly united to the nasal bone by collagenous connective tissue fibers. The perpendicular plate of the ethmoid bone and the vomer are united to the nasal bone by taut collagen fiber bundles. The anteroinferior edge of the septum is not fixed to bone or cartilage but lies in free contact with the membranous septum. The lower edge of the septum lies on the premaxilla, in front of the alae. Here the cartilage has a perichondrial layer and a fascial cap. The nasal crest of the palatine process of the maxilla is also ensheathed by periostial structures resembling fascia, and by connective tissue from the septal cartilage. Some fibers adopt a figure of eight between the cartilage and the bone and form a type

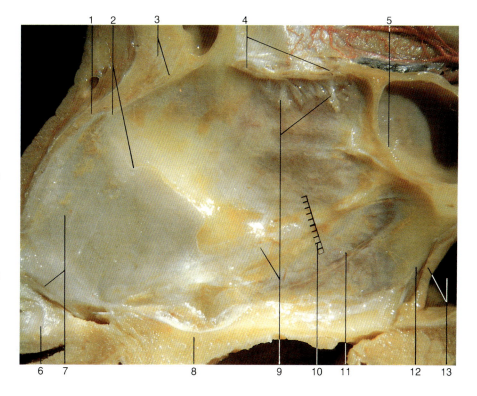

Fig. **46** Elements of the nasal septum
 1 Nasal bone
 2 Anterior edge of the perpendicular plate
    of the ethmoid bone
 3 Nasofrontal suture and nasal spine of the
    frontal bone
 4 Cribriform plate
 5 Anterior wall of the sphenoidal sinus
 6 Medial crus of the greater alar cartilage
 7 Septal cartilage
 8 Hard palate
 9 Olfactory filaments and posterior process
    of the septal cartilage
10 Vomer with a millimeter strip
11 Nasopalatine nerve
12 Posterior edge of the vomer
13 Mucosa retained on the medial edge of
    the choana, and the pharynx

of joint capsule. Fatty tissue also lies in the anterior part of the septum between the bone and the cartilage, allowing the septum to move relative to the neighboring cartilages (Aymard, 1917). The thickness of the posterior segment of the septal cartilage in the newborn and at the age of 3 months is the same as in adults (2.1–2.5 mm) (Kowatscheff, 1942). The bones and cartilage forming the nasal septum are covered by a layer of periostium and perichondrium, over which lie the submucosa and the mucosa of the nasal cavity and of the vestibule. Joseph (1967) measured the thickness of the nasal septum and its mucosal covering in 300 patients at the nasal valve: it measured 5–8 mm in leptorrhine noses, 10–13 mm in platyrrhine noses and 4–8 mm in children (quoted by Klaff, 1970).

Tubercles of the Septum

According to Zuckerkandl (1893) the anterior septal tubercle (septal intumescence) was first described by Morgagni (1681–1771): it forms the entrance to the olfactory cleft. The septum is markedly thickened in some subjects in this area lying between the two middle conchae (Fig. **47**).

The tubercle of the posterior septum. Almeida (1975) described an adenovascular body of the posterior part of the nasal septum present in about 60% of living subjects. The adenovascular body occupies between one-fifth and one-sixth of the surface of the nasal septum. Smooth, trabecular and folded protuberances can be seen in this area. This area atrophies in old age (Wustrow, 1951). The protrusion contains seromucinous glands and numerous vessels (Almeida, 1975), and lies in the region of the choanal crest which is present in 54% of subjects (Perovic, 1959–1960). The terms posterior "hypertrophic septum", "septal caudae" and "septal wings" are also used.

Septal angle. The angle between the lower edge of the septal cartilage and the anterior edge (in the region of the dorsum of the nose) lies between 25° and 30° (Masing, 1964). The surface area of the septum measures 30–35 cm^2 (Gherardi, 1939).

Paraseptal Cartilages

(Fig. 45)

Paraseptal cartilages have been known since 1700 (Morrison, 1970). They arise from an anterior and a posterior cartilaginous center which soon fuse. In man the paraseptal cartilages lie lateral to the anterior part of the nasal septum, and below Jacobson's organ (Fawcett, 1911). (Unfortunately, the paraseptal cartilage is also described as Jacobson's cartilage.) The cartilage always lies below Jacobson's organ, but never has any direct connection to it. In the 65 mm embryo the paraseptal cartilage lies lateral to the lower, thickened, end of the septal cartilage, and immediately behind the anterolateral process of the septum (the ventrolateral process of Spurgat or the ventral process of Zuckerkandl). The paraseptal cartilage is a thin bar of cartilage lying lateral to the septum. In front, it narrows to form two processes which reach the anterolateral process of the septum. A further process runs laterally and upwards, below the nasal introitus, towards the alar process of the lateral nasal capsule forming a V-shaped cartilaginous

structure with its apex pointing downwards. The posterior process ossifies, and unites with a connective tissue anlage joining the posterior copula and the lateral nasal capsule. The posterior paraseptal cartilage does not ossify but is converted into connective tissue in the 150 mm foetus, whereas the connective tissue bridges between the anterior and posterior paraseptal cartilages ossify and unite with the vomer (Fawcett, 1911). The ossified paraseptal cartilage does not fuse with the vomer, but forms an independent ossicle which unites with the vomer only during the perinatal period (Augier, 1931). Augier found ossification of the paraseptal cartilage in the 60 mm embryo, but Eloff (1952) could not find it in embryos smaller than 100 mm. Also, union of an ossification center of the cartilage with the vomer (Fawcett, 1911) is not visible before the 100 mm stage. In the 108 mm embryo, connective tissue ossification can be recognized entirely independent of the anterior paraseptal cartilage, immediately posterior to the posterior

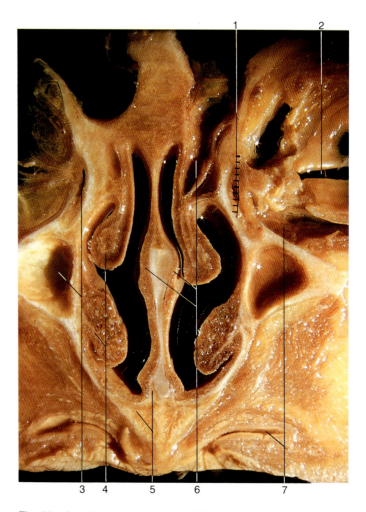

Fig. **47** Anterior intumescence of the septum in frontal section from behind
1 Lacrimal sac with a millimeter strip
2 Palpebral celft
3 Lacrimal sac and the maxillary sinus
4 Middle and inferior nasal conchae
5 Incisive bone and ala for the lower edge of the septum
6 Frontonasal duct and septal intumescence
7 Origin of the inferior orbital part of the orbicularis muscle and the vestibule of the mouth

end of the latter cartilage. Its anterior end overlaps the posterior extent of the paraseptal cartilage. This connective tissue bone is the paraseptal ossicle described by Augier (Eloff, 1952). In 145 and 150 mm embryos a large bony plate can be recognized at the posterior end of each anterior paraseptal cartilage lying on each side of the vomer (Fawcett, 1911). This bony plate inserts into the posterior end of the anterior paraseptal cartilage that ossifies perichondrally and endochondrally (Eloff, 1952). In the 200 mm foetus the posterior ossification center of the anterior paraseptal cartilages has become smaller. The vomer has proliferated into the membrane which embraces the anterior paraseptal cartilage and its posterior ossification center. The paraseptal cartilage in adults is shown in Figs. **47–49.** A paraseptal ossicle was demonstrated in a 265 mm embryo; it had not fused with the anterior paraseptal cartilage and could only be demonstrated on the right side.

Nasal Septum as a Growth Center

The growth of the human nose, nasal cavity and face depends largely on the nasal septum (Scott, 1953, 1956, 1957, 1958, 1959, 1963). Experimental resection of the nasal septum in rabbits confirms this (Sarnat and Wechsler, 1966).

Jennes (1954) and Fischer (1957) demonstrated the importance of the septal cartilage in the growth and shape of the nose (Farrior and Connolly, 1970). Two theories (Moss, 1976) attempt to explain the role of the septal cartilage in the growth of the nose and of the middle third of the face:

1) The growth of the septal cartilage influences the growth of the middle third of the facial skeleton in an inferior direction.

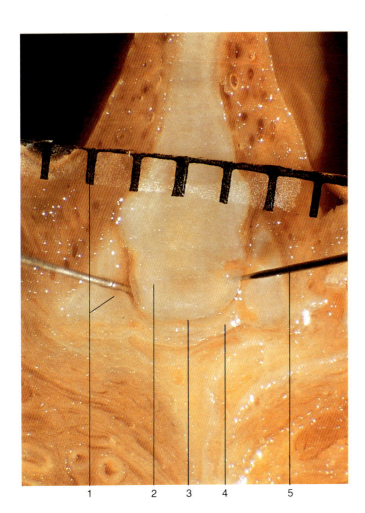

Fig. **48** Pseudoarthrosis of the septal cartilage in frontal section from in front
1 Paraseptal cartilage with a millimeter strip
2 Inferior end of the septal cartilage
3 Pseudoarthrosis
4 Connective tissue bridges of the paraseptal cartilages and anterior nasal spine
5 Pointer displaying the paraseptal cartilage

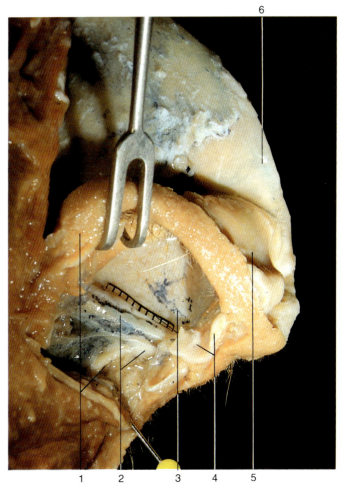

Fig. **49** Paraseptal cartilage (Jacobson's cartilage) in lateral view
1 Lateral edge of the nares retracted superiorly, and the subnasal punctum
2 Paraseptal cartilage and anterior nasal spine
3 Septal cartilage with a millimeter strip
4 Medial crus of the greater alar cartilage
5 Lateral crus of the greater alar cartilage
6 Lateral nasal cartilage

2) The growth of the septal cartilage and the nasal septum is dictated by changes of the bony central part of the face.

Pirsig (1975) observed increased regeneration of septal cartilage around the anterior diminished free end of the septal cartilage in an adolescent who had undergone a septoplasty 14 months previously. He also demonstrated that early resection of the center of the septal cartilage in childhood often provokes renewed deviations of the septum (Pirsig, 1977). There are various zones of growth activity within the septal cartilage, particularly at its anterior end (Vetter et al., 1983, 1984). There is thus an age-dependent part of the septum for the synthesis of the matrix, lying in the supramaxillary zone. Vetter et al. (1984) measured the cell thickness of chondrocytes of the nasal septum in 12 adolescents and 12 adults, using small pieces of cartilages taken during septoplasty. The cells were always thickest at the anterior end of the septal cartilage. The cells were particularly thick in adults between 18 and 52 years, less so in the supramaxillary zone, and even less in the central area of the septum (with the exception of specimens from adults). The thickness of the chondrocytes of the posterior part of the nasal septum was much less than those of the anterior part.

Septal Dislocation in the Neonate

Metzenbaum (1936) was the first to describe dislocations of the nasal septum in the newborn (Jeppesin and Windfeld, 1972). It is said that the septum is dislocated during rotatory movements in the mother's pelvis; the dislocation should be recognized and reduced as rapidly as possible.

Fig. **50 a–d**   Cleft palate with a deviated septum. Frontal section through the head of a boy aged 56 months

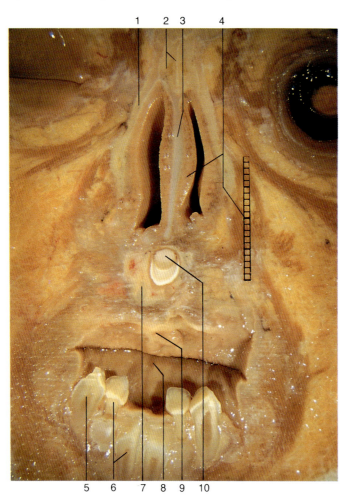

Fig. **50 a**   Section 25 mm behind the apex of the nose as seen from behind
 1 Frontal process of the maxilla
 2 Internasal suture and nasal bone
 3 Correctly developed septal cartilage
 4 Anterior intumescence of the septum with a millimeter strip
 5 Canine tooth
 6 Inferior incisor teeth
 7 Incisive bone
 8 Lower lip
 9 Upper lip with furrows
10 Pulp of the permanent incisor tooth

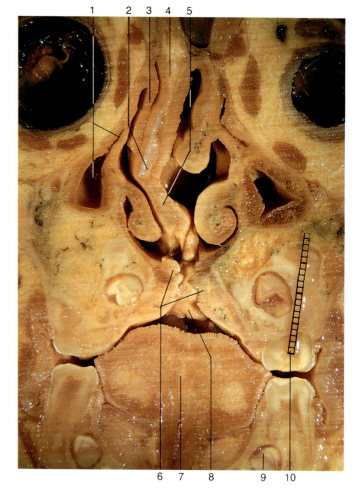

Fig. **50 b**   Section 32 mm behind the tip of the nose seen from behind
 1 Maxillary ostium and maxillary sinus. The mucosa is thickened
 2 Septal cartilage deviated to the left
 3 Left medial nasal concha
 4 Ossified perpendicular plate
 5 Vomer with no attachment to the palate
 6 Palatal cleft
 7 Tongue
 8 Area which has been corrected by surgery
 9 Anlage of a permanent tooth
10 First deciduous molar with a millimeter strip

Interuterine dislocations of the nasal septum lead to later abnormalities of growth of the external nose (Pirsig, 1977). Many authors have found slight deformities and dislocations in up to 21% of subjects.

Septal Deviations

(see Figs. **8** and **50**)

Theile (1855) found septal deviations in the bony nose of 22% of subjects; like us, Zuckerkandl (1893) found that the deviation of the nasal septum was more often to the left side; he found S-shaped deformities also. Deviations of a lesser degree were generally found in the lower part of the bony septum, behind the anterior nasal spine, usually associated with thickening of this part of the septal cartilage. Thickenings of the septum in the region of the posterior (sphenoidal) process of the cartilage can develop into formal ridges in about 30% of cases (Zuckerkandl, 1892). Usually the opposite side of the nasal septum is then grooved. In 63% of cases the septal deviation lies in the perpendicular plate (Stier, 1895). The vomer alone is bent in only 1% of cases, the perpendicular plate and the vomer are both deviated in 26% with equal frequency to the left and right sides. In 12% of cases the perpendicular plate and the vomer are deviated in opposite directions, the plate always to the left side, and the vomer to the right. In 11.1% of cases the perpendicular plate, the vomer and the nasal crest were deviated, the deviation being twice as often to the right as to the left. Stier (1895) found a straight septum

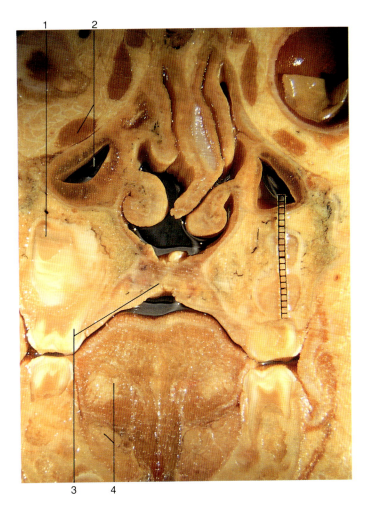

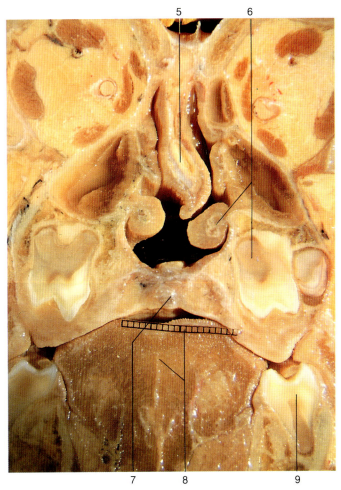

Fig. **50c** Section behind the cleft demonstrated from in front
1 Anlage of the first permanent molar tooth
2 Inferior rectus muscle and maxillary sinus
3 Second deciduous molar tooth and uncorrected palatal cleft
4 Tongue and sublingual gland

Fig. **50d** Section behind the cleft viewed from in front
5 Septal cartilage and nasal septum with no connection to the soft palate which has been surgically corrected
6 Anlage of the first permanent molar and the inferior concha
7 Repaired soft palate
8 Body of the tongue with a millimeter strip
9 Second deciduous molar tooth

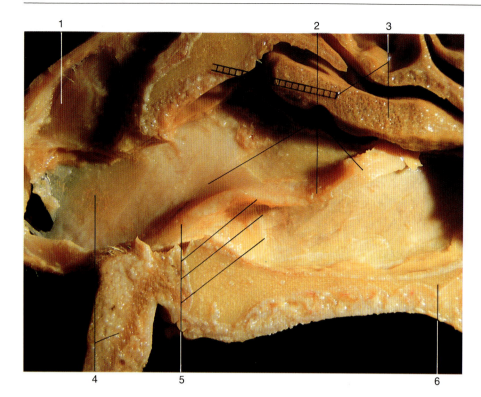

Fig. **50e**   Septal deviation with extremely large premaxillary wing. Paramedian sagittal section seen from the left side
1 Nasal ala retracted superiorly
2 Cartilaginous part of the deviation in the region of the posterior process of the cartilaginous septum
3 Medial nasal concha with a millimeter strip
4 Septal cartilage and the upper lip
5 Extremely large premaxillary wing with a dorsal suture
6 Hard palate

in 21% of men, compared with 72% in women; he postulated that the more frequent deviations in men were caused by previous injury. He found fractured nasal bones in 15% of cases. Obliquely placed nasal bones associated with a crooked vomer and nasal crest were also found. Welcker (1882) found this type of deviation of the nasal bones in 5.5% of cases. McKenzie found bony septal deviations in about 75% of 2152 skulls (Thomson and Negus, 1948). Stier (1895) found deviations in 65%. Fig. **50** shows that a septal deviation can be present, even in the presence of a cleft palate.

Scoliotic Nose. Isolated correction of the external part of a scoliotic nose is usually futile: both the external nose and the septum must be corrected (Naumann 1966).

Types of Septal Deviation

Gray (1965) distinguishes two types of septal deviation:

1) A cartilaginous type in which the anterior part of the septal cartilage is bent upon itself or dislocated out of the nasal crest.
2) A cartilaginous-bony type in which the nasal crest, the vomer, the perpendicular plate and the neighboring cartilage are deformed.

Combinations of both types are frequent.

Causes of Septal Deviation

Anton (1893) demonstrated deviations in 16% of neonates. Both he and Gruenwald (1925) made the following observations:

1) Deviations can be due to unequal growth of the part of the skeleton forming the septum.
2) Deviations may be due to unequal development of the premaxilla and closure of the palate due to the fact that the tongue is displaced downwards first on one side and then the other so that the palatal shelves of the right and left sides grow into the horizontal plane at different times.
3) The more frequent forms of septal deviation are due to unequal growth at puberty. In particular, the incisor or molar teeth initially erupt on one side in more than 50% of cases.
4) Gruenwald (1925) reported subluxation of the parts of the skeleton forming the septum.
5) If the septum is deviated, the middle concha on the concave side undergoes compensatory growth.
6) In children with septal deviation or kinks of the cartilaginous septum, the vomer or the nasal crest, the normal transmission of pressure is lost. The deviation due to birth trauma becomes more pronounced during growth.
7) Septal deviations of various types can be present during fetal life (Boyden, 1948; Patrzek, 1890).
8) Many septal deviations are due to trauma, which may be slight and without other sequelae, and which include a greenstick fracture in adolescents (Naumann, 1987).
9) Septal deviations may arise in cleft palate also (Fig. **50b**).

Removal of the Septum in Childhood

Reidy (1968) removed the thickened septal cartilage in children, particularly of children with clefts. Nasal growth was not retarded in any of the children. Other experienced authors emphasize the supportive function of the nasal septum, and claim that removal of the anterosuperior part of the septum leads to a duckbill nose.

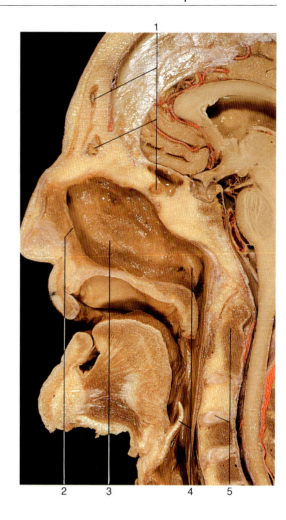

Fig. **51** Absent nasal concha and the bony nasal septum
1 Minimal pneumatization
2 Posterior edge of the cartilaginous septum covered during life with normal mucosa
3 Lateral wall of the nose with absent conchae
4 Torus tubarius and epiglottis
5 Dens of the axis and intervertebral disc between C3 and C4

Absence and Perforation of the Septum

Heymann (1900) described absence of the cartilaginous septum. McLaughlin (1949) reported an absent septal cartilage with retarded growth of the nose and the upper lip: the septum had probably been injured during birth and had then suffered further damage due to inflammation.

Absence of the Posterior Part of the Nasal Septum

(Fig. **51**)

McKenzie (1923) observed a defect of the vomerine segment of the nasal septum. Our material also contained a case with absence of the vomerine segment, the perpendicular plate and the nasal concha (Lang and Kley, 1981).

Perforations

Zuckerkandl (1893) found 8 perforations of the cartilaginous septum in 150 bodies. We also found such perforations. Forced respiration in these cases causes a whistling sound. Previously these lesions were usually due to syphilis.

Membranous Septum (Mobile Septum)

The soft part of the septum between the anteroinferior edge of the septal cartilage and the columella is the membranous septum; it is between 6 and 10 mm long. The mobile, lower segment of the septum consists of the membranous septum and the columella.

Aplasia

Menzel reported absence of the columella in a 15-year-old patient (Stupka, 1938). Both nasal vestibules formed a single cavity, and the anterior edge of the columella was formed by the anterior edge of the septal cartilage. The point of the nose was prolapsed.

Folds, Polyps and Pneumatization of the Septum

Folds

Czermak and Semmelleder were the first to demonstrate the septal folds and their marked individual variations (Kallius, 1905). They run obliquely from posterosuperior to anteroinferior, and form 5–9 mucosal swellings which are most pronounced between the 4th and 9th fetal month. Generally they atrophy in the 9th fetal month, but can be demonstrated in 31% of cases after the tenth year of life. They may undergo marked hypertrophy in disease. We found one 5 mm long mucosal fold projecting downwards. The narrow border between the lateral wall of the septum and the mucosal fold was covered with respiratory epithelium. Numerous lymphoepithelial organs are found on the septal surface and the inner surface of the fold.

Polyps

Multiple polyps have been described arising from the nasal septum (Brandenburg, 1935).

Hematomas and Abscesses

(Fig. **52**)

According to Hirschfeld, 75% of abscesses of the nasal septum are due to trauma (Rosenvold, 1944). Subperichondrial or subperiostial hematomas follow fractures of the nasal cartilage or the nasal bone: breech of the septal mucosa allows secondary infection to develop. One case of a fracture of the cartilaginous septum was found in our material (Fig. **52**). Intracranial extensions of a septal abscess had been described on only 17 occasions up to 1944.

Expansion of the Nasal Septum

Numerous surgeons state that thickening of the nasal septum on one or both sides is usually due to organization of a septal hematoma by connective tissue.

Pneumatization

(Fig. **54**)

Pneumatization of the nasal septum was found rarely in our material; it was combined with pneumatization of the crista galli, mostly through the frontal sinus. Krmpotic-Nemanic (1977) reported septate septal sinuses, and showed that the sphenoid sinus can project into the nasal septum. Similar findings were reported by Onodi (1893) and Schaeffer (1920). Schwartz showed septate septal sinuses by radiology in more than 2% of cases. Similar recesses of the ethmoidal sinus were also found in our material.

Nerves

Nervus Terminalis

A nerve plexus lies in the septal olfactory region in which the actual nerve cells are embedded. A slender nerve arises from this plexus and enters the cranial cavity through a foramen in the cribriform plate, behind the crista galli, and there connects with the terminal ganglion. From this point arise fine fibers which enter the anterior edge of the medial olfactory stria of the brain (De Vries, 1905); Johnston, 1914; Larsell, 1950).

Vomeronasal Nerve

(Fig. **55**)

The vomeronasal nerve and organ can be demonstrated after the 6th fetal week, and are clearly developed by the 5th fetal month (Fleischer, 1877; Klaff, 1970; Hedewig, 1980). The vomeronasal organ is initially open towards the nasal cavity, but soon closes; it atrophies in the human after birth. However, Merkel was able to demonstrate it in 2 men (Fig. 173 in Lang, 1985).

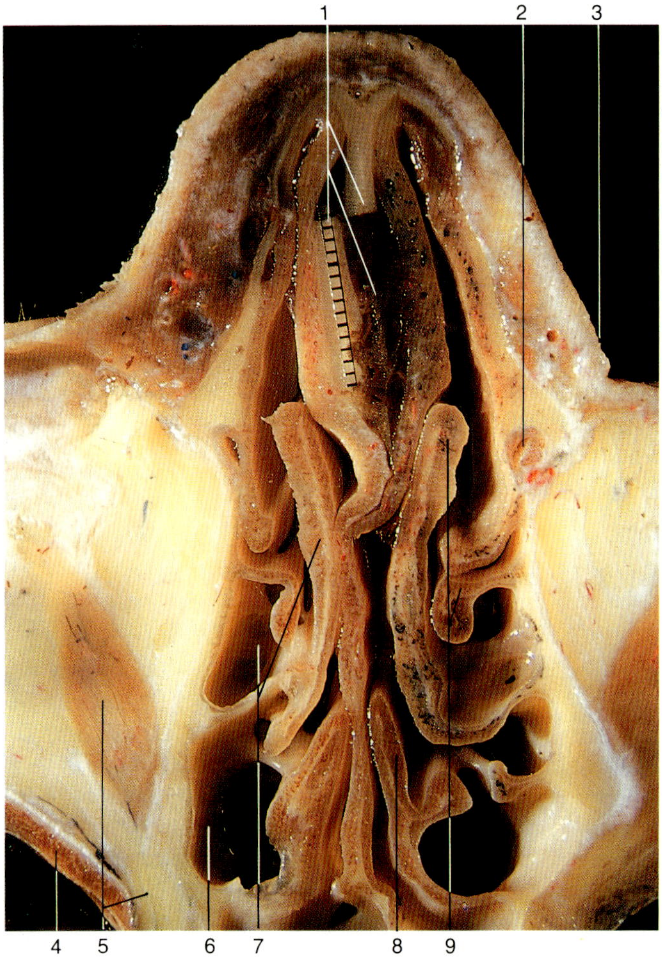

Fig. **52** Fracture of the septal cartilage showing a transverse section from below
1 Fractured ends of the septal cartilage with a hematoma and a millimeter strip
2 Nasolacrimal duct
3 Upper part of the nasal ala
4 The greater wing of the sphenoid bone
5 Inferior rectus muscle and fat at the medial end of the superior orbital fissure
6 Posterior ethmoidal cell
7 Anterior ethmoidal cell and middle nasal concha
8 Superior nasal concha
9 Middle nasal concha and uncinate process

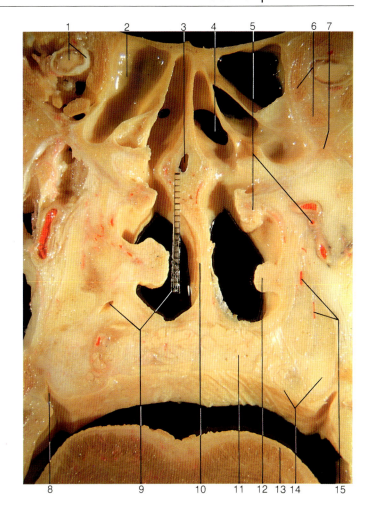

Fig. **53** Septal recess of the sphenoid sinus in frontal section from in front
1 Optic nerve and dura mater of the optic nerve
2 Posterior ethmoidal cells
3 Septal recess of the sphenoidal sinus
4 Ostium of the left sphenoidal sinus (note the right-sided ostium)
5 Middle concha and pterygoid segment of the maxillary artery
6 Medial and inferior rectus muscles
7 Orbital muscle
8 Oral vestibule
9 Major palatine artery and millimeter strip
10 Posterior segment of the nasal septum
11 Palatine glands
12 Posterior end of the inferior concha
13 Dorsum of the tongue
14 Oral mucosa and atrophic alveolar process
15 Palatine arteries

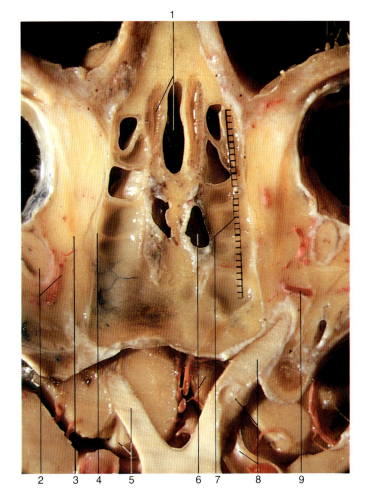

Fig. **54** Pneumatization of nasal septum in transverse section as seen from below
1 Mucosa of the roof of the nasal cavity, crista galli pneumatized from the frontal sinus, and the nasal septum
2 Optic nerve and right ophthalmic artery
3 Medial rectus muscle
4 Orbital plate of the ethmoid bone
5 Optic nerve and olfactory tract
6 Section of olfactory fossa and rectal gyrus
7 Superior ethmoidal cells with a millimeter strip
8 Infracanalicular segment of the optic nerve, and pit produced by a subdural hematoma arising from the internal carotid artery and the anterior cerebral artery
9 Ophthalmic artery and anterior clinoid process

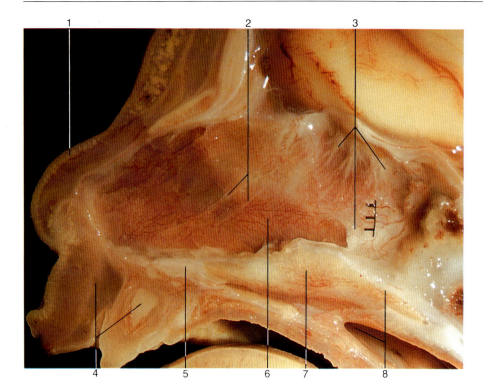

Fig. **55** Jacobson's organ and vomeronasal cartilage, with the vomer in situ from
the medial side in a 40 cm fetus
1 Dorsum of the nose and nasal bone
2 Vomeronasal nerve
3 Olfactory filaments and perichondrium of
  the septum in situ. Millimeter strip
4 Upper lip and anlage of incisor tooth
5 Vomeronasal cartilage
6 Septal surface of the nasal mucosa, with
  the perichondrium removed
7 Vomer in situ
8 Ala of the vomer, lateral edge and
  choana

Olfactory Region

The olfactory region lies on the upper part of the nasal septum and the lateral wall of the nose. Sensory and supporting cells may be distinguished in this area. Fibers of the sensory cells (olfactory neurosensory cells) conduct the sensation of smell. The peripheral processes are provided with kinocilia, the central non-myelinated axons unite with other central processes of the olfactory cells to form the olfactory filaments. They are ensheathed by Schwann cells, and pierce the cribriform plate to reach the olfactory bulb. The surface area of the olfactory region is about 370 mm^2 on each side, part lying on the septum, and part on the superior concha (Von Brunn, 1892). The olfactory region shrinks with increasing age. See also pages 1 and 13.

Nasal Vestibule

(Fig. **56**)

The vestibule of the nasal cavity is that area lying on the lateral wall of the nose between the nares and the limen nasi. Normally the greater ala of the lateral cartilaginous crus overlaps the lower edge of the lateral nasal cartilage. This causes a swelling within the nasal cavity (the limen nasi) overlying the cartilage. The alar sulcus lies on the external surface at this point. In rare cases the limen nasi is bounded inferolaterally by the posterior edge of the lateral crus itself. Accessory pieces of cartilage often lie in this area.

On the septal side of the nasal cavity the *medial intumescence* (the superior edge of the medial crus of the greater alar cartilage) forms the boundary between the nasal vestibule and the nasal cavity.

The medial wall of the nasal vestibule is formed by the mobile septum consisting of the columella (which contains no cartilage) in the medial part of the vestibule overlying the medial crura of the alar cartilage (Fig. **27 b**).

The covering of the vestibule of the nose consists of thin external skin with vibrissae (but without arrector pilorum muscles) and sweat and sebaceous glands. The vibrissae point externally and inferiorly. The transition to the respiratory zone does not end at the skeletal part of the posterior boundary of the vestibule. The squamous epithelial zone is always greatest in the anterosuperior segment of the vestibule, laterally it follows the piriform aperture approximately, but does not reach this zone completely. In adults the area of the vestibule lies between 485 and 1375 mm^2 (Hoffmann and Lang, 1969). The surface area of the left nasal vestibule is significantly greater than that of the right. During ageing the area of the vestibule increases at the expense of the respiratory region of the nasal cavity.

6.5 glands are found per mm^2 in the anterior part of the vestibule, and 8.5 glands in the posterior part, in subjects between the ages of 60 and 95 (Tos and Mogensen, 1976).

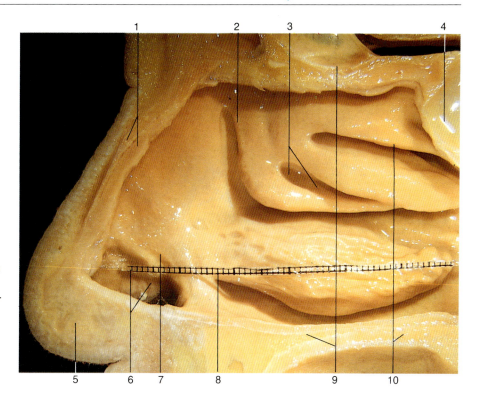

Fig. **56** Lateral wall of the nasal cavity, nasal vestibule and longitudinal cleft in the medial nasal concha

1 Nasal bone resting on the lateral nasal cartilage
2 Anterior insertion of the middle nasal concha
3 Longitudinal cleft
4 Septum of the sphenoidal sinus
5 Columella (mobile part of the septum)
6 The nasal vestibule, and a millimeter strip
7 Limen nasi
8 Anterior insertion of the inferior nasal concha, and a millimeter strip
9 Dura mater, olfactory fossa and hard palate
10 Superior nasal concha and palatine glands

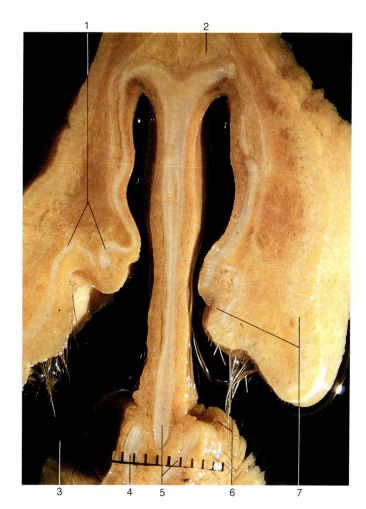

Fig. **57** Frontal section of the nasal valve seen from in front
1 Greater alar cartilage and the lower edge of a crumpled lateral nasal cartilage
2 Nasal bone
3 Nares
4 Medial crus of the greater alar cartilage
5 Lower end of the septal cartilage with a millimeter strip
6 Vibrissae and medial part of the internal nostril
7 Nasal ala and internal nostril

Kiesselbach's Plexus

(Fig. **58**)

At the junction between the squamous epithelium of the vestibule and the respiratory epithelium of the nasal cavity lies a strip about 1.5 mm wide covering a region of capillary loops that are unusually wide and long. This area is known as Kiesselbach's plexus. Even mild trauma to this area can cause bleeding, particularly in childhood. The long capillary loops of Kiesselbach's plexus appear to be particularly suitable for secreting a profuse fluid stream which guarantees the regular nourishment of the epithelium, and prevents drying of the surface between the keratinized skin of the vestibule and the mucosa covered with mucus of the respiratory region. Kiesselbach (1884) stated that the plexus that he described had previously been stated by Michel and Woltolini to be the most frequent source of nose bleeding. He stated that this area lies in the lower and central part of the cartilaginous septum. Boysen-Moeller (1965) applied the term 'corpus cavernosum of the septum' or Kiesselbach's ridge to this area. However this term is also used to describe the anterior tubercle of the septum. The latter ridge is a useful landmark for access to the middle meatus: it is present in the neonate. Its height depends on the shape of the lateral nasal wall. Posteriorly the ridge extends between the middle and inferior conchae. Anteriorly the corpus cavernosum of the septum extends as far as Kiesselbach's triangle. In this area the mucosa is thin,

highly vascular and fixed firmly to the perichondrium. The blood supply for these vessels is derived from the ascending branch of the anterior palatine artery, the posterior septal rami, the anterior ethmoidal artery and the superior labial artery.

The nares (anterior nostrils) form the entrance to the vestibule; their area lies between 50 and 130 mm^2 (Naumann and Naumann, 1977). The skin of the vestibule behind the nares is very thin, being very firmly attached to the lateral wall and to the inner surface of the lateral crus of the greater alar cartilage (Kallius, 1905). It then continues on the anterior edge of the lateral nasal cartilage. Because these two cartilages overlap the lateral nasal cartilage usually projects into the nasal cavity. At this point the mucosa forms a pouch facing anteriorly, termed the apical recess (Koerner, 1938 and von Brunn, 1892). It is bounded above by the limen nasi and below by the projection of the lateral crus of the alar cartilage. Cottle (1955) describes this space as the cul-de-sac; he also states that the lateral cartilage forms an angle of about 10° with the nasal septum. The nares in the white races have a long anteroposterior diameter, whereas they are more transverse in the black races. In the white races an elliptical nostril is the most frequent, and it is relatively narrow; in the black races the nostril is wider and rounder. We found an apical nasal recess in injection preparations, bounded by the medial and lateral crura of the greater alar cartilage, and extending inferiorly as far as the soft triangle. The base lay close to the nasal apex, the tip pointed posteriorly. The mean distance from the nares

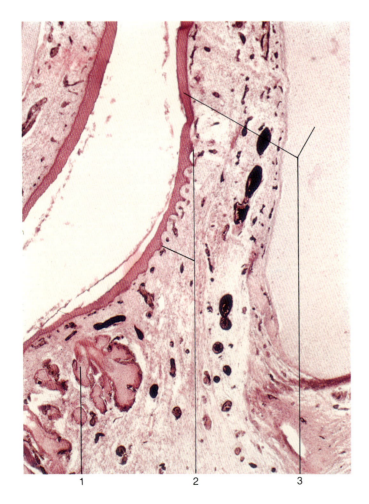

Fig. **58** Injected specimen of Kiesselbach's plexus in a neonate
1 Sebaceous gland in the nasal vestibule
2 Area of long, wide capillaries extending into the epithelium
3 Nasal septum and respiratory region

was 3.7 mm; the recess was 3.9 mm wide, 3.9 mm deep and 8.6 mm long. In the same transverse plane as the apical recess of the vestibule lies an indentation on the posterior wall of the vestibule at a mean distance of 4.2 mm from the nares: we have termed this the posterior recess. The mean width, length and breadth of the posterior recess were 3.9 mm, 3.7 mm, and 2.4 mm, respectively.

Limen Nasi

(Fig. 56)

The limen nasi is about 10 mm long; it is wide and superficial anteriorly, but narrows as it runs backwards towards the anterior end of the middle concha (Kallius, 1905). It lies upon the upper edge of the lateral crus of the greater alar cartilage; occasionally detached pieces of cartilage take part in its formation.

Medial Intumescence and the Internal Nostril

The medial crus of the greater alar cartilage narrows the vestibule on the medial side. An occasional sharp mucosal fold on the medial wall of the vestibule is due to widening of the septal cartilage. This area has been termed the medial boundary of the internal nasal ostium by several authors. The long axes of the external and internal nostril lie neither in the same direction nor in the same plane. The long axis of the nares is always rotated medially compared with the long axis of the internal ostium; in Europeans it runs in an apicomedial, posterolateral, direction. It forms a wide angle of variable size with the median sagittal plane. Several systems of folds take part in the lining of the nasal vestibule: a sharp fold runs from the lower edge of the septal cartilage to the medial wall of the vestibule, and then continues backwards to form the lower boundary of the posterior vestibular recess. The vestibular recess is enclosed above by a fold which is a continuation of the limen nasi. Connective tissue that is inserted into the septal cartilage is found in this fold.

Surface Area of the Nasal Vestibule

In our material the surface area of the entire vestibule measured between 485 and 1375 mm^2; the left vestibule had a mean area about 60 mm^2 greater than the right. The mean area of the nasal vestibule in adults was 852.2 mm^2, and in neonates 150 mm^2. Usually the mucosal boundary followed the edge of the piriform aperture, but never reached it completely. With advancing age the surface area of the nasal vestibule increases at the expense of the mucosal area of the nasal cavity (Lang and Hoffmann, 1969).

Nasal Vestibule and the Internal Naris (Nasal Valve, Airstream)

The cross-sectional area for respiratory air at the limen nasi is 20–60 mm^2. The inspired air passes through this region at a high flow rate, but then disperses and slows down as the cavity opens up beyond the nostril. The area of the central part of the nose is 100–300 mm^2, whereas it is 100–250 mm^2 at the choana (Naumann and Naumann, 1977). It was found that the nasal airstream in cadavers passed mainly through the middle meatus (Scheff, 1895). The nasal vestibule lies like a buttress oblique to the nasal cavity (Legler, 1967, 1968; Bachmann, 1969). The plane of the internal ostium of the vestibule lies in roughly the same plane as the tympanic membrane relative to the sagittal plane of the body. In contrast Zuckerkandl's internal ostium lies perpendicular to the axis of the nasal cavity. The nasal isthmus (Zuckerkandl, 1892) is a curved surface. The vestibule has a curved central axis which forms an angle of 100°–130° with the axis of the nasal cavity when viewed from the side (Bachmann, 1969). When viewed from the front it forms an angle between 15° and 30°. The surface area of the internal ostium is 1.4–1.6 times greater than that of the external ostium (Schmidt, 1968).

Floor of the Vestibule

The floor of the vestibule in white adults usually lies at a lower level than the piriform aperture. Occasionally the lower edge of the aperture is bounded by a bony ledge measuring 3–8 mm. The sharp edge of the piriform aperture usually present in the white races is absent in negroes (Holl, 1882; Cottle, 1955). The aperture may have a single or double edge (prenasal sulcus) or the edge can be absent and be replaced by a prenasal plane.

Jacobson's Torus

(Fig. 97)

The vomeronasal organ in man was investigated in particular by Koelliker in 1883, and by His in 1885 (Merkel, 1892). The organ cannot be demonstrated in all adults and neonates (Merkel, 1892). The nasal mucosa immediately above the nasal opening of the incisive canal bulges over a length of 4 (2–7.9) mm; Koelliker (1883) termed this area Jacobson's torus. It slopes upwards from in front backwards, and enfolds the duct of Jacobson's organ which has a diameter of 1–1.5 mm anteriorly and 0.5–1.0 mm posteriorly. Jacobson's organ was further investigated by Koelliker (1883), Peter (1913), Hedewig (1980) and others.

Vestibular Cysts

Zuckerkandl (1882) was the first to describe cysts of the nasal vestibule. Arnoldi (1929) reviewed 22 cases in the literature. These cysts arise from ectodermal tissue of the embryonal development of the face in the region of the lateral nasal cleft (Klestadt, 1926). Others feel that a displaced nasolacrimal duct or cysts of the nasopalatine duct are responsible for the genesis of these cysts (Breuggermann, 1920). Montreuil (1949) described three further cysts of this type.

Karmody and Gallagher (1972) reported 130 cases of these cysts. They arise from the floor of the nasal vestibule, extend anteriorly and elevate the nasal alae. If large they displace the anterior end of the inferior concha. They are found in adults, more often in women than in men, and more often in negroes than in white races.

Nasal Cavity

Floor

The anterior segment of the floor of the nasal cavity is formed by the premaxilla and the maxilla, and the posterior quarter by the horizontal plate of the palatine bone. The mean width of the floor is 15.9 mm in neonates, 22.4–24.0 mm at 5 months, and 25.5 mm at 1 year (Kowatscheff, 1943). Fig. **59** illustrates the postnatal growth of the floor of the nasal cavity (Lang and Baumeister, 1982). The mean length of the floor of the nasal cavity between the nasospinale and the posterior nasal spine is 36 mm in 3–9 month old children, 43 mm in 3 year olds, and 45 mm in 5 year old girls (Rosenberger, 1934).

Sutures

The suture between the palatine process of the maxilla and the horizontal plate of the palatine bone may be straight, convex anteriorly or convex posteriorly. Often the two sutures do not meet at the same point in the midline. In 0.15% of cases a process arising from the two palatine processes of the maxilla projects between the horizontal plates of the palatine bone, forming a complete posterior palatine process. The two palatine bones then do not meet.

Incisive Canal

About 12 mm (8–18) behind the anterior end of the floor of the nasal cavity lies a small pit in the mucosa of the nasal cavity, immediately adjacent to the nasal septum. This pit marks the upper end of the incisive canal which contains the terminal branches of the nasopalatine nerve, the greater palatine artery, and a short mucosal canal (Stenson's organ). The incisive canal has a length of 17.6 (8–26) mm measured from the oral cavity in adults; posteriorly its length is 11.6 (6–10) mm (Hassmann, 1975). In our material the incisive canal did not grow significantly after the second year of life. The axis of the canal forms an angle of 70° (57°–89.5°) with a plane through the eye and the ear.

Teeth Projecting into the Nasal Cavity

Zuckerkandl (1893) discovered occasional incisor teeth lying in the nasal cavity; like normal teeth, their crowns lay upwards. He also described a canine tooth that had penetrated into the nasal cavity. Nichol found a bicuspid whose crown projected superiorly towards the orbit, whereas its apex pointed inferiorly. Albini (1747) described canine teeth with their crown at the inferior orbital margin.

Roof

(Fig. **60**)

The upper part of the nasal cavity is termed variously the olfactory cleft, the nasal carina (Merkel, 1892) or the subfrontal space. For many years it has been divided into a nasal part lying anteriorly, an ethmoidal part centrally and a sphenoidal part posteriorly. The nasal spine of the frontal bone and the nasal bone form the roof of the nasal part. In the ethmoidal segment lie the ethmoidal foramen and the cribroethmoidal foramen (in the most anterior part), through which pass nerves and vessels. The sphenoethmoidal recess lies in the posterior segment (Meyer, 1956). It plays the same role for the posterior paranasal sinuses as the semilunar hiatus plays for the anterior (Mink, 1915). A well-developed sphenoethmoidal recess was only present in 48% of our specimens (Lang and Sakals, 1981). The number of ethmoidal foramina, the upper and lower lengths of the cribriform plate and the distance between the posterior surface of the anterior wall of the frontal sinus and the anterior edge of the cribriform plate are shown in Fig. **95.**

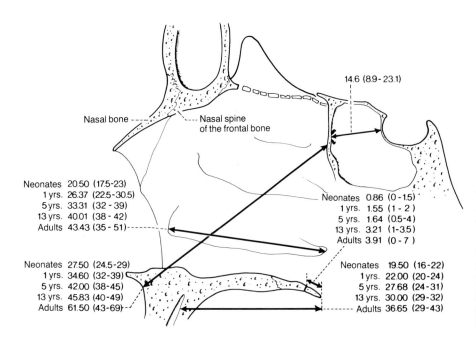

14.6 (8.9- 23.1)

Nasal bone

Nasal spine of the frontal bone

Neonates 20.50 (17.5-23)
1 yrs. 26.37 (22.5-30.5)
5 yrs. 33.31 (32 - 39)
13 yrs. 40.01 (38 - 42)
Adults 43.43 (35 - 51)

Neonates 0.86 (0 -15)
1 yrs. 1.55 (1 - 2)
5 yrs. 1.64 (0.5-4)
13 yrs. 3.21 (1-3.5)
Adults 3.91 (0 - 7)

Neonates 27.50 (24.5-29)
1 yrs. 34.60 (32-39)
5 yrs. 42.00 (38-45)
13 yrs. 45.83 (40-49)
Adults 61.50 (43-69)

Neonates 19.50 (16-22)
1 yrs. 22.00 (20-24)
5 yrs. 27.68 (24-31)
13 yrs. 30.00 (29-32)
Adults 36.65 (29-43)

Fig. **59** Length of the inferior nasal concha, the distance between the subspinale and the ostium of the sphenoid sinus, and that between the aperture and the anterior wall of the pituitary fossa. The length of the lower surface of the hard palate between the incisive canal and the posterior edge of the posterior nasal spine, the length of the latter, and the postnatal growth in length of several of these parameters are also given. (Lang and Baumeister, 1982; Krauss, 1987)

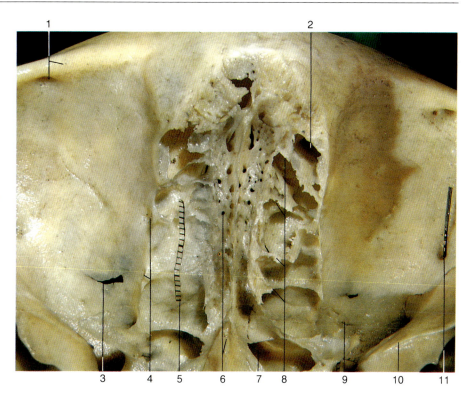

Fig. **60**   Cribriform plate, superior ethmoidal cells and the surrounding area from below

1 Supraorbital margin and foramen
2 Frontonasal duct
3 Rarefaction of the orbital roof
4 Anterior and posterior ethmoidal foramina
5 Roof of the ethmoidal cells formed by the frontal bone with a millimeter strip
6 Cribriform plate and vomer
7 Medial edge of the ostium of the sphenoidal sinus
8 Walls of the superior ethmoidal cells
9 Suture between the lesser wing and the frontal bone
10 Upper edge of the inferior orbital fissure
11 A pointer in the meningo-orbital foramen leading to the anterior wall of the middle cranial fossa

Lateral Wall of the Nasal Cavity

General Observations

The ethmoid bone, the maxilla, the palatine bone, the lacrimal bone, the inferior concha and medial surface of the medial pterygoid plate all contribute to the formation of the lateral wall of the nasal cavity (Fig. **61**). Anteriorly a small area is contributed by the nasal bone. Two, and rarely three, ethmoidal conchae project into the cavity. Below them lies the inferior nasal concha, an independent bone with a complex area of attachment to the skeleton of the lateral wall of the nose. Medial to the conchae lies a single air space termed the common nasal meatus. The air spaces under the conchae are termed the superior, middle and inferior meatus, respectively. They communicate with the common nasal meatus at the lower edge of each concha.

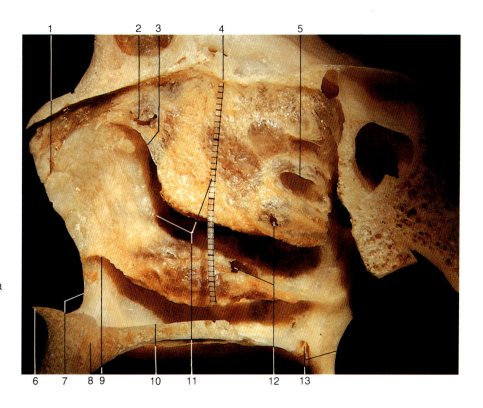

Fig. **61**   Osteology of the lateral wall of the nose

1 Nasomaxillary suture
2 Agger nasi
3 Anterior edge of the middle concha
4 Cribriform plate curving inferiorly
5 Very small superior nasal concha
6 Anterior nasal spine
7 Piriform aperture at its greatest width
8 Incisive canal
9 Anterior attachment of the inferior concha
10 Lateral surface of the nasal crest of the maxilla
11 Lacrimal bone with a millimeter strip
12 Rarefied middle and inferior conchae
13 Lesser palatine foramen and medial pterygoid plate

Early Development of the Paranasal Sinuses and Nasal Conchae

(Fig. **62**)

The frontal sinus, the ethmoidal cells and the maxillary sinus first develop as mucosal clefts in the cartilaginous anlage of the ethmoid bone. The sphenoid sinus arises from the posterior blind end of the ethmoidal segment of the nasal cavity in the cartilaginous anlage of the body of the sphenoidal bone during the third to fourth fetal months (von Mihalcovics, 1896; Peter 1925; van Gilse, 1926). This paleosinus grows posteriorly, inferiorly and medially towards Bertini's ossicle (sphenoidal concha) (van Gilse, 1926).

In the 55 mm embryo (i. e. during the third fetal month) a mucosal bud sprouts from the medial meatus to form the anlage of the maxillary sinus (Richter, 1932). At the same time, a bud arises anteriorly and superiorly from the same area to form the anterior ethmoidal cells, and a small posterosuperior bud of the nasal meatus forms the anlage of the posterior ethmoidal cells. At the beginning of the fourth fetal month the mucosal buds of the anlage of the ethmoidal cells develop as a vesicle and are surrounded by embryonal connective tissue with blood vessels; in the

fifth fetal month the cartilaginous capsule medial to the maxillary cavity disappears. Fleischmann (1903) states that the anterior ethmoidal cells belong to the procribrium, the central and posterior cells to the mesocribrium and the postremal cells to the metacribrium. The tissue of origin of the anterior and middle ethmoidal cells lies above the inferior concha, that of the posterior cells above the middle concha, and that of the most posterior cells above the superior concha. From the latter arise the postremal cells. Schaeffer (1916) demonstrated the frontal recess lying under the middle concha at the end of the third and the beginning of the fourth fetal month. The cartilaginous lateral nasal wall at this time forms several thickenings which project into the middle meatus as partly ossified folds. Between the folds lie small grooves or gutters between 0 and 5 in number; they are the anlage of the frontal sinus, of the anterosuperior ethmoidal cells and of the maxillary sinus. The frontal sinus is a direct extension of the frontal recess from one or other group of anterior ethmoidal cells. The anterior ethmoidal cells have already sprouted in the ninth fetal month, in the region of the orbit. Ossification of the walls of the ethmoidal sinus begins in the eighth fetal month. Onodi stated that the anterior end of the ethmoid bone in the neonate is 1–5 mm long, and its posterior end 2.5–5 mm long (Richter, 1932). The height of the ethmoid bone anteriorly is 1–3 mm and posteriorly 4.5–5 mm; its width anteriorly is 1.3 mm, and posteriorly 1.5–2 mm. Frontal, orbital and infundibular ethmoidal cells can be demonstrated in the first year of life (Richter, 1932). Later, new cells grow towards the cribriform plate and the orbit. In the third year of life the shape of the ethmoidal cells has changed from a round or oval cavity to a more angular form. Later their party walls become thin. An anterior ethmoidal cell expands on each side to form the anlage of the frontal sinus. The frontal sinus on one or both sides may be double or triple (Schaeffer, 1916).

Ethmoidal Infundibulum

(Fig. **63**)

The ethmoidal bulla and the uncinate process meet anteriorly, both in neonates and adults.

Boyer was the first to use the name infundibulum in 1805 (Zuckerkandl, 1893). The cells opening into the infundibulum are therefore called Boyer's cells in the French speaking countries. The medial wall of the infundibulum is usually formed by the lateral wall of the middle concha; its lateral wall is the anterior and superior region between the ends of the uncinate process and the ethmoidal bulla (or the lateral torus). Posteroinferiorly, the infundibulum merges with the semilunar hiatus.

Frontal Recess

The term frontal recess was previously used only with reference to the developmental period. The frontal sinus arises by growth of the frontal recess of the ethmoidal infundibulum into the frontal bone (Killian, 1895/1896; Peter, 1913; Gruenwald, 1925); this is termed direct formation of the frontal sinus. Extension of ethmoidal cells from the recess into the frontal bone is described as indirect formation.

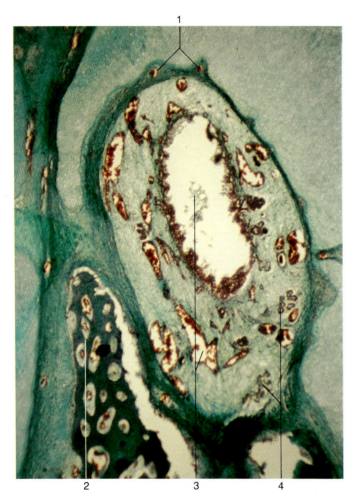

Fig. **62**   Anlage of the sphenoidal sinus in a 39 cm fetus
1 Lytic buds in the sphenoid cartilage
2 Anlage of the vomer
3 Anlage of blood vessels of the sphenoidal sinus
4 Glandular anlage

Frontonasal Duct and Frontal Ostium

Whether the channel draining the frontal cavity is termed a duct or an ostium depends on the definition used. We define a channel longer than 3 mm as a duct and a shorter channel as an ostium. Between the superior ends of the uncinate process and the ethmoidal bulla (or the lateral torus) there usually lies a transverse ledge of bone forming the medial boundary of the frontonasal duct. Often a transverse bony ledge lies at the posterior extent of the duct between the two structures (Fig. **64**).

The frontal ostium is first formed by apposition of the frontal bone onto the ethmoid bone. The typical form of the frontonasal duct arises by slight expansion of the infundibulum which migrates towards the frontal sinus with the frontal ostium (Hajek, 1909). If it does not expand and flatten in an anterosuperior direction but narrows and deepens a frontonasal duct is formed. Normally the medial wall of the frontonasal duct is formed by the middle concha. If the latter is pneumatized by the ethmoidal cells (conchal bulla) it bounds the ductal zone.

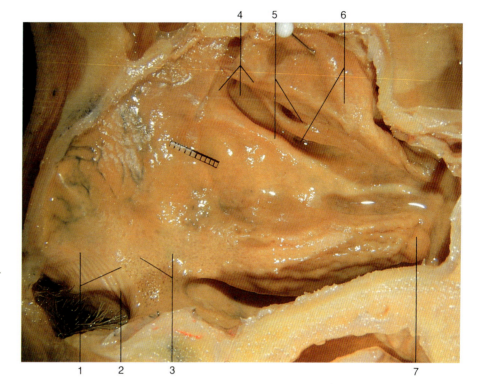

Fig. **63** Ethmoidal infundibulum and semilunar hiatus seen from the medial aspect
1 Limen nasi
2 System of folds at the nasal vestibule
3 Opening of seromucinous ducts
4 Ethmoidal infundibulum
5 Uncinate process and the ethmoidal bulla (the non-pneumatized part forms the lateral torus)
6 Middle nasal concha reflected superiorly, and the semilunar hiatus in the region of the ostium of the maxillary sinus
7 Posterior end of the inferior nasal concha with polypoidal change

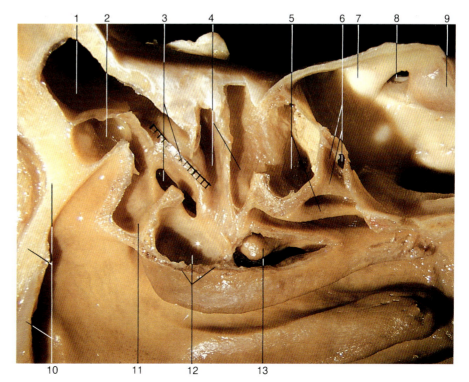

Fig. **64** Frontonasal duct and anterior ethmoidal cells seen from the medial surface. The middle and superior conchae have been opened
1 Frontal sinus
2 Nasal cells and anterior ethmoidal cells (threshold cells)
3 Infundibular and lacrimal cells, and entrance to the frontonasal duct with a millimeter strip
4 Anterosuperior ethmoidal cells
5 Posterosuperior ethmoidal cells and the superior concha
6 Supreme concha, sphenoethmoidal recess and the ostium of the sphenoidal sinus
7 Medial wall of the optic canal
8 Infraoptic recess
9 The floor of the sella
10 Nasion, nasal bone and septal cartilage
11 Agger cell
12 Anterior conchal sinus and cut edge of the middle concha
13 Ethmoidal bulla

Frontal Infundibulum

Killian (1895) termed the superior entrance of the frontal sinus into the frontonasal duct (and into the ostium leading to the nasal cavity) the frontal infundibulum, a term which has also been used by others (Messerklinger, 1967, 1970).

Nasal Conchae

General Remarks

Santorini in 1775 described three nasal conchae on the medial surface of the ethmoid bone. The superior ethmoidal concha is now termed the supreme nasal concha; it is present in 60–67% of subjects (van Alyea, 1939; Schaeffer, 1920). In our material a well-developed supreme nasal concha was present in only 17% of subjects (Lang and Sakals, 1981). Messerklinger (1977) also showed that the presence of a supreme concha in adults was exceptional. Pedziwiatr (1972) found furrows on the medial surface of the lateral nasal wall in the 4 and 5 month old fetus, indicating the formation of three or four conchae. The inferior nasal concha develops as an independent bone.

Ossification of the Lateral Wall of the Nasal Cavity

Ossification can be shown by dissection of the maxilla in the 16 mm embryo (Woo, 1949; Dixon, 1952), and by radiology in the 54 mm fetus (O'Rahilly and Meyer, 1956). Ossification of the palatine bone begins in the 27 mm fetus (Woo, 1949). The inferior concha is ossified in the 139 mm fetus (Noback, 1944), and the ethmoid bone and the conchae in the 175 mm (6 months old) fetus (Richter, 1932; Noback, 1944). The palatine bone ossifies from below upwards in the 50 mm fetus (Vidic, 1971). In the 63 mm fetus further ossification occurs in parts of the maxilla in the direction of the roof of the nasal cavity, and of the perpendicular plate of the palatine bone up to the level of the medial concha. In the 160 mm fetus the nasal capsule begins to ossify in its middle third, to form the central and posterior segment of the inferior and middle conchae. In the 220 mm fetus ossification centers appear in all parts of the cartilage of the central segment of the lateral wall of the nasal cavity (Vidic, 1971). The anterior segment is still cartilaginous. In the 263 mm fetus the lateral wall of the nasal cavity is almost completely ossified. Similar results were reported by Peter (1925) who found that the middle concha was ossified in the fifth month, and the superior in the seventh fetal month.

Basal Lamillae of the Ethmoidal Labyrinth
(Fig. 65)

The basal lamillae of the ethmoidal labyrinth were first described many years ago (Seydel, 1891; Hajek, 1909). These bony partitions between the ethmoidal cells extend from the lateral wall of the nasal cavity to the orbit. The first basal lamella is a continuation of the uncinate process: it can be seen lying laterally and anterosuperiorly in Fig. 65. Behind it lies the frontonasal duct, and behind that the second basal lamella arising from the ethmoidal bulla. This lamella forms the boundary between the nasal part of the frontal sinus and the ethmoidal labyrinth. If this lamella lies posteriorly then the frontal sinus and its duct are longer and wider; conversely if the bulla lies anteriorly the frontal sinus and duct are shorter and narrower. The third basal lamella is the continuation of the attachment of the middle concha. Unlike the others this lamella usually reaches the orbital plate of the ethmoid bone laterally. The anterior ethmoidal labyrinth is enclosed between the second and third lamillae. The fourth basic lamella arises at the attachment of the superior concha. If a supreme concha is present a fifth basal lamella arises from it and extends laterally.

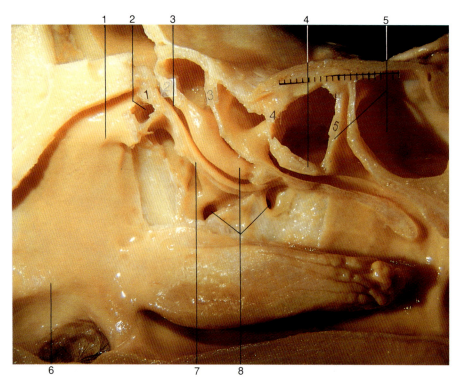

Fig. 65 Basal lamillae of the ethmoidal labyrinth
1 Agger nasi
2 Opened lacrimal cells
3 Frontonasal duct
4 Cut edge of the superior nasal concha
5 Posterior boundary of a posterosuperior ethmoidal cell and the sphenoidal sinus. A millimeter strip lies superiorly. The basal lamillae 1–4 are marked with numbers, and correspond to the usual description. The fifth lamella is the posterior wall of a posterior ethmoidal cell in front of the sphenoethmoidal recess
6 Limen nasi
7 Uncinate process with its lower part removed
8 Ethmoidal bulla, with maxillary and accessory maxillary ostia

Size and Position of the Conchae
(Figs. 66–69)

We investigated the conchae both in the dried bone (Lang and Baumeister, 1982) and when covered by mucosa (Lang and Sakals, 1981). Figs. 66–69 show our results with respect to the length, height and position of the conchae in the adult. The height of the nasal cavity, too, was measured in different parts, with and without a mucosal covering

(Figs. 70–72) (Lang and Sakals, 1981; Lang and Baumeister, 1982). The length of the floor of the nasal cavity in adults measured between the subspinale and the staphylion was 41 (33–57) mm, whereas between the anterior and posterior nasal spine (Fig. 73) it measured 51.6 mm, a value considerably lower than the 60–65 mm reported by Mihalkovics (1896). The paramedian length in adults in our material was 42.6 mm in men, and 40.1 mm in women; the highest value was 54 mm. We are unaware of any compar-

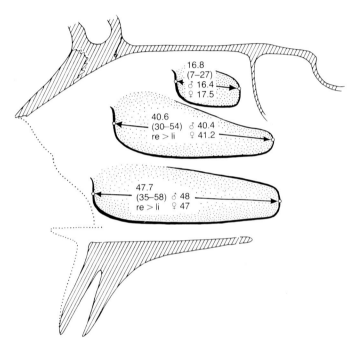

Fig. **66** Length of the nasal conchae in adults (adapted from Lang and Sakals, 1981)

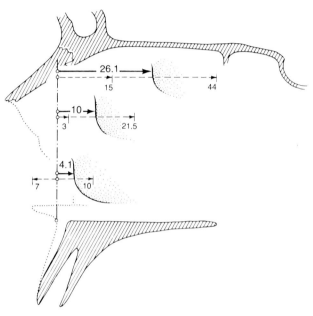

Fig. **68** Distance of the anterior edges of the nasal conchae from a vertical line passing through the subspinale. Mean values are given in thick print, and the range in thin figures (Lang and Sakals, 1981)

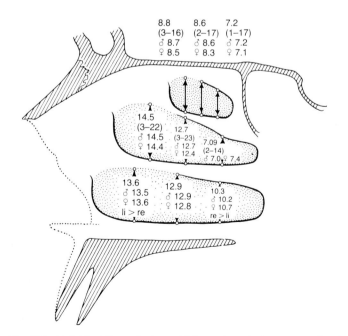

Fig. **67** Height of the anterior, middle and posterior segments of the nasal conchae (Lang and Sakals, 1981). The height of the anterior end of the middle nasal concha was not measured from the lateral edge of the cribriform plate above, but to the conchal region lying further inferiorly

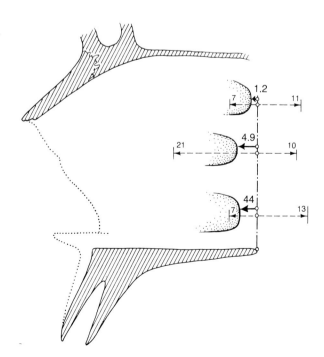

Fig. **69** Distance of the posterior edges of the nasal conchae from a vertical line drawn through the hard palate (Lang and Sakals, 1981)

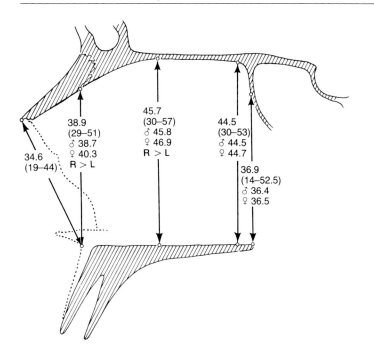

Fig. **70**   Mean values for the nasal cavity at various points. The sex and right to left differences are shown (Lang and Sakals, 1981)

Fig. **72**   Postnatal development in height and width of the nasal ▶ cavity (Lang and Baumeister, 1982). The distances between the lower edges of the middle and inferior nasal concha and the floor of the nasal cavity, the total height of the nasal cavity, and its breadth at several points are shown

Ethmoidal canal		Dehiscences
Anterior	2.04	(1.1 - 4.0)	92.8 %
Tertiary	1.02	(-1.1-3.25)	38.8 %
Posterior	1.51	(0.84-3.1)	58.9 %
	mm	Lang & A. Haas 1986

Neonates 19.21 (17 - 21)
9 months 24.38 (23 - 25)
3 yrs. 30.08 (26 - 33)
5 yrs. 34.57 (32 - 37)
8 yrs. 38.00 (33 - 43)
Adults 45.73 (38 - 52)
mm

Lang & Baumeister 1982

19.53 (12-23) Hajnis et al. 1967

Neonates 1.35 (0.5-2)
9 months 3.95 (3 - 5)
3 yrs. 4.18 (3 - 7)
5 yrs. 4.57 (4 - 6)
8 yrs. 5.18 (4.5-7)
Adults 6.79 (3 - 9)
mm

Neonates 8.50 (7 - 10)
9 months 9.56 (9 - 13)
3 yrs. 13.40 (11 - 17)
5 yrs. 15.23 (13 - 19)
8 yrs. 18.06 (15 - 21)
Adults 21.53 (16 - 27)
mm

Neonates 6.16 (4 - 8)
9 months 8.75 (7 - 10)
3 yrs. 10.10 (9 -11.5)
5 yrs. 11.43 (9.5-15)
8 yrs. 13.06 (12 -14.5)
Adults 17.86 (13 - 24)
mm

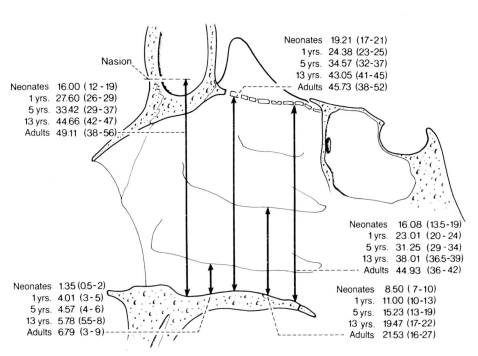

Nasion

Neonates 19.21 (17 - 21)
1 yrs. 24.38 (23 - 25)
5 yrs. 34.57 (32 - 37)
13 yrs. 43.05 (41 - 45)
Adults 45.73 (38 - 52)

Neonates 16.00 (12 - 19)
1 yrs. 27.60 (26 - 29)
5 yrs. 33.42 (29 - 37)
13 yrs. 44.66 (42 - 47)
Adults 49.11 (38 - 56)

Neonates 16.08 (13.5 - 19)
1 yrs. 23.01 (20 - 24)
5 yrs. 31.25 (29 - 34)
13 yrs. 38.01 (36.5 - 39)
Adults 44.93 (36 - 42)

Neonates 1.35 (0.5 - 2)
1 yrs. 4.01 (3 - 5)
5 yrs. 4.57 (4 - 6)
13 yrs. 5.78 (5.5 - 8)
Adults 6.79 (3 - 9)

Neonates 8.50 (7 - 10)
1 yrs. 11.00 (10 - 13)
5 yrs. 15.23 (13 - 19)
13 yrs. 19.47 (17 - 22)
Adults 21.53 (16 - 27)

Fig. **71**   Distance separating the floor of the nasal cavity from the nasion, the distance between the lower edge of the bony inferior nasal concha and the floor of the nose, the height of the nasal cavity at several points, the distance of the lower edge of the middle nasal concha from the floor of the nose, and the height of the nasal cavity at several points during the postnatal period (Lang and Baumeister, 1982)

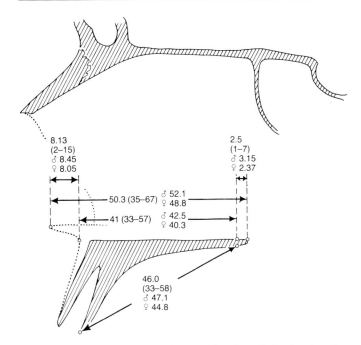

8.13
(2–15)
♂ 8.45
♀ 8.05

2.5
(1–7)
♂ 3.15
♀ 2.37

50.3 (35–67)   ♂ 52.1
                ♀ 48.8

41 (33–57)   ♂ 42.5
                ♀ 40.3

46.0
(33–58)
♂ 47.1
♀ 44.8

Fig. **73** Length of the anterior nasal spine of the hard palate from various different landmarks. Sex differences are also shown (Lang and Sakals, 1981)

able figures for the position of the nasal conchae. The measurements of length and height of the conchae agree with the relatively rough results of previous investigators, with a few exceptions. Zuckerkandl (1893) reported particularly numerous variations in the shape of the conchae. These included curves, pneumatization, conchae projecting far medially, unusual grooves on the surface of the concha and variation in the number of the ethmoidal conchae

(Zuckerkandl, 1892). Messerklinger (1973), using endoscopy on humans, found only one superior concha as a rule. It ended freely or merged into the posterior wall of the sphenoethmoidal recess. The anterior end of the middle concha may be slender or lobular. A small ridge is occasionally found in the underlying nasal cavity. It does not reach the level of the concha, and may be regarded as a rudiment of the second ethmoidal concha (Zuckerkandl, 1892).

Inferior concha: Perovic (1940) investigated the inferior concha thoroughly. He was the first to describe the medial protrusion of the anterior segment of the inferior concha, which he called the pars evoluta (Fig. **8**). He called the posterior segment of the inferior concha the pars involuta. In his series the greatest length of the pars evoluta varied between 8 and 16 mm. Anteriorly the inferior concha is attached to the conchal crest of the maxilla. Von Spee (1901) described a projection at the posterior end of the conchal crest at the point where it joins the lacrimal margin. This is the lacrimal prominence. Perovic found this projection in 88% of cases.

Variations of the Conchae

Supreme nasal concha: In the material described by van Alyea (1939) the supreme concha was pneumatised in 57% of cases. The cells drained into the supreme meatus.

Middle concha:

a) Extreme furrow formation (Fig. **74**): A groove was found in the medial concha in the fifth month in 50% of subjects, in 29% in the sixth and seventh fetal month, and in 36% in the ninth and tenth fetal months, compared with 13.6% of children but only 6% of adults (Grünwald, 1917). Messerklinger (1977) also observed these grooves, and emphasized that the posterior end of the groove occa-

Fig. **74** Deep clefts in the middle nasal concha
1 Deep cleft in the middle nasal concha, with a millimeter strip
2 Small superior nasal concha
3 Sphenoethmoidal recess and ostium of the sphenoidal sinus
4 Limen nasi
5 Incisive canal
6 Inferior nasal concha
7 Hard palate
8 Inferior nasal meatus
9 Sphenoidal sinus and ostium of the pharyngotympanic tube

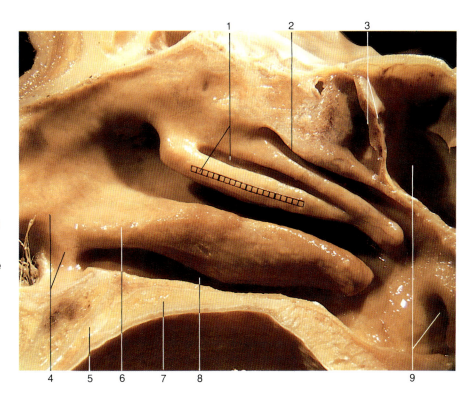

sionally cuts across the posterior end of the concha which then appeared swallow-tailed. One middle concha demonstrated two sagittal and one frontal groove, and was divided into four parts. We also found this type of furrow in our material on the medial and inferior surfaces.

b) *Lobules on the middle concha* are often found at the anterior end of the concha in the fetus, and more rarely in the adult. They resemble the concha of lower mammals and apes in shape.

c) *Pneumatization* (Figs. **64, 75–77**): numerous investigators have found pneumatization of the middle concha, the so-called conchal sinus. This conchal sinus may be found in both the posterior and anterior segments of the middle concha in about 8% of cases (Grünwald, 1925). Zuckerkandl (1893) found a bony vesicle 23 mm long and 13 mm wide in the anterior end of the concha. He therefore termed it a bullous concha. This type of concha can extend almost as far as the piriform aperture. Particularly wide conchae were found in Zuckerkandl's material (1893). In our material we found medial conchae completely bounding the middle meatus laterally, and which also fusing with the lateral nasal wall.

Zuckerkandl termed these vesicular expansions of the middle concha the anterior ethmoidal tubercle.

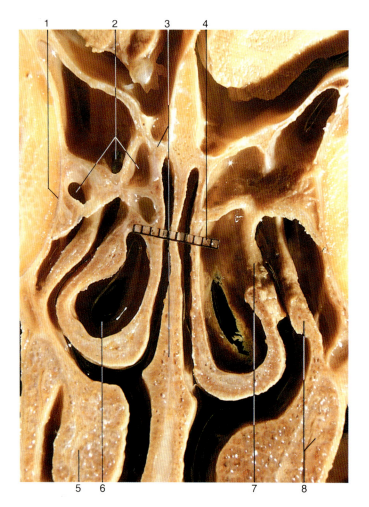

Fig. **75** Pneumatization of the middle nasal concha (bullous concha, conchal sinus) in frontal section seen from behind
1 Medial wall of the orbit
2 Ethmoidal cells
3 Cribriform plate and nasal septum
4 A millimeter strip
5 Inferior nasal concha
6 Pneumatized middle nasal concha
7 Ostium of the bullous sinus of the middle nasal concha on the right side
8 Uncinate process and nasolacrimal duct in cross-section

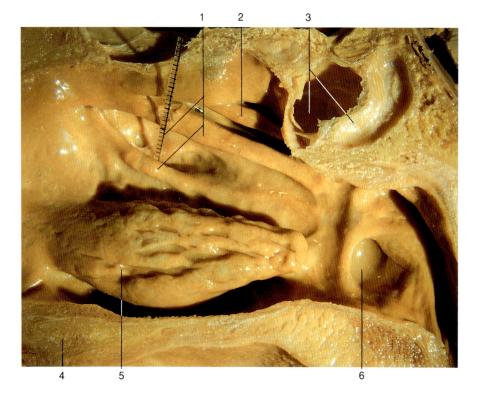

Fig. **76** Rudimentary middle nasal concha
1 Rudiments of the middle nasal concha, millimeter paper
2 Superior nasal concha
3 Sphenoidal sinus with oblique septum
4 Hard palate
5 Inferior nasal concha with grooving
6 Very wide pharyngeal opening of the pharyngotympanic tube

Leicher (1928) showed that the upper and lower limits of the height of the nasal concha are inherited recessively.

Inferior concha: the inferior concha may be curved convex laterally, as may the superior concha (Zuckerkandl). It may also be notched.

Absence of the Conchae

We observed one case of absence of the conchae, the vomer and the perpendicular plate (Lang and Kley, 1981). Zuckerkandl (1892) records a defect of the septum and of the concha in his Table 16, Fig. 3. Remnants of the superior ethmoidal concha alone were present in a case of syphilis. In our preparation there was no evidence of prior inflammation (Lang and Kley, 1981).

Bony Bridges

Messerklinger (1972) observed occasional bony bridges between the posterior ends of the middle and inferior conchae, at the level of the medial surface of the conchae or lateral to it. The medial meatus then ended blindly in a recess.

Precautions during Surgery

(Fig. **78**)

The anterior part of the medial concha joins the lateral edge of the cribriform plate at the base of the skull. This area has also been termed the *conchal lamina.* The base of the skull above the middle concha should be approached with the greatest care: the surgeon should always make great efforts to preserve a rim of both mucosa and bone at its base during ethmoidectomy (Kuemmel, 1913). Conchotomes are very dangerous instruments in the hands of a beginner, and especially in the hands of those who are unfamiliar with the anatomy (see also Fig. **79**). The posterior border of the attachment of the conchal lamina to the cribriform plate lies at the level of the posterior third of the crista galli in the frontal plane.

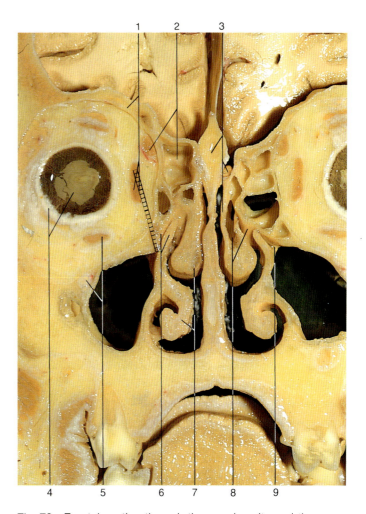

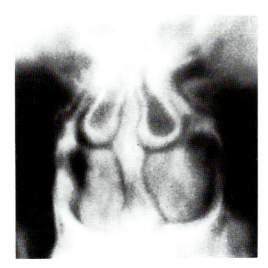

Fig. **77** Tomogram of a bullous concha (supplied by the ENT Clinic of the University of Würzburg)

Fig. **78** Frontal section through the nasal cavity and the paranasal sinuses viewed from in front
1 Orbital roof and medial rectus muscle with a millimeter strip
2 Superior oblique muscle and anterior ethmoidal canal
3 Pneumatized crista galli, olfactory bulb in the olfactory fossa and the conchal lamina
4 Sclera and remnants of the retina
5 Infraorbital nerve and inferior rectus muscle
6 Semilunar hiatus, in section, and uncinate process
7 Middle and inferior nasal conchae
8 Conchal sinus and ethmoidal bulla
9 Maxillary ostium

Paranasal Sinuses

General Observations

The paranasal sinuses comprise the maxillary, sphenoidal, frontal, and the ethmoidal sinuses (Nomina Anatomica, 1983). The ethmoidal sinuses are subdivided into the anterior, middle and posterior sinuses or cells, The sprouting nasal sinuses do not conform to bony boundaries, as suggested by the terms maxillary, sphenoidal and frontal sinus. Furthermore the superior ethmoidal cells are usually limited superiorly by the frontal bone, and other ethmoidal cells by the lacrimal bone, the nasal bone or by the maxilla. It is difficult to interpret previous findings because of the variable nomenclature for the sinuses, their ducts and their site of origin. For example, Peter (1913) wrote "the morphology of an ethmoidal cell is determined not only by its position but also by its opening". Moreover, terms for the ethmoidal cells depending on the position within the bone (for example, agger cells) have become accepted. Finally, eponyms are used in clinical practice for certain cells, for example Haller's cells and Onodi's cells. The access to the medial meatus is termed the atrium of the middle meatus. This area lies below the agger nasi (q.v.) and at the anterior end of the middle nasal turbinate.

Middle Nasal Meatus and the Paranasal Sinuses Arising from It

The middle nasal meatus is bounded above by the attachment of the medial nasal concha, below by the attachment of the inferior nasal concha, and laterally by the middle turbinate. The middle nasal concha is part of the ethmoid bone: its anterior part is attached above to the skull base, lateral to the cribriform plate. Posteriorly the turbinate is attached to the lateral nasal wall in the region of the ethmoid bone and the perpendicular plate of the palatine bone. At that point lies a medial conchal crest. The sphenopalatine foramen lies immediately posterior, superior and inferior to the posterior attachment of the medial concha; it varies in shape and is often subdivided. The perpendicular plate of the palatine bone is indented superiorly to form the sphenopalatine notch; it then gives off the orbital process to the posterior segment of the floor of the orbit, and the sphenoidal process to the inferior surface of the sphenoidal bone. In 71% of cases, round or oval dehiscences for the passage of nerves or blood vessels to the lateral wall of the nose are present in the perpendicular plate and below the notch for the sphenopalatine foramen. In 18% of subjects, similar openings are found in the middle meatus (and less often in the inferior meatus), and in 17% posterior to the insertion of the middle turbinate (Nikolic and Jo, 1967) (Fig. **79**). The lateral wall of the nasal cavity in front of the perpendicular plate is formed mainly by the ethmoid bone, whereas posteriorly it is formed by the medial pterygoid plate. Beneath the central segment of the middle concha the uncinate process projects from anterosuperior in a posteroinferior direction (Fig. **80**). It unites with the neighboring bones in various ways. The uncinate process forms the immediate continuation of the agger nasi, and demonstrates numerous variations of position, breadth, thickness and connections with neighboring bones. It limits the semilunar hiatus below and medially. Usually the upper edge of the uncinate process is concave, and its lower edge convex. A maxillary process arises from the superior border; it curves laterally and upwards towards the roof of the maxillary sinus. If this connection is absent, a bony process arises from the roof of the maxillary sinus, and unites with the uncinate process either directly or by a mucosal band (Zuckerkandl, 1893). The inferior process arises from the inferior edge of the uncinate process to join the inferior turbinate. Posteriorly the uncinate process either lies free or is attached to the perpendicular plate of the palatine bone. Zuckerkandl (1893) described several variations:

1) Narrow uncinate processes which form two processes, one to the inferior turbinate, the other to the superior wall of the maxillary sinus.
2) The posterior end of the uncinate process may be broad and occasionally united with the palatine bone and the inferior turbinate by five thin processes.
3) The uncinate process may be connected with the palatine bone and the roof of the maxillary sinus by a broad plate.

Many other variations have been described.

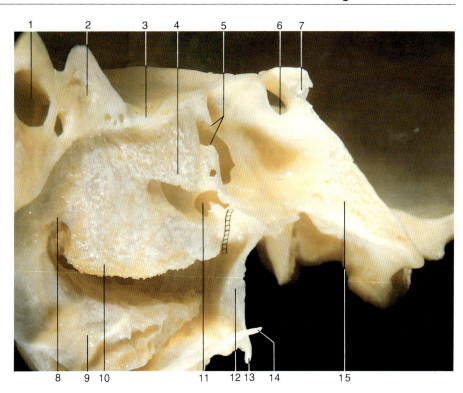

Fig. **79** Bones of the lateral nasal wall and the neighboring structures, seen from in front and medial
 1 Frontal sinus
 2 Crista galli
 3 Cribriform plate
 4 Superior nasal concha
 5 Bony aperture of the sphenoidal sinus
 6 Pituitary fossa
 7 Dorsum sellae
 8 Agger nasi
 9 Inferior nasal concha
10 Medial nasal concha
11 Sphenopalatine foramen placed superiorly and partly divided into two compartments by a bony spur
12 Medial pterygoid plate
13 Hamulus
14 Posterior nasal spine
15 Clivus

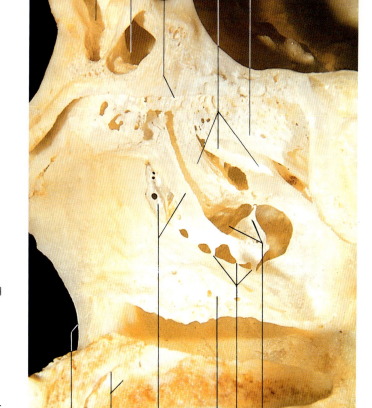

Fig. **80** Bones of the semilunar hiatus
 1 Frontal sinus
 2 Frontal bulla
 3 Cribriform plate
 4 Crista galli
 5 Ethmoidal bulla and posterior attachment of the middle nasal concha
 6 Superior nasal concha
 7 Piriform aperture
 8 Incisive canal
 9 Lacrimal bone and uncinate process
10 Inferior nasal concha
11 Lower attachment of the uncinate process
12 Posteroinferior end of the semilunar hiatus and upper attachment of the uncinate process

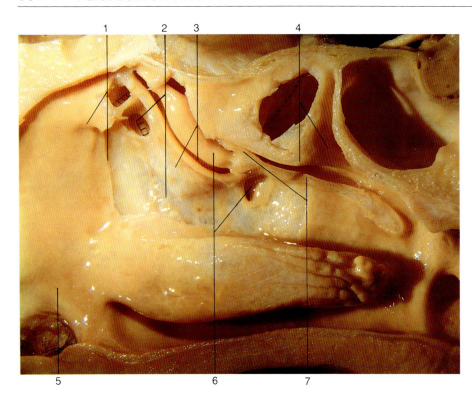

Fig. **81** Ethmoidal bulla, uncinate process, anterior fonticulus and accessory ostium of the maxillary sinus

1 Agger nasi and region from which the mucosa has been removed
2 Lacrimal cell and anterior nasal fontanelle
3 Uncinate process and semilunar hiatus
4 Area from which the superior nasal concha has been removed, and the sphenoethmoidal recess
5 Limen nasi
6 Ethmoidal bulla and accessory ostium at the posterior nasal fontanelle
7 Posterior end of the inferior nasal concha and the region from which the middle nasal concha has been removed

Ethmoidal Bulla

(Figs. **81, 82, 86**)

A long bony bar usually projects above the uncinate process, running from anterosuperior to posteroinferior. In our material the ethmoidal bulla was 18 (9–28) mm long, and 5.4 (2–13) mm high. Zuckerkandl (1893) recorded lengths between 20 and 26 mm. The term bulla indicates that this part of the bone is pneumatized; it was first used by Zuckerkandl. Soemmering (1809) and Grünwald (1925) termed the bulla the lateral torus. This structure is pneumatized in only 62% of cases, and the term ethmoidal bulla is correct only in these cases (Grünwald, 1925). In our material the bulla was pneumatized in 70% of cases; in the rest a lateral torus extended to the junction of the medial and inferior orbital walls. A smaller segment of the anterior part of the lateral wall of the middle meatus is formed by the lacrimal bone. Usually this arches forward in a medial direction. The frontal process of the maxilla projects upwards in front of the lacrimal bone, forming the lateral wall of the middle meatus. Immediately in front of the attachment of the medial nasal concha lies the agger nasi. The uncinate process forms one body with the agger nasi: the free part is the agger and the covered part is the uncinate process (Zuckerkandl, 1893). The agger nasi is always well formed in the fetus and in young children (Mihalkovics, 1896).

Fonticuli

The medial wall of the maxillary sinus may demonstrate defects, anteriorly and inferiorly (particularly posterior to the inferior process) due to variations in the union of the uncinate process with the neighboring bones. These defects are termed the anterior and posterior fontanelles. The mucosa of the nasal cavity and the maxillary sinus are continuous at these points.

Accessory Ostia

(see Fig. **81**)

The mucosa of the neighboring spaces can disappear from these fonticuli, producing accessory ostia of the maxillary sinus. The incidence of these openings varies widely, from 9.5% (Zuckerkandl, 1893; Lang and Sakals, 1982), to 23% (van Alyea, 1936). In our recent material we included even the smallest ostia, and then found an incidence of 28%. The size of the accessory ostia varied between a pinhead size and 10.5 × 6.5 mm (Myerson, 1932). The wide variation probably depends on age changes: accessory openings can develop even in advanced age. Myerson (1932) found accessory ostia most often (51%) in the posterior nasal fontanelle behind and below the main ostium of the maxillary sinuses. In 23% they lay further posteriorly, in 14% inferiorly and in about 11% superiorly.

Ethmoidal Infundibulum

(Figs. **82, 86**)

Initially a frontal recess arises from the frontal cells in the superior part of the medial meatus. The frontal recess itself may extend widely and grow into the frontal bone (direct formation of the frontal sinus) (Killian, 1895–1896; Peter, 1913). Anterior ethmoidal cells also sprout from the recess; they too can grow into the frontal bone (indirect formation

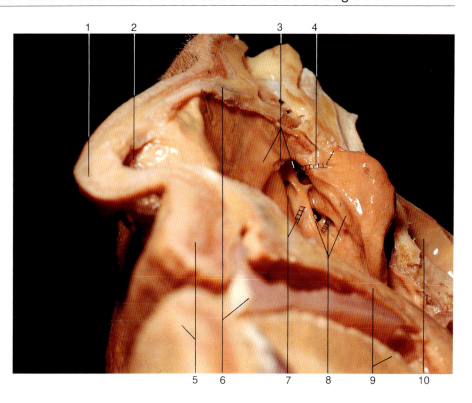

Fig. **82** Ethmoidal infundibulum and ostia of the paranasal sinuses containing millimeter strips. The middle nasal concha has been retracted medially and upwards. The view is of the median sagittal plane from medial and below

1 Tip of the nose
2 Nasal vestibule
3 Agger nasi, cut edge of the middle nasal concha, and the ethmoidal infundibulum
4 Millimeter strip in the nasofrontal duct
5 Upper and lower lips
6 Nasal bone and false teeth
7 Uncinate process and a millimeter strip in the maxillary ostium
8 Ethmoidal bulla, millimeter strip in the middle ethmoidal cells, and middle nasal concha retracted upwards
9 Hard palate and tongue
10 Sphenoidal sinus

of the frontal sinus). Rarely (in 1.5% of our material) another ethmoidal cell may grow into the frontal bone.

The name ethmoidal infundibulum (Figs. **82, 86**) is used to describe a niche in the medial meatus lying below the middle nasal concha and in front of the ethmoidal bulla. The medial wall of the infundibulum is usually the lateral wall of the middle nasal concha. If the latter is pneumatized (a bullous concha) then the conchal cell borders on the ethmoidal infundibulum. The lateral boundary of the ethmoidal infundibulum is the anterior region between the upper end of the uncinate process and the ethmoidal bulla (or lateral torus). Usually a transverse bony bar lies medially between the two structures. Often a similar bony bar also lies further posteriorly, forming the posterior boundary of the nasal ostium (or duct) of the frontal sinus. The following structures open into the ethmoidal infundibulum: the duct of the frontal sinus, the anterosuperior ethmoidal cells, the lacrimal, agger, frontal, and nasal cells – the latter either directly or via other cells. The infundibulum was first given this term by Boyer in 1805; in French-speaking countries the cells opening into this area are therefore known as Boyer's cells (Zuckerkandl).

Frontal Ostium and Frontonasal Duct

(Figs. **83, 84**)

The round or oval ostium of the fronto-nasal duct lies in the anterosuperior part of the ethmoidal infundibulum. In about 80% of our material we found a frontonasal duct 5.1 (2–11.2) mm high and 2.6 (0.75–6.4) mm deep. About 20% of our subjects demonstrated a frontal ostium (in accordance with our definition). Zuckerkandl (1893) found that the ostium lay 2–10 mm from the semilunar hiatus, and that the anterior end of the short semilunar hiatus was

copula shaped if the frontonasal duct was absent. Fig. **85** shows details of further connections of the frontonasal duct to the agger cells, to the opposite side, medially to the semilunar hiatus, towards the semilunar hiatus, and other types of drainage ducts of the frontal sinus (Lang and Haas 1988). In our previous material, the frontal sinus opened in front of the semilunar hiatus in about 50% of cases, in 22% at its anterior end, in 26% in the anterior quarter and in 2% above it (Fig. **85**). If the duct was absent, Hajek described this condition as a frontal recess of the infundibular area; the cells opening in this recess are then termed the cells of the frontal recess. Most often, three or four anterior, superior and medial ethmoidal cells arise from this type of recess. Killian (1895) termed the superior opening of the frontal sinus into the frontonasal duct the frontal infundibulum.

Frontal Cells (Frontal Bulla)

(Fig. **86**)

Ethmoidal cells projecting into the frontal cavity were termed frontal bullae by Zuckerkandl (1893). Sieur and Jacob (1901) found this type of cells in 8–9% of cases; Onodi (1912) cited Zuckerkandl as having found them in 6 of 30 preparations, and they were also present in 20% of Onodi's 300 specimens. Van Alyea (1941) found adjoining cells that he did not define exactly in 50% of cases; 16.5% lay close to the ostium of the frontal sinus. Dixon (1958) and Prott (1974) found them in 8% of cases in the posterior wall of the frontal sinus; Nikolic also found them in 15.3% of 1100 preparations (Salinger, 1965). We found frontal cells (frontal bullae) of varying degrees of development in 17% of our material.

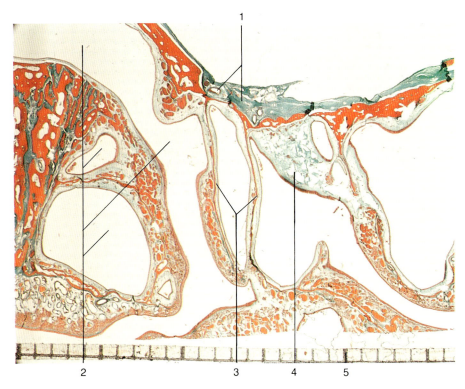

Fig. **83** Paramedian sagittal section through the ethmoidal labyrinth. The thin bony walls should be noted

1 Anterior ethmoidal artery and dura mater of the olfactory fossa
2 Nasofrontal duct, anteromedial ethmoidal cells and agger cells (below)
3 Walls of an anterior ethmoidal cell with mucosa
4 Ethmoidal cell with horizontal section of the mucosa
5 Millimeter strip

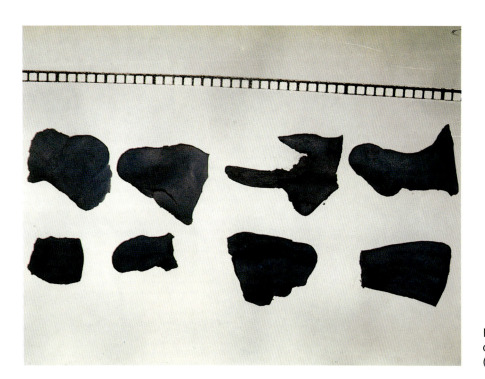

Fig. **84** Various shapes of the frontal infundibulum (Killian) and of the frontonasal duct (casts made by Haas)

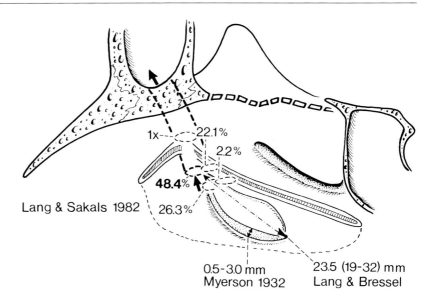

Fig. **85**   Directions of the opening of the fronto-nasal duct and the frontal ostium (Lang and Sakals, 1982). In one of the 100 dissections the frontonasal duct opened at the conchal lamina of the middle nasal concha. The length of the uncinate process measured in a straight line in our material is given, and also the width of the semilunar hiatus adapted from Myerson (1932). The length of the uncinate process when covered by mucosa and measured in a straight line was reported by Lang and Bressel (1988)

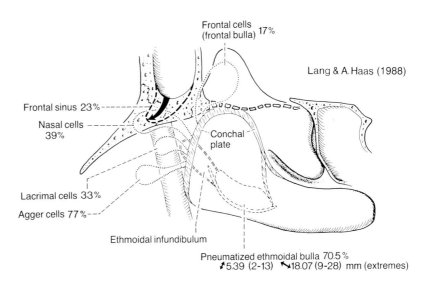

Fig. **86**   In our material there was marked inferior extension of the floor of the frontal sinus in 23% of cases, and ethmoidal cells growing into the nasal bone were present in 39% of cases. The figure also shows the height and length of the ethmoidal bulla. The bulla was pneumatized in about 70% of cases, and in the remainder a solid bone plate was present. The hatched area is the conchal lamina at the lateral edge of the cribriform plate, and its fairly frequent area of attachment of the ethmoidal bulla (Lang and Haas, 1988; Lang and Bressel, 1988)

Frontal Sinus

Opening

(Fig. **87**)

Diameter: The largest and smallest diameter of the duct of the frontal sinus (measured on 60 specimens) was 5.1 (2.0–11.25) mm, and 2.6 (0.8–6.4) mm respectively. The anteroposterior diameter measured on a further 42 specimens was 2.4 (1–5) mm, and the mediolateral depth was 3.1 (1–6) mm.

The length of the *frontonasal duct* (measured on 66 specimens) was 6.2 (3.2–14.9) mm. Based on our definition, a frontonasal duct was present in 77% of cases, and an ostium of the frontal sinus in 23%.

Opening of the frontonasal duct (Fig. **88**): The frontonasal duct, when present, opens into the semilunar hiatus in 67% of cases: in 59% into its anterior segment, in 2% via an orbital recess of the frontal sinus, in 2% the main ostium drained in the usual manner, but there was an additional second duct of the frontal sinus leading to the semilunar hiatus, and in 4% an accessory nasofrontal duct led to the semilunar hiatus.

The opening of the frontonasal duct lay outside the semilunar hiatus in the other 33% of cases, being anterior to the semilunar hiatus in 24%, anterior and lateral to it in 2%, in the region of an agger cell in 4% and superior to the anterior end of the medial nasal concha, but still within the middle meatus, in 4%.

Angle of the frontonasal duct with the Frankfurt horizontal: The frontonasal duct runs from above and in front in a posteroinferior direction. We used angled telescopes to inspect the ostia, and found that the angle between the frontonasal duct and the Frankfurt horizontal was 116.3° (100°–134°).

In 23% of cases we found a *frontal ostium* (Fig. **89**) which met our criteria. Probing showed that the ostium led to the anterior part of the semilunar hiatus in 47% of cases; in 40% the opening lay in front of the semilunar hiatus, in 7% lateral to it, and in 7% the ostium opened into an anterior ethmoidal cell.

If the data for the ostia and the frontonasal duct are combined, then the opening lay in the semilunar hiatus in 62% of cases: in 56% of cases it opens in the anterior part of the semilunar hiatus, in 1.5% the channel ran anteriorly and laterally via an orbital recess of the frontal sinus, in 1.5% there was a main channel and an accessory duct to the anterior segment of the semilunar hiatus, and finally in 3% the hiatus was reached via an accessory canal of the frontonasal duct. In the remaining 38% of cases, the opening of the frontonasal duct (or the frontal ostium) pointed in a posterior and inferior direction, but not to the semilunar hiatus. 27% of frontal ducts opened in front of the semilunar hiatus, 1.5% lateral to it, and 1.5% anterior and lateral to it; 3% ended in an agger cell, 1.5% in an anterior ethmoidal cell, and finally 3% opened superior to the anterior pole of the medial nasal concha but into the middle meatus.

In 23% of cases the frontal sinus had an inferior indentation that reached the nasal bone.

The "Dangerous" Frontal Bone

If the anterior end of the olfactory fossa protrudes forwards into the frontal sinus great care must be paid to this area during operations on the frontal sinus (see Fig. 69 in Lang, 1983). The superior segment of the septum of the frontal sinus often deviates markedly from the midline – its lower segment almost never.

Hypoplasia and Aplasia

The frontal sinuses are aplastic in 17% of various European races, in 12% of the continental European races, in 35% of other races, and in 52% of Eskimos (Turner and Porter, 1921). In another series the right frontal sinus was aplastic in 3.2% of cases, the left side in 2.7%, and both sides in 17.5% (Stern, 1939). Nowak and Mehls (1977) found the frontal sinus to be aplastic on the right side in 4.2% in men and on the left in 3.6%. In women the right sinus was not developed in 4.1% of cases and the left in 2.8%. Radiology showed bilateral absence of the frontal sinus in 4.8% of cases, and a single frontal sinus in 2.5% of cases (Gulisano et al., 1978). Asymmetry of the frontal sinuses is commoner in dolichocephalic than in brachocephalic or mesocephalic subjects. The wide variation in incidence of absent frontal sinuses (2%–20%) is partly explained by unsatisfactory methods of investigation. Both frontal sinuses are aplastic in 38.8% of adolescents with a cleft of the secondary palate, the left side is aplastic in 6% and the right side in 11% (Nowak and Mehls, 1977).

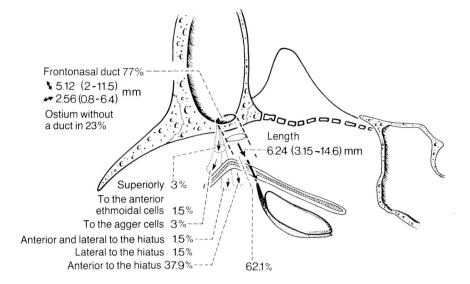

Frontonasal duct 77%

↘ 5.12 (2-11.5)
↗ 2.56 (0.8-6.4) mm

Ostium without a duct in 23%

Length
6.24 (3.15-14.6) mm

Superiorly   3%
To the anterior ethmoidal cells   1.5%
To the agger cells   3%
Anterior and lateral to the hiatus   1.5%
Lateral to the hiatus   1.5%
Anterior to the hiatus 37.9%   62.1%

Fig. **87**   Data from our more recent material on the opening of the frontal sinus (Lang et al., in press). The widths of the frontonasal duct, the ostium of the frontal sinus, the area of the opening of the duct and the length of the frontonasal duct are given. A frontonasal duct, defined in accordance with our criteria, was present in 77% of cases

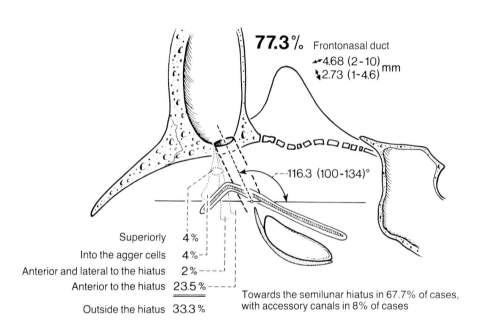

77.3% Frontonasal duct
↗ 4.68 (2-10)
↘ 2.73 (1-4.6) mm

116.3 (100-134)°

Superiorly   4%
Into the agger cells   4%
Anterior and lateral to the hiatus   2%
Anterior to the hiatus 23.5%

Outside the hiatus 33.3%

Towards the semilunar hiatus in 67.7% of cases, with accessory canals in 8% of cases

Fig. **88**   Frontonasal duct, showing the incidence of occurrence, the angle formed with the Frankfurt horizontal and the direction of opening of the ostium (Lang et al., in press)

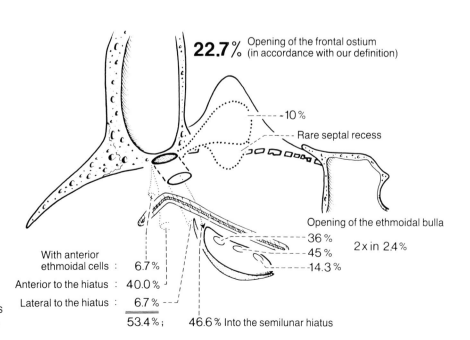

22.7% Opening of the frontal ostium (in accordance with our definition)

10%

Rare septal recess

Opening of the ethmoidal bulla
36%
45%   2x in 2.4%
14.3%

With anterior ethmoidal cells :   6.7%
Anterior to the hiatus :   40.0%
Lateral to the hiatus :   6.7%
53.4% ;   46.6% Into the semilunar hiatus

Fig. **89**   Frontal ostium defined by our criteria: incidence and direction of opening. The area of the ethmoidal bulla in which the opening lay is also shown in those cases in which the bulla was pneumatized (70.5%) (Lang and Bressel, 1988)

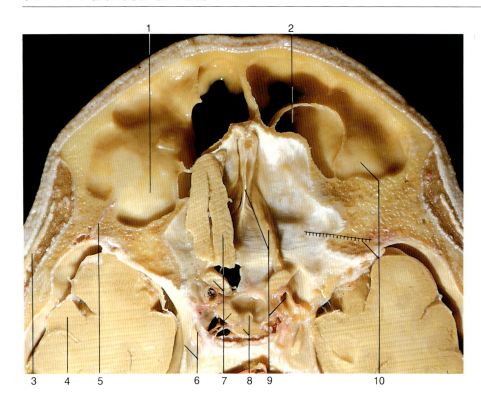

Fig. **90** Pneumatization of the roof of the orbit shown in transverse section from above
1 Large frontal sinus on the left side
2 Anterosuperior ethmoid cell in the orbital roof (a frontal bulla by our criteria)
3 Temporal muscle
4 Temporal lobe pole
5 Meningo-orbital ramus
6 Anterior petroclinoid fold and oculomotor nerve
7 Gyrus rectus , optic nerve and section of the anterior lobe of the pituitary gland
8 Infundibulum and section of the posterior lobe of the pituitary gland
9 Falx cerebri, olfactory tract and section of the internal carotid artery
10 Frontal sinus on the right side with a millimeter strip

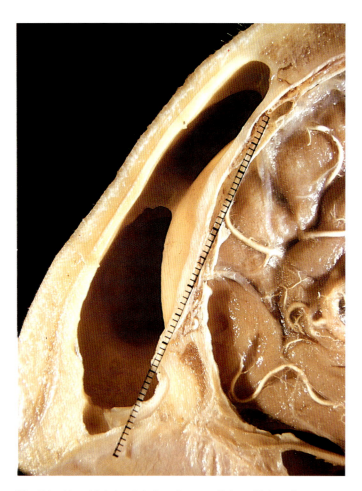

Fig. **91** Very high frontal sinus in a medial sagittal section

Supernumerary Frontal Sinuses (Anterosuperior Ethmoidal Cells in the Orbital Roof, Frontal Bulla)

(Fig. **90**)

Frontal sinuses divided into three or more chambers have been described by several authors, but have very rarely been named. Boege (1903) found two frontal sinuses on one side in 1.5% of his material, Onodi (1895) described fronto-orbital cells in 10% of his material, and Gruenwald (1925) in 3%. Jovanovic (1961) reported an incidence of 21% but did not give an accurate definition. This extra sinus lay in the medial third or quarter of the orbital roof, and was present in 17% of cases, being commoner on the left side than the right. We found this cell in 17% of our material.

Size

(Figs. **91, 92, 93**)

The frontal sinus reaches a height of 24.3 (5–66) mm within the frontal bone (Millosslawski, 1903). The lateral wall of the frontal sinus lies 29.0 (17–49) mm from the midline in adults (Lang and Haas, 1979). The longitudinal extent of the frontal sinus between the anterior and posterior end (in the orbital roof) was 20.5 (10–46.5) mm (Figs. **92** and **93**). Flesch (1876) described one frontal sinus which extended posteriorly as far as the optic canal; the roof of the orbit was completely duplicated. Witt (1908) found a duplicate orbital roof in almost 40% of his skulls (23% on both sides and 16% on one side). He described frontal bullae up to 1 cm deep and 1 cm wide in the septum of the frontal sinus. Guiseppe (1942) demonstrated agenesis of the frontal sinus in most specimens with a persistant frontal suture (Salinger, 1948). Marcus (1933) described a frontal sinus extending laterally in the orbital roof as far as the lateral canthus.

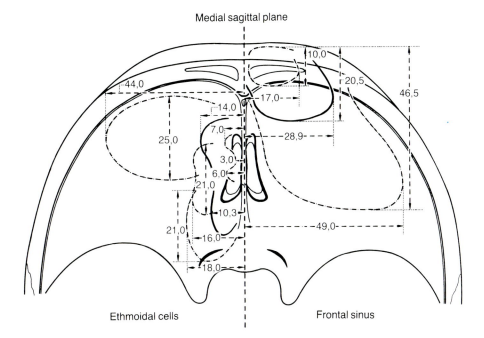

Medial sagittal plane

Ethmoidal cells

Frontal sinus

Fig. **92** Superior ethmoid cells and frontal sinus in the orbital roof (Lang and Haas, 1979). The thick continuous line shows the mean values in mm, the interrupted lines show minimal and maximum values in our material

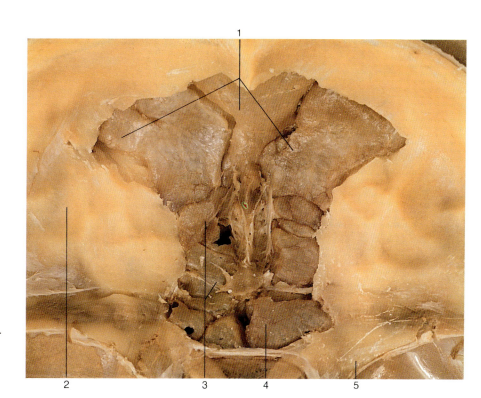

Fig. **93** Paranasal sinuses exposed from above
1 A tripartite frontal sinus
2 Orbital part of the frontal bone
3 Superior ethmoidal cells (middle and posterior)
4 Sphenoidal sinus
5 Lesser wing of the sphenoidal bone

Thickness of the Wall of the Sinus and the Floor

The bone of the anterior wall of the frontal sinus just lateral to the septum was 4.0 (0.5–12.5) mm thick in 77 specimens, being 4.6 (1.7–12.5) mm thick in men, and 3.7 (1.2–7.7) mm thick in women. Its posterior wall at a similar point was 1.9 (0.1–4.8) mm thick, being 2.1 (0.3–4.05) mm thick in female specimens and 1.9 (0.45–3.75) mm thick in male skulls. The position of the floor relative to the nasion could only be determined in 29 specimens: it lay 3.1 mm below the nasion.

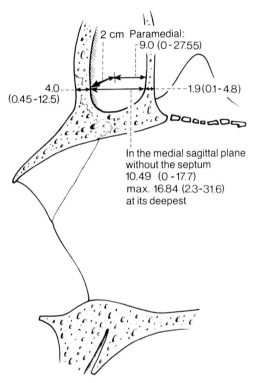

Fig. **94**   Thickness of the anterior and posterior walls of the frontals sinus in the midline (MS) and 2 cm from the midline

Anteroposterior Depth

(Fig. **94**)

The anteroposterior depth of the frontal sinus (when present) of 69 skulls divided through the midline, was 16.8 (2.3–31.6) mm, being 17.3 (4.6–31.6) mm, and 14.8 (2.3–27.7) mm in men and women, respectively. The anteroposterior extent measured just lateral to the septum (on 58 specimens) was 10.5 (0–17.7) mm, being 11.0 (4.6–17.6) mm and 8.3 (0–17) mm in men and women, respectively. Usually the burr holes for trephining the frontal sinus are made 2 cm lateral to the midline. The depth of the sinus at this point (on 57 specimens) was 9 (0–27.6) mm, being 10.3 (0–27.6) mm and 6.4 (0–18.7) mm in men and women, respectively.

The distance between the posterior surface of the anterior wall of the frontal sinus and the anterior edge of the cribriform plate (in 65 specimens in which the frontal sinus was developed) was 12.7 (4.7–21.3) mm (Fig. **95**), being 13.0 (4.7–21.3) mm and 10.8 (6.3–17.0) mm and in men and women, respectively.

Defects of the Frontal Sinus and Orbital Roof

The wall between the frontal sinus and the roof of the orbit may rarely show defects (Hajek, 1909; Fig. 38 in Lang, 1983).

Postnatal Growth

Expansion of the sinus into the frontal bone begins in the 3½ year old child (Onodi, 1911). Growth proceeds slowly up to the age of 11, and then more quickly. Szilvassy (1981) investigated the frontal sinus by radiology in children aged between 3 and 17 years. The mean area of the frontal sinus in the occipitofrontal view, with a focus film distance of 1 meter perpendicular to the Frankfurt horizontal, was 0.7 cm² in 3-year-olds, 1.1 cm² in 5-year-olds, 3.1 cm² in 7-year-olds, 5.1 cm² in 9-year-olds and 9.3 cm² in 12- to 17-

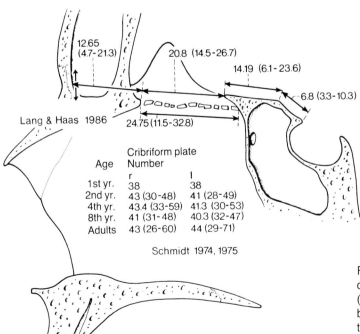

Age	Cribriform plate Number r	l
1st yr.	38	38
2nd yr.	43 (30-48)	41 (28-49)
4th yr.	43.4 (33-59)	41.3 (30-53)
8th yr.	41 (31-48)	40.3 (32-47)
Adults	43 (26-60)	44 (29-71)

Schmidt 1974, 1975

Fig. **95**   Distance between the posterior edge of the anterior wall of the frontal sinus and the anterior edge of the cribriform plate (Lang and Haas, 1988); length of the superior surface of the cribriform plate (Schmidt, 1974, 1975), length of the lower surface of the cribriform plate, length of the planum sphenoidale and the prechiasmatic sulcus (Lang and Brueckner, 1981)

year-olds. The mean value for boys was higher than that for girls in the 3–5 year-old age group, but less in 7–10 year-olds. In 12–17-year-old boys it again exceeded the values for girls.

Koch (1930) stated that the sinus reaches its final form at the age of 20; Stern (1939) thought that the pneumatization only reaches its maximal extent in the 40th year of life, whereas Finby and Kraft (1972) showed a continuing increase in height and depth of the frontal sinus after the age of 40.

Meningocephalocele

Richter (1951) reported one case of meningoencephalocele presenting within the frontal sinus in a 24-year-old woman with a 5-year history of perennial catarrh. A watery nasal discharge indicated a CSF leak. The frontonasal encephalocele penetrates between the cribriform plate and the frontal bone or between the nasal bone and the nasal cartilage; also it can present as a nasoethmoidal cell in the inner canthus (von Meyer, 1890; Fenger, 1895).

Mucocele

Cysts covered by mucosa and filled with mucus are termed mucoceles. There was also one case of retained mucus in the frontal sinus in our material.

Empyema of the Frontal Sinus

An empyema of the frontal sinus usually pierces the floor of the frontal sinus at the inner canthus, less often the posterior wall bounding the anterior cranial fossa, and more rarely, the septum of the frontal sinus. If the sinuses are well developed in a vertical extent the abscess may also penetrate through the forehead. Of a total of 17 penetrating empyemas of the frontal sinus, 5 invaded the anterior wall, 3 the floor, 1 the posterior wall, 3 both the floor and the posterior wall, 1 the cribriform plate, 2 the superomedial angle of the orbit and 1 each the posterior and anterior wall (Richter, 1958). Johnson (1948) reported that 8.8% of patients admitted to hospital for frontal sinusitis had an osteomyelitis. This was 2½ times more frequent in men than in women, and twice as common on the left side as on the right.

Trauma

Fenton (1944) reported trauma of the frontal sinuses. Kley (1968) distinguished between fractures of the anterior wall and floor of the frontal sinus, fractures of the orbital plate of the ethmoidal bone and fractures of the anterior wall of the sphenoid sinus approaching the base of the skull, but not causing a fracture of the skull base itself. However, if the fracture line passes through the posterior wall of the frontal sinus, the roof of the ethmoidal sinuses or the roof and posterior wall of the sphenoid sinus then the anterior cranial fossa and hypophyseal fossa are breached. Direct fractures should be distinguished from indirect stress fractures (Kley, 1968). In 62% of fractures of the anterior cranial fossa there was no radiological evidence of a fracture, nor in 40% of fractures affecting the ethmoidal sinuses or the roof of the ethmoids (Beckmann, 1962).

A tear of the dura mater must be closed with fascia to stop the cerebrospinal fluid leak.

Blindness After Irrigation of the Frontal Sinus

Blindness after surgery on the paranasal sinuses is very rare. Sudden unilateral blindness followed irrigation of the frontal sinus of a 54 year old woman. A large dehiscence of the floor of the frontal sinus allowed the sterile physiological saline solution to escape and compress the central retinal vein, artery and causing thrombosis (Thompson et al., 1980).

Eosinophilic Granuloma

Zehm (1965) described an eosinophilic granuloma of the frontal bone, and showed that bony changes in the orbit had led to displacement of the bulb, and thus to a disorder of vision.

Drainage of the Frontal Sinus

(Figs. **96–99**)

Kressner (1950) describes median and contralateral drainage of the frontal sinus. In unilateral disease the septum of the frontal sinus is completely removed providing drainage into the healthy frontal sinus (contralateral drainage).

Trephine of the Frontal Sinus

Frontal sinus (Beck's) trephine may be used with good results for acute, subacute and chronic frontal sinus infection with early orbital complications. The thickness of the anterior and posterior walls of the frontal sinus, its depth in the midline (without the septum) and 2 cm lateral to the midline are shown in Figs. **94** and **95**.

Dawes (1961) reviewed the methods of access to the frontal sinus, and illustrated the pathways of infection of the frontal sinus thoroughly.

Obliterative Frontal Sinusitis

Skillern (1936) reported partial or complete obliteration of the frontal sinus and chronic disease of the sinus: obliterative sinusitis is due to thickening of the bone, mainly of the anterior wall of the frontal sinus. He claimed that radical operation above the supraciliary ridge was successful.

Osteoma

Osteomas are relatively unusual, being commonest in the frontal sinus; their origin is controversial. Kling (1950) described four men and one woman, aged between 32 and 39. Their symptoms included frontal headache irradiating to the occiput, and tension of the posterior cervical muscles. In his view, erosion of the frontal sinus by an osteoma must always be dealt with surgically.

Lacrimal Cells (Ethmolacrimal Recess)

The anterior ethmoidal cell that arises from the region of the frontonasal duct was termed the ethmolacrimal recess by Gruenwald (1925) and as a terminal cell by Heymann and Ritter (1908), who found it in 25% of cases. Our results are shown in Fig. **86**.

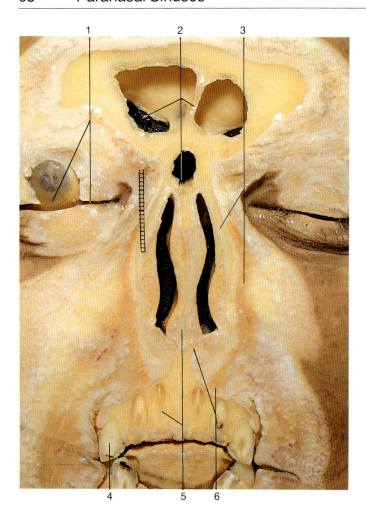

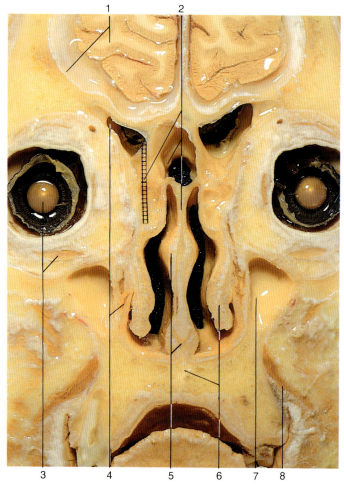

Fig. **96** Frontal sections through the frontal sinus and the surrounding area, seen from in front (Figs. **96–99** are a series of sections through the head of a 35-year-old man)
1 Section of iris and eyelid
2 Right frontal sinus, septum and anterior ethmoidal cells (nasal cells)
3 Frontal process of the maxilla and levator labii superioris alaeque nasi muscle
4 Canine teeth
5 Septal cartilage and first incisor tooth
6 Ala of the premaxilla and the incisive muscle (part of the orbicularis oris muscle)

Fig. **97** Frontal section through the frontal sinus and the surrounding area, seen from behind
1 Anterior cranial fossa and the frontal bone
2 Anterior ethmoidal cell and perpendicular plate with a millimeter strip
3 Lens and inferior oblique muscle
4 Left frontal sinus and nasolacrimal duct
5 Thickened mucosa of the nasal septum (anterior septal intumescence, Jacobsen's torus) and vomer
6 Inferior nasal concha and nasomaxillary suture
7 Anterior wall of the maxillary sinus
8 Buccinator muscle

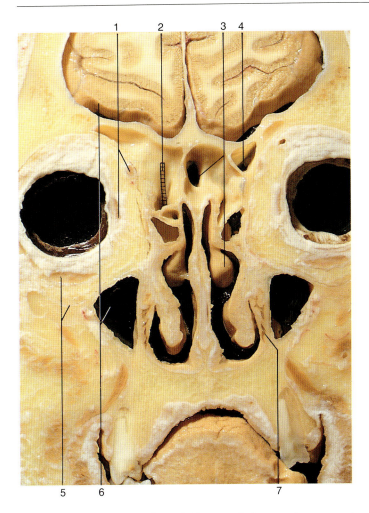

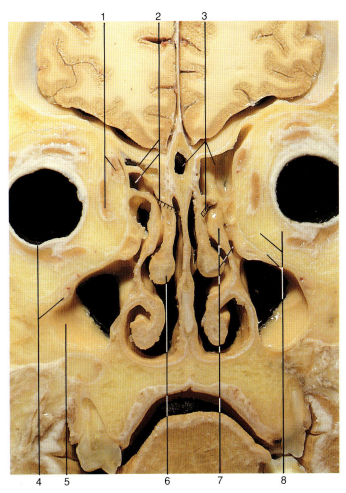

Fig. **98** Frontal section through the nasal sinus and paranasal sinus as seen from the front
1 Medial rectus and superior oblique muscles
2 Millimeter strip in the frontonasal duct
3 Nasal cell, and entrance to anterior edge of the middle nasal concha
4 Left frontal sinus
5 Inferior oblique muscle and floor of the orbit
6 Orbital part of the frontal lobe and maxillary sinus
7 Left nasolacrimal duct

Fig. **99** Frontal section through the nasal cavity and paranasal sinuses from behind
1 Medial rectus and superior oblique muscles
2 Anterosuperior ethmoidal cells with a millimeter strip in the frontonasal duct
3 Pneumatized crista galli, anterosuperior ethmoidal cell and a millimeter strip in the right frontonasal duct
4 Sclera and infraorbital nerve and artery
5 Maxillary sinus
6 Middle nasal concha and septal cartilage
7 Ethmoidal bulla and semilunar hiatus
8 Periorbital fascia and septa in the orbital fat

Semilunar Hiatus and Middle Nasal Concha

(Fig. **100**)

The anterosuperior end of the semilunar hiatus lies between the ethmoidal bulla and the uncinate process, and is usually covered by the middle nasal concha. In one series of 111 specimens, the anterior end of the hiatus lay in front of the anterior end of the middle nasal concha in 2% of cases; in these cases the middle nasal concha was underdeveloped. In 5% it lay at the same level as the anterior attachment of the middle concha, in 43% between 1 and 10 mm behind the attachment, and in 47% of cases 11–20 mm behind it. In one case (0.9%) the anterior end of the semilunar hiatus lay 23 mm posterior to the anterior attachment of the turbinate. The length of the semilunar hiatus lay between 14 and 22 mm and its medial-lateral extent between 0.5 and 3.0 mm (Myerson, 1932). In one case (0.9%) the ethmoidal bulla and the uncinate process had not developed. A mucosal fold ran downwards from the anterior segment of the lateral wall of the middle nasal meatus, arising from the posterior edge of the lacrimal bone. The anterior segment of this fold fused with the lateral nasal wall, whereas the posterior part projected freely into the middle nasal meatus. Several similar variants were also found in our material.

Middle Ethmoidal Cells, Frontal Bullae, Ethmoidal Bulla and Infundibular Cells

The ethmoidal bulla in our material was 18 (9–28) mm long, 5.4 (2–13) mm high, and pneumatized in 70% of cases. 1–3 ethmoidal cells drain above the ethmoidal bulla and within the attachment of the middle concha. Killian termed these the middle ethmoidal cells or superior intermediate cells of the middle nasal meatus. In about 70% of cases one of these cells pneumatizes the ethmoidal bulla itself. Its ostium usually lies at the antero-superior part of the bulla (Fig. **86** and Fig. **89**).

Grünwald (1925) termed those ethmoidal cells which lie within the bony septum between two others and which do not reach the periphery of the ethmoid at any point as *intermediate cells*.

Haller's Cells (1743)

(Fig. **101**)

In 4% of cases a process (lateral crus) arises from the dorsal area of attachment of the middle nasal concha, and then runs downwards and laterally towards the orbital cavity; this process can be pneumatized. Haller's cells are found in such cases (Grünwald, 1925). These Haller's cells can restrict access to the maxillary sinus or the anterior ethmoidal cells during endonasal procedures (Messerklinger, 1980). Haller's cells may lie lateral to the infundibulum; they then open into the middle nasal meatus. Stupka (1938) thought that Haller's cells arose from a cell protruding from the ethmoidal bulla between the layers of the orbital floor, bulging the roof of the maxillary sinus. They project below the floor of the orbit over a variable distance. Schlungbaum (1921) described a bipartite antral cavity: the smaller anterior chamber opened into the middle nasal meatus and the posterior chamber into the superior nasal meatus. The latter could of course be regarded as a posterior ethmoidal cell projecting downwards. However, several authors feel that in this type of bipartite antral cavity a semilunar hiatus with the same boundaries and the same elements as that of the middle nasal meatus is present in the superior nasal meatus. It is said to be bounded by the posterior maxillary process of the palatine bone and the maxillary process of the medial nasal concha (Krmpotic-Nemanic et al., 1985). Two antral cavities of this type can become diseased independently and must be irrigated or drained independently. A second type of secondary maxillary sinus is classified as a Haller's cell if it is due to a posterior ethmoidal cell projecting far forwards in an inferior direction under the floor of the orbit. The transmaxillary route for opening and clearance of the ethmoidal cells is easier in such cases (Krmpotic-Nemanic et al., 1985). If Haller's cells are particularly well developed they border the orbit on one side, and the medial part of the superior wall of the maxillary sinus on the other (Terrahe and Muendnich, 1973). The maxillary sinus then does not meet the ethmoidal labyrinth or the orbit (maxilloethmoidal angle) in the frontal plane at an acute angle, but appears to be flattened out in this area by the Haller's cells. The medial wall of the maxillary sinus may be displaced laterally if the nasal cavity and the ethmoidal labyrinth are well developed. There is then a danger of injury to the orbit during transmaxillary ethmoidectomy.

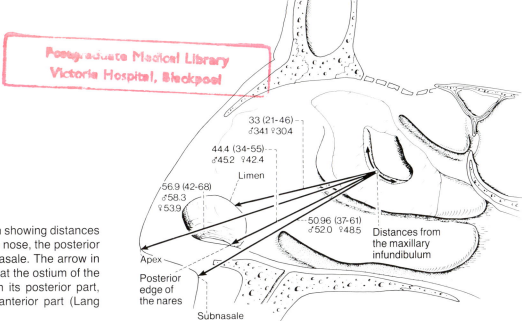

33 (21-46)
♂341 ♀30.4

44.4 (34-55)
♂45.2 ♀42.4

Limen

56.9 (42-68)
♂58.3
♀53.9

50.96 (37-61)
♂52.0 ♀48.5

Distances from
the maxillary
infundibulum

Apex

Posterior
edge of
the nares

Subnasale

Fig. **100** Maxillary infundibulum showing distances from the limen nasi, the tip of the nose, the posterior edge of the nostril and the subnasale. The arrow in the semilunar hiatus indicates that the ostium of the maxillary sinus may lie either in its posterior part, centrally or occasionally in its anterior part (Lang and Bressel, 1988)

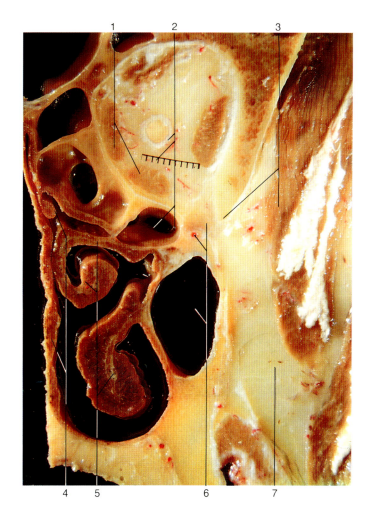

Fig. **101** Haller's cell lying far laterally (frontal section from behind).
1 Medial and inferior rectus muscle
2 Dura mater of the optic nerve, millimeter strip and Haller's cell lying lateral to the inferior rectus muscle
3 Greater wing of the sphenoid bone (superior edge of the inferior orbital fissure) and temporal muscle
4 Superior nasal concha and nasal septum
5 Middle and inferior nasal conchae
6 Orbitalis muscle, infraorbital artery and maxillary sinus
7 Fatty tissue

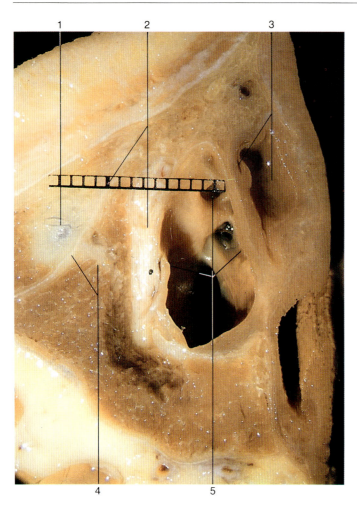

Maxillary Sinus

Postnatal Growth

(see Table **13**)

In our material (Lang and Papke, 1984) the maxillary sinus was 2.5 mm wide in one 39 cm fetus. Onodi stated that the maxillary sinus is 5.3 mm high, 10 mm long and 3.5 mm broad in the newborn (Peter, 1938). At this age it does not yet reach the infraorbital canal laterally. In a four year old boy in our material the maxillary sinus was 7 mm wide, 17 mm long and 12 mm high (Fig. **102**). The infraorbital canal and sulcus lay immediately lateral to its lateral wall. In our adult material the anterior segment of the maxillary sinus was 26.2 (16.4–37.9) mm broad on the right, and 26.9 (16.1–39.8) mm on the left side (Fig. **103**). Its medial side was 38.4 (30.1–49.2) mm long on the right side, and 39.1 (31.1–45.8) mm on the left. The cavity was 40.0 (29.3–56.2) mm high on the right side and 40.8 (31.3–56.9) mm on the left (Fig. **104**) (Lang and Papke, 1984).

◀ Fig. **102** Infraorbital canal exposed from the roof of the maxillary sinus: transverse section in a 4-year-old boy
1 Zygomatic bone
2 Infraorbital nerve dissected, with a millimeter strip
3 Inferior nasal meatus and nasolacrimal duct
4 Zygomaticomaxillary suture and the maxilla
5 Maxillary ostium and medial and lateral wall of the maxillary sinus

Age	Mean size Width in mm	Mean size Height in mm	Minimal size Width in mm	Minimal size Height in mm	Maximal size Width in mm	Maximal size Height in mm	n
0–12 months	12	12.5	7	8	17	17	28
13–18 months	13	13.5	7	10	19	19	48
19–24 months	16	16	9	10	20	22	54
3 Years	18	18	14	12	29	24	110
4 years	19.5	19.5	14	14	27	27	98
5 years	20.5	20	14	14	27	27	157
6 years	21.5	22	15	14	31	29	147
7 years	22.5	23	17	19	31	29	98
8 years	23	24	18	19	31	30	72
9 years	25	26.5	18	20	31	30	48
10 years	27	27	19	19	31	33	48
11 years	28	29	20	21	32	33	38
12 years	28	29	21	22	34	35	18
13 years	28	30	22	26	34	35	12
14 years	28.5	30	22	27	35	38	24
Roof segment in adults	26.4	40.4	10.1	29.3	39.8	56.9	50

Table **13** Size of the maxillary sinus in radiological views (from Menger, Kocoglu and Kocoglu 1969). 85 cm focus–film. (Anatomic measurements after Lang and Papke)

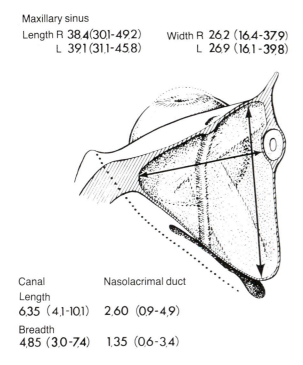

Maxillary sinus
Length R 38,4(30,1-49,2)   Width R 26,2 (16,4-37,9)
       L 39,1(31,1-45,8)   L 26,9 (16,1-39,8)

Canal	Nasolacrimal duct
Length	
6,35 (4,1-10,1)	2,60 (0,9-4,9)
Breadth	
4,85 (3,0-7,4)	1,35 (0,6-3,4)

Fig. **103** Length and breadth of the roof of the maxillary sinus, and of the nasolacrimal duct and canal (Lang and Papke, 1984)

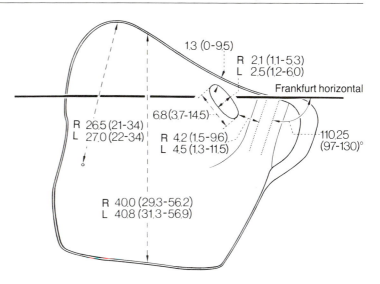

1,3 (0-9,5)
R 2,1 (1,1-5,3)
L 2,5 (1,2-6,0)
Frankfurt horizontal
R 26,5 (21-34)
L 27,0 (22-34)
6,8 (3,7-14,5)
R 4,2 (1,5-9,6)
L 4,5 (1,3-11,5)
110,25
(97-130)°
R 40,0 (29,3-56,2)
L 40,8 (31,3-56,9)

Fig. **104** The maxillary sinus in a paramedian sagittal section. Entry of the posterosuperior alveolar nerve, height of the maxillary sinus, width of the maxillary ostium, its distance from the roof of the maxillary sinus, distance between the maxillary ostium and the frontonasal duct, width of the maxillary ostium and angle of the nasolacrimal duct with the Frankfurt horizontal (data should be read off from left to right). Differences between the right and left sides are also shown (Lang and Papke, 1984)

Recesses

A *palatine recess* can extend towards the hard palate, occasionally within a few millimeters of the median sagittal plane. An *infraorbital recess* projects anteriorly to the right and left of the infraorbital canal. A prelacrimal recess is almost always present (Fig. **105**). A *zygomatic recess* extends into the zygomatic bone. A *recess of the palatine bone* can project into the maxillary sinus if the orbital process of the palatine bone reaches the sinus (Hajek, 1909). The *alveolar recess* is larger in brachycephalic than in dolicocephalic skulls (Mündnich, 1937). It is present in 40% of cases, but in only 25% of cases when the canine fossa is deep (Salinger 1939).

Fig. **105** Roof of the maxillary sinus with the prelacrimal recess, as seen from below in a transverse section
1 Sulcus and infraorbital canal
2 Millimeter strip in the frontonasal duct
3 Maxillary recess and roof of the inferior nasal meatus
4 Lateral wall of the maxillary sinus
5 Temporalis muscle
6 Millimeter strip in the maxillary ostium
7 Sphenoidal sinus and ostium
8 Middle nasal concha, nasal septum and septum of the sphenoidal sinus

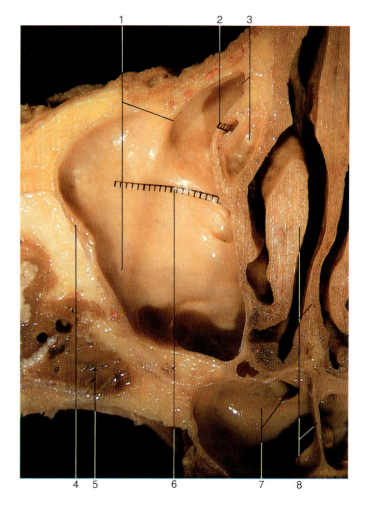

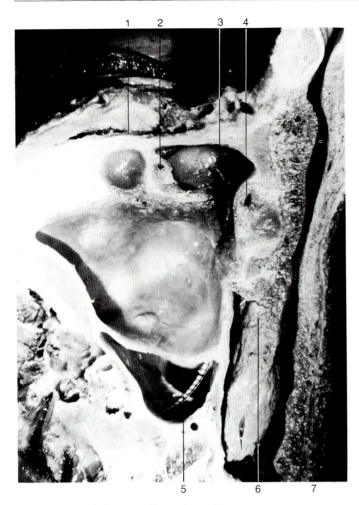

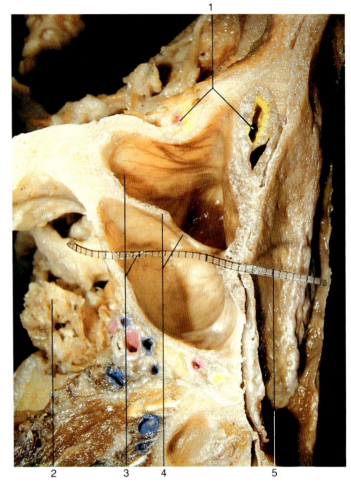

Fig. **106**   Roof of the maxillary sinus with a transverse septum
1 Lower eyelid
2 Infraorbital artery
3 Millimeter strip in an anterior diverticulum of the anterior part of the sinus
4 Nasolacrimal duct
5 Inferior nasal concha
6 Nasal septum
7 Millimeter strip in the posterosuperior part of the sinus, and opening of the posterior ethmoidal bulla

Fig. **107**   Frontal septum of the maxillary sinus shown in transverse section from below
1 Infraorbital artery and nasolacrimal duct
2 Temporalis muscle retracted
3 Anterior and posterior segment of the maxillary sinus with a millimeter strip
4 Partial septum with a foramen in its medial part covered by mucosa
5 Inferior nasal concha

Septa

(Figs. **106–108**)

Septa of the sinus can also be regarded as walls of Haller's cells. The maxillary sinus may be completely partitioned in 1–2.5% of cases (Gruber, 1848, 1850; Yoshinaga, 1909). Abbada (1937) reported a sagittal bony septum about 2 mm in diameter in the maxillary sinus of a 17-year-old boy (Salinger, 1939). Furthermore, frontal lobuli can occur with or without a connection with the main sinus (Fig. 8 in Lang and Sakals, 1982, and Fig. 13 in Lang and Papke, 1984). We found duplication of the maxillary sinus of varying arrangements and shapes, and reduplication of the maxillary sinus connected to the main sinus, in 6% of our

cases (Lang and Papke, 1984). The two sinuses probably arise from two anlages of the middle nasal meatus. In one of our cases the posterior sinus opened behind the ethmoidal bulla, and could therefore be classified as an exceptional form of a Haller's cell. In one 49-year-old woman, the connection with the nasal cavity lay above the middle nasal concha so that the posterior antral cavity could be classified as a posterior ethmoidal cell growing downwards. The party wall may be eroded with progressive pneumatization, producing a defect in the party wall of a bipartite maxillary sinus (Stupka, 1938). Such a specimen was present in our material in a 60-year-old man. Bullous, mainly elliptical, posterior, ethmoidal cells could be shown in the region of the maxillary sinus in 6% of our cases.

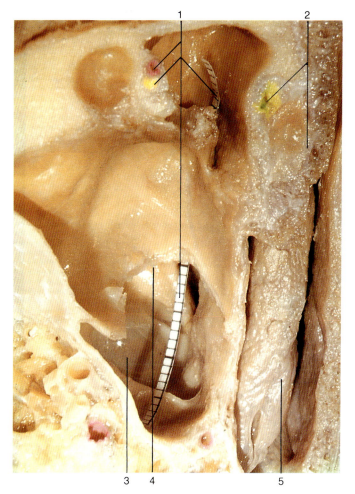

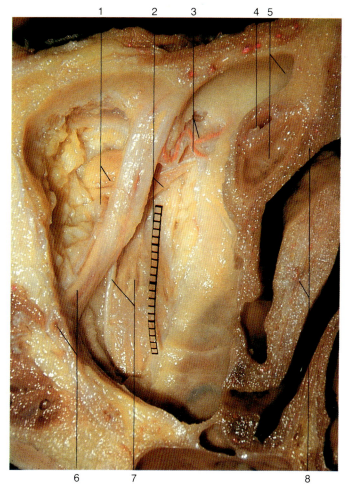

Fig. **108** Transverse section of the maxillary sinus from below.
1 Millimeter strip in the upper part of the sinus, and the infra-orbital artery and nerve
2 Nasolacrimal duct and inferior nasal concha in section
3 Upper part of the maxillary sinus
4 Part of the septum removed
5 Middle nasal concha

Fig. **109** Roof of the maxillary sinus removed showing a view from below.
1 Inferior oblique muscle and nerve entering it
2 Inferior oblique muscle, posterior edge and millimeter strip
3 Intra-extraorbital arterial anastamosis
4 Nasolacrimal duct
5 Prelacrimal recess and roof of the inferior nasal meatus
6 Infraorbital nerve and artery (sulcus region)
7 Inferior rectus muscle and muscular ramus to the inferior oblique muscle
8 Middle and inferior nasal concha

Roof and Neighboring Structures

(Fig. **109**)

In our series of 117 adult specimens aged between 37 and 90 years, the roof of the maxillary sinus was 0.4 (0.1–7.0) mm thick medial to the infraorbital canal, and 0.5 (0.1–1.1) mm thick lateral to it. In about 14% of cases the infraorbital canal demonstrated dehiscences, varying in size from 3–11 mm. The thickness of the roof of the maxillary sinus increases towards the orbital margin (Fig. **110**) (Lang and Papke, 1984).

Blow-Out Fractures

Lang (1889) was the first to describe a fracture of the orbital floor, producing double vision and limitation of upward movement of the eye (Rowe, 1975). Smith and Regan (1957) introduced the term "blow-out fracture" for this injury. Retrobulbar fat and orbital contents are compressed by a sudden marked pressure on the bulb, and then burst through the least resistant part of the orbit. Although the medial wall of the orbit is not thick it is buttressed by the intermediate septa of the ethmoidal cells. Therefore, a typical blow-out fracture affects the floor of the orbit. The orbital periosteum, the fatty tissue and the inferior rectus muscle and its sheath can be displaced through the fracture line, and become clamped in the cleft. Shortening of the

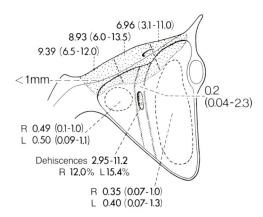

Fig. **110**   Thickness of the roof of the maxillary sinus lateral and medial to the infraorbital sulcus and canal. The lower part of the wall of the canal shows dehiscences in 14% of cases. Its length is 3.0–11.2 mm. The anterior part (infraorbital margin) of the roof of the maxillary sinus which is more than 1 mm thick is also shown (Lang and Papke, 1984)

muscles or their sheath incarcerated in the fracture line causes the retraction phenomenon: the eyeball cannot be rotated passively upwards, and the patient also complains of vertical diplopia. Occasionally the medial wall of the orbit also bursts (Edwards and Ridley, 1968). In one case, an eyeball subluxated into the nasal cavity could perceive light transmitted through the nostril (Straub, 1972).

Boenninghaus (1969) was the first to report a blow-out fracture of the orbital roof due to trauma to the eyeball, with simultaneous fracture of the orbital plate of the ethmoid bone.

Fig. **111** provides details of the structures related to the maxillary sinus.

Mucosal Folds

(Fig. **112**)

Mucosal folds arising from the floor of the maxillary sinus, and bony ridges of varying height were found in 56% of our material. The haustra were 7.8 mm high and 2.9 mm thick, and on occasions surrounded fairly high niches. In 10% of our cases the bony ridges and mucosal folds were higher than 13 mm.

Height of the Floor

At the end of the second year of life the floor of the maxillary sinus lies somewhat lower than the insertion of the inferior nasal concha. At the age of seven it lies roughly at the height of the inferior nasal meatus, and at the age of nine at the level of the floor of the nasal cavity. Later the floor of the maxillary sinus can sink further and invade the hard palate in a medial direction, forming the palatine recess. In 26% of cases the floor of the maxillary sinus lies below the floor of the nasal cavity, at the same level in 28% of cases, and higher in 6% of cases. In the next commonest type the anterior half of the floor of the maxillary sinus lay deeper than the floor of the nose, whereas the posterior part lay in this plane. Numerous other variations including differences between the left and right sides, were found (Hajnis et al., 1967).

The Maxillary Sinus and the Teeth

(Fig. **113**)

Runge, in 1928, investigated the relation of the maxillary sinus to the teeth by both anatomical dissection and by radiology (Peter, 1938). The first dentition had no influence on the direction of growth and form of the maxillary

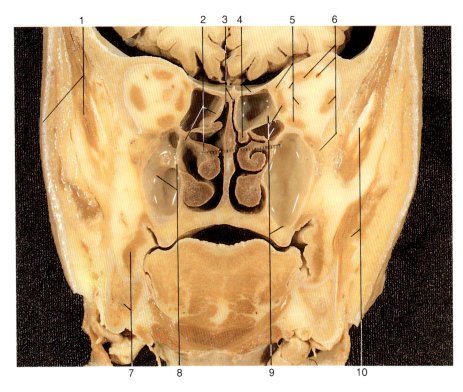

Fig. **111**   Frontal section through the head in the posterior third of the orbit
 1 Skin and temporalis muscle
 2 Middle nasal concha with connections to the orbit and the sphenoidal plane, with a millimeter strip
 3 Domes of the nasal cavity of unequal width
 4 Sphenoidal plane and superior nasal concha
 5 Superior oblique muscle, optic nerve, inferior rectus muscle and ophthalmic artery
 6 Superior rectus muscle, ophthalmic vein, lateral rectus muscle and orbitalis muscle
 7 Buccinator muscle and inferior alveolar nerve in an edentulous mandible
 8 Posterior wall of the maxillary sinus, and a large accessory ostium
 9 Ethmoidal cells, medial rectus muscle and a deep floor of the maxillary sinus
10 Tendon of the temporalis muscle and masseter muscle

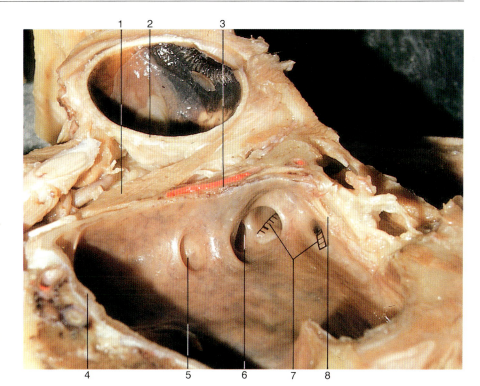

Fig. **112** Anterosuperior mucosal niche of the maxillary sinus, paramedian sagittal section from lateral and below
1 Inferior rectus muscle
2 Ocular bulb
3 Infraorbital artery and nerve
4 Posterior wall of the maxillary sinus
5 Posterior mucosal diverticulum
6 Maxillary ostium
7 Millimeter strip in anterosuperior mucosal diverticula
8 Exposed infraorbital nerve

sinus, since the dental follicles of the deciduous teeth were separated from the floor of the sinus by a thick bony layer. In the seventh month of life a bony layer 1.5–2.0 mm thick lies over the deciduous molars. The saccule of the canine tooth lay 1.5–4.0 mm from the maxillary sinus in the first to the fifth year of life. Between the ages of six and eleven almost all tooth buds lateral to the incisor teeth (with the exception of that of the first molar) lie in immediate relation to the mucosa of the maxillary cavity. The first molar tooth is related to the mucosa from the fourth year of life, and the second molar tooth from the fifth year of life, although the second molar tooth can be separated by a bony layer 1–2 mm thick. The canine tooth between the ages of six and eleven almost always reaches the floor of the maxillary sinus. Usually its root then lies in front of the anterior wall of the maxillary sinus over a distance of 7.1 mm (Bonsdorff, 1925).

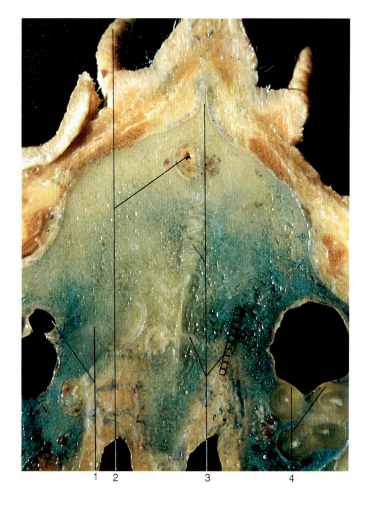

Fig. **113** Roots of a third molar, with four roots (variation) projecting into the maxillary sinus. Transverse section from below
1 Section through the right maxillary sinus and maxilla
2 Nasal ala, and Stenson's duct in the incisive canal
3 Anterior nasal spine and sagittal and transverse sutures of the hard palate. Millimeter strip
4 Anterior root of the third molar (variation) with no bone cover encroaching upon the left maxillary sinus

The floor of the maxillary sinus has a minimum thickness of 0.5 mm over the first premolar in 5% of cases, over the second premolar in 20% of cases, over the first molar in 27% of cases, over the second molar in 46% of cases, and over the third molar in 30% of cases (Harrison, 1961). The floor of the maxillary sinus may be perforated by the roots of the second premolar, as well as the first, second and third molars. Defects are most common over the first molar, being found in 2.2% of cases, and then over the root of the second molar in 2%. The third molar and second premolar are less often the origin of an oroantral fistula which is most frequent when the floor of the maxillary sinus is low-lying. The authors have only seen tooth roots projecting into the maxillary sinus in two cases (1.8%).

Hajek (1909) termed those maxillary cavities which do not reach the level of the floor of the nose as "narrow" maxillary sinuses. In his material the alveolae of the molar and canine teeth were the most frequent to project into the antral cavity, followed by that of the premolar teeth.

Diseases: Mayer states that Highmore (1651) extracted an upper molar and showed that pus drained from the opened antral cavity. He emphasized that the site of the three molars must be assessed carefully before draining the maxillary sinus, and that it is possible to penetrate the canine fossa by drilling in a vertical direction if the maxillary sinus is small. The maxillary sinus should not be affected if it is opened by extraction of a tooth, but an emphysema of dental origin should be treated by rhinological principles (Peter and Sicher, 1920). On the other hand, direct or indirect damage to the teeth can follow operations on the maxillary sinus. Paresthesia of the teeth and tooth retention apparatus due to radical operations on the maxillary sinus was reported by Port in 1908, and by Guhraurer in 1914 (Schicketanz and Schicketanz, 1961). We investigated the point of entry of the posterosuperior alveolar rami, the medial superior alveolar nerve and the nasodental nerve into the maxillary sinus (Lang and Papke, 1984). The nasodental nerve runs towards the attachment of the inferior nasal turbinate, supplies the nasolacrimal duct and then turns downwards at the piriform aperture (see Fig. **114**).

The infraorbital nerve should be preserved during Caldwell-Luc antrostomy. If the mucosa of the alveolar recess alone is removed disorders of sensation are 10% less common than after complete removal of the mucosa (Grosse-Helleforth and Duecker, 1976).

Holzmann (1931) found loss of reaction or hypoesthesia after Caldwell-Luc antrostomy in the following proportions: in 35% of the second premolar teeth, 25% of the first premolar teeth, 27% of the canine teeth, 30% of the second incisors and 17% of the first incisors. Damage to the teeth was found in 22% of patients undergoing Caldwell-Luc antrotomy, most frequently to the canine tooth and then with decreasing frequency to the first premolar, the

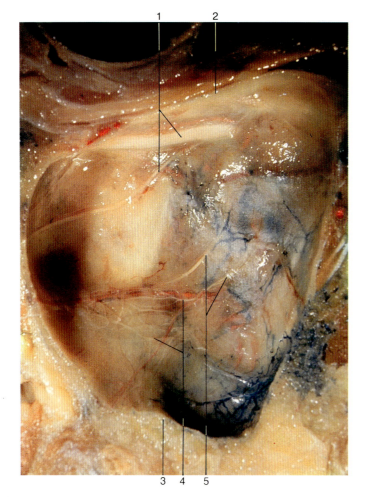

Fig. **114** Posterior superior and middle superior alveolar branches of the infraorbital nerve: paramedian sagittal section from the medial side.
1 Infraorbital nerve lying in its canal with the middle superior alveolar branch
2 Roof of the maxillary sinus
3 Floor of the maxillary sinus
4 Neural plexus and sinus mucosa
5 Posterior superior alveolar branch

second premolar, the incisors, the first molar and then the third molar. Injuries to the teeth, most frequently the incisors, were found in 15% of cases after Denker's operation, most frequently to the incisors (Schicketanz and Schicketanz, 1961).

Draf (1982) also showed that transient paresthesia in the region of the incisor and canine teeth as well as post-operative surgical emphysema and phlegmon of the cheek can follow antroscopy, but severe bleeding only occurred once in 1000 cases. Hall and Thomas (1938) reported 12 patients with spontaneous bleeding into the maxillary sinus as a complication of hyperplastic maxillary sinusitis, the incidence being 1:1400 patients.

Brusis (1979) proposed the following steps for the prevention of neuralgia after operations on the maxillary sinus:

1) A vertical incision lateral to the canine tooth.
2) Creation of a small posterior window in a part of the anterior wall of the maxillary sinus that is relatively poor in nerves.
3) Resection solely of the diseased mucosa.

Drainage in the Treatment of Maxillary Sinusitis

Zuckerkandl showed as long ago as 1893 that the maxillary sinus can be drained either through the often relatively thick wall of the inferior meatus, or into the middle meatus at the fontanelles (Figs. **65** and **115**). Good reviews are available of intranasal endoscopic antral operations, of the procedure via the fontanelles, and all the surgical approaches to the maxillary antrum and the other paranasal sinuses (Wigand and Steiner, 1977; Wigand et al., 1978; Straatman and Buiter, 1981; Draf, 1982). The approach through the canine fossa for chronic maxillary sinusitis was first described by Caldwell in 1893 and by Luc in 1895. Petersen (1973) described a method for puncture of the maxillary sinus through the canine fossa.

Rare Complications of Disease of the Maxillary Sinus

Proptosis of the right eye, and ptosis of the right upper eyelid has been reported in a 43-year-old man with a mucocele of the maxillary sinus. The symptoms resolved after removal of the mucocele (Parker, 1961).

Tovi et al. (1983) reported a parapharyngeal abscess in a 45-year-old woman after maxillary sinusitis following a dental extraction. The pterygopalatine and intratemporal fossae can also be affected.

Resistance of the ostium of the maxillary antrum after irrigation of the maxillary sinus: Drettner (1965) reported his findings after 100 irrigations on 57 patients. Obstruction of the ostium is commoner in chronic than in acute sinusitis. The resistance of the ostium falls during the healing phase of acute sinusitis but remains high in chronic sinusitis. The measurements were carried out using hydrostatic pressures.

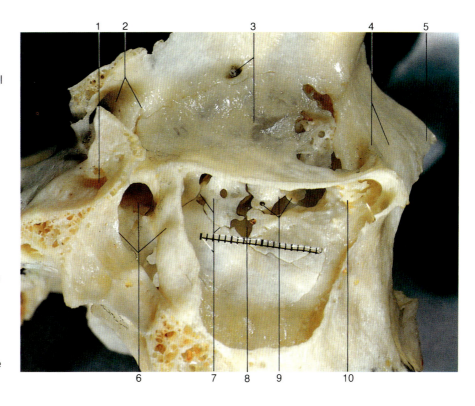

Fig. **115** Medial wall of the maxillary sinus with numerous fonticuli. Paramedian sagittal section through the skull seen from the lateral surface
1 Intracranial opening of the foramen rotundum
2 Optic canal and suture between the lesser wing and the frontal bone
3 Single ethmoidal canal (shown by a probe), and orbital plate of the ethmoidal bone
4 Frontal process of the maxilla and anterior lacrimal crest
5 Nasal bone
6 Sphenopalatine foramen and sphenomaxillary fissure
7 Process of the ethmoidal bone running to the orbital process of the palatine bone and to the maxilla (millimeter strip)
8 Posterior nasal fontanelle
9 Uncinate process and anterior nasal fontanelle
10 Bony excrescences on the lateral surface of the nasolacrimal canal

Maxillary Infundibulum and the Ostium of the Maxillary Sinus
(Fig. **116**)

Initially a large round or oval bony defect lies on the medial side of the antral cavity. It was called the maxillary hiatus by Henle (Zuckerkandl, 1893). The hiatus may be rhomboid, semicircular, egg-shaped, bean-shaped or triangular (Perovic, 1954). Initially the antral opening lies in front and above. Subsequent growth of the sinus is accompanied by proliferation and resorption. A short, wide gutter projects between the maxillary hiatus and the frontal process of the maxilla; it is called the sulcus for the lacrimal bone. This groove is limited behind by the edge of the maxillary sinus curving in a nasal direction and in front by the sharp edge of the frontal process. The superior edge of the maxillary hiatus may be either angular or broad, and occasionally split into two laminae (Zuckerkandl, 1893). A small infundibulum leads into the mucosal ostium of the maxillary sinus.

Position: In Myerson's (1932) material the *ostium* of the maxillary sinus lay at the posterior end of the semilunar hiatus in 23% of cases. In our material the ostium of the maxillary sinus lay in the posterior quarter in 2%, in the third quarter in 48%, in the second quarter 28% and in the anterior quarter in 22% (Lang and Sakals, 1982). The ostium of the maxillary sinus lay horizontally in one of Myerson's cases, and was 2.5 × 3.5 mm wide. The ostium of the maxillary sinus in Myerson's (1932) material was completely independent of the ethmoidal bulla and of the uncinate process in 5% of cases.

Shape: According to Zuckerkandl (1882) the ostium of the maxillary sinus is usually an elliptical cleft with a long sagittal axis, but it can also be circular or kidney-shaped. In his material the smallest ostium had a diameter of 3 mm, the largest a diameter of 19 mm and a width of 5 mm.

Usually it was between 7–11 mm long and between 2–6 mm wide. Occasionally the ostium is divided into two parts by a mucosal membrane. The ostia may be as long as 18 mm (Turner, 1902; Schaeffer, 1920) or even 20 mm. The ostium forms a short canal running downwards and backwards into the maxillary sinus (Skillern, 1913). Simon (1939) found the ostium to have a mean width of 5.5 (1.0–15.5) mm. Ostia longer than 3 mm can be classified as canals and those which are shorter as ostia. Simon classified 83% as canals, and 17% as ostia.

Direction of the canal (Fig. **116**): The *infundibulum* originates in the semilunar hiatus. From it the ostium (or the canal) passes inferiorly and laterally: in 56% in a posteroinferior direction, but more anteriorly in 44%. Duplicate ostia are found in 2% of cases, and duplicate or accessory ostia or canals with two separate openings into the middle nasal meatus in 1% (Simon, 1939). Two main maxillary ostia were also found in our material (Figs. 15 and 16 in Lang and Papke, 1984).

When viewed from outside the maxillary sinus, the ostium (or the laterally directed funnel-shaped opening of the canal) of the maxillary sinus is usually a long ellipse directed laterally and anteriorly. In our material the lumen was 6.8 (3.7–14.5) mm wide; the opening of the duct was 2.3 (1.1–6.0) mm wide. It lay 1.6 (0–9.5) mm from the superior wall of the maxillary sinus (Lang and Papke, 1984). The distance of the maxillary ostium from the nasolacrimal duct was 4 (1.3–11.5) mm.

Endoscopic Findings

Messerklinger (1970) demonstrated many variations of the maxillary sinus by endoscopy, and reported that the middle meatus is exceedingly complex (1970, 1972). He observed nipple-shaped protrusions of the mucoperiostial layer of the fontanelle into the middle meatus, particularly in chronic maxillary sinusitis. Like Zuckerkandl (1893) he

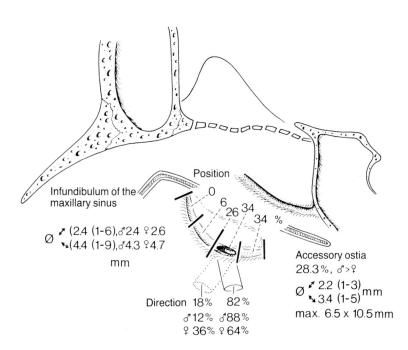

Fig. **116** Infundibulum and ostium of the maxillary sinus, position in the semilunar hiatus and direction of the short canal posteroinferiorly or anteroinferiorly. The diameter of the infundibulum, the number of the ostia and their width are also shown. In our more recent material, in contrast with earlier investigations, this type of infundibulum could not be demonstrated in the anterior part of the semilunar hiatus (Lang and Bressel, in press)

termed this region the area of the anterior and posterior nasal fontanelle. Draf (1983) illustrated various maxillary ostia (large and triangular, narrow and slit-like, with acute mucosal swelling, mural polyposis, etc). The results of ultrasound were reported by Mann (1984).

Maxillary Sinusitis

Erbs showed purulent maxillary sinusitis in 142 of 496 children submitted to autopsy (Muehler, 1971). The proportion was higher in sucklings than in older children. A simultaneous bronchitis was also frequent.

Inhibition of Pneumatization

Differences between the right and left sides are rarer in the maxillary sinus than in the frontal sinus. Rudimentary sinuses have been described, usually lying posteriorly and superiorly at some distance from the teeth (Zuckerkandl, 1893; Gruber, 1848). Benjamins saw a case with complete absence of the maxillary sinus, the middle turbinate, the ethmoidal labyrinth and the frontal sinus (Stupka, 1938). Stupka also reported that Lang had seen one case with complete aplasia of the paranasal sinuses. Our material included one maxillary sinus only 10 mm broad and 18 mm long: its medial wall was 3.5 mm thick, the turbinates and the nasal septum were aplastic (Lang and Kley, 1981).

Pneumosinus Dilatans

Pneumosinus dilatans has been reported in the frontal sinus, and more rarely in the maxillary sinus (Wolfensberger, 1984). This author used manometry to demonstrate a one-way valve between the nasal cavity and the maxillary sinus. The disease is characterized by bone destruction, and by expansion of a normally aerated paranasal sinus. The facial contours change slowly; the patient complains of mild pain and a feeling of pressure. The frontal sinus is most often affected, followed by the ethmoids and then by the sphenoids. Pneumosinus dilatans of the maxilla was reported in a 15-year-old boy whose eyeball was gradually displaced upwards by 3 mm.

Ethmoidal Cells Arising from the Superior (and Supreme) Nasal Meatus

(Fig. 117)

The *posterior ethmoidal cells* of the superior nasal meatus in the neonate are 4 mm high, 2.5–5 mm long and 1.5–2 mm broad (Koch, 1930); our values were higher. Three ethmoidal cells generally develop from the superior nasal meatus (Zuckerkandl, 1893; Hajek, 1909; Gruenwald, 1925; Peter, 1938). One grows superolaterally, the other posterosuperiorly, and another sometimes grows into the ethmoidal bulla. A supreme nasal meatus was present in one-third of Peter's cases; in these subjects cells were present which had extended backwards and upwards in 75% of cases. In the material described by Van Alyea (1939) cells arising from the superior nasal meatus were found in 96%. In one of the four specimens without this type of cell a large cavity was present whose ostium opened into the supreme nasal meatus; the second case showed two cells of this type. In the other two specimens, posterior ethmoidal cells had not developed (on both sides in one head).

In 38 of the 100 specimens investigated by Van Alyea, cells were present arising from the supreme nasal meatus. He found two cells of this type in five of his specimens. Overall, 43% of this specimens demonstrated *postremal ethmoidal cells* (Gilbert et al., 1958).

Fig. **117** Ethmoidal labyrinth opened from the orbit with the intervening walls in situ
1 Anterior ethmoidal cell with a millimeter strip in the ostium, lateral to the frontal sinus
2 Horner's muscle (tensor tarsi) and lacrimal sac opened from the lateral side
3 Posterior ethmoidal cell, superior oblique muscle and nasociliary nerve
4 Ophthalmic artery and posterior ethmoidal cell with a millimeter strip leading towards the ostium
5 Posterior ethmoidal cell, millimeter strip, ostium opened up immediately above the middle nasal concha, and the middle nasal concha
6 Middle ethmoidal cell, millimeter strip, foramen immediately above the lateral torus
7 Millimeter strip in the ostium of the maxillary sinus, and the maxillary sinus
8 Orbital part of the orbicularis oculi muscle and the origin of the inferior oblique muscle

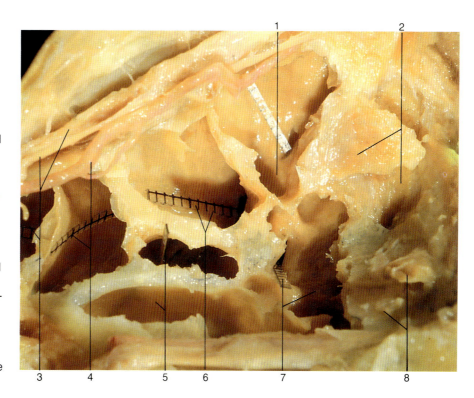

Ethmoidal Bulla and Posterior Ethmoidal Labyrinth

Van Alyea (1939), too, showed that bulla cells often pneumatize a large part of the ethmoidal labyrinth. These medial ethmoidal cells can extend anteriorly into the infundibulum, and posteriorly behind the posterior ethmoidal cells. These bullae contacted the sphenoid sinus via cells sprouting posteriorly; in 2% these bullar cells were large and in 2% they were small. Altogether, the posterior labyrinth was pneumatized in 11% by bullar cells.

Dehiscences of the Ethmoidal Cells

Dehiscences of the ethmoidal cells have a particular clinical significance. Tonndorf investigated 100 human skulls, including fetal skulls, and showed that the cribriform foramina opened into a frontal recess, that is lateral to the middle nasal concha, in 10 cases (Stupka, 1938). The superomedial wall of the ethmoidal cell which bounds the olfactory groove is rarefied in 38% of cases, and dehiscent in 14% (Ohnishi, 1981). We did not observe these dehiscences in our material. Rarefactions were shown along the course of the anterior ethmoidal nerve in 35% of cases, and bony defects in 11%. They were much commoner in our material (v.i.). The anterolateral part of the roof of the ethmoidal sinus was rarefied in 14% of cases. Rarefaction was found in the posterior ethmoids (that is the region of the posterior ethmoidal nerve) in 26% of cases, and bony defects in 14% of older subjects. The dehiscences in the orbital plate of the ethmoid bone in old age may be due to excessive pneumatisation (Stupka, 1938).

Ethmoidal Canals, Level of the Cribriform Plate and Dehiscences

(Figs. **118–121**)

The position of the ethmoidal canals in relation to the cribriform plate is important in diagnosis, in intranasal ethmoidectomy and in closure of CSF fistulae. The vertical position of the anterior ethmoidal canal was determined on 54 subjects. This canal runs medially and anteriorly through the ethmoidal labyrinth, lying between 2 (1.1) mm below and 4 mm above the cribriform plate.

Dehiscences of the walls of the anterior ethmoidal canal 6.9 (1.8–13.5) mm long were found in 93% of cases. Vessels and nerves pass through these dehiscences to the ethmoidal cells.

Tertiary ethmoidal canals were present in 33% of the material, lying 1 (1.1–3.3) mm above the cribriform plate. In 39% of cases there were dehiscences 2 (0.75–3.8) mm long in the walls of the tertiary ethmoidal canals.

Posterior ethmoidal canals could be found in all specimens. The greatest part of their course lay 1.5 (0–3.1) mm above the cribriform plate, running in an anteromedial direction. Dehiscences 3.6 (1.1–7.7) mm long were found in these canals in 59% of cases.

In our material the orbital opening of the posterior ethmoidal canal lay not less than 2 mm from the orbital aperture of the optic canal, not only medially but also from above and laterally (Fig. 173 in Lang, 1983). Fig. **122** shows details of the width, length and shape of the ethmoidal canals. The arteries of the ethmoidal canals and their branches are shown in Fig. **123**.

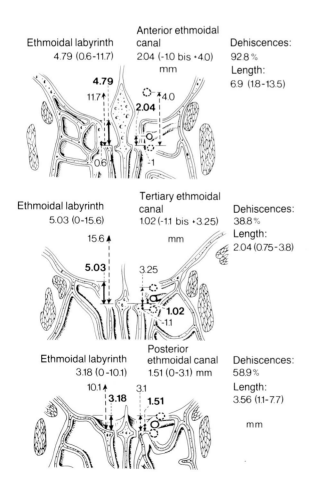

Fig. **118** Height of the ethmoidal canal relative to the cribriform plate, dehiscences in the anterior, posterior and tertiary ethmoidal canal, and depth of the olfactory fossa (Lang and Haas, 1988)

Fig. **119** Ethmoidal arteries after removal of the superior ethmoidal cells. Left side of a 72-year-old female specimen from the right and below
  1 Pons
  2 Medial wall of the right sphenoid sinus
  3 Bifurcation of the basilar artery and posterior lobe of the pituitary gland
  4 Optic nerve, and anterior lobe of the pituitary gland
  5 Anterior cerebral artery
  6 Left sphenoidal sinus and frontal lobe
  7 Posterior ethmoidal artery, and a millimeter strip
  8 Anterior ethmoidal artery with a dehiscent canal
  9 Clivus
  10 Soft palate
  11 Branch of the sphenopalatine artery
  12 Hard palate and tongue
  13 Ethmoidal bulla, inferior edge and semilunar hiatus
  14 Millimeter strip in the nasofrontal duct, and an agger cell

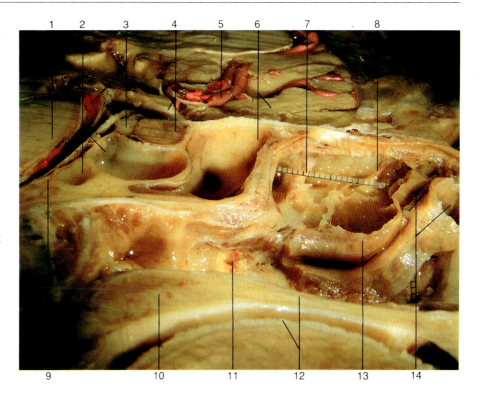

Fig. **120** Olfactory fossae of unequal depth, ethmoidal arteries and a septal deviation
  1 Orbital part of the frontal lobe and roof of the orbit
  2 Superior oblique muscle, ophthalmic and anterior ethmoidal arteries
  3 Anterior ethmoidal canal with a high ethmoidal labyrinth on the right side
  4 Crista galli and left olfactory bulb
  5 Anterior ethmoidal artery, orbital and canal areas in the lower lying ethmoidal labyrinth
  6 Superior oblique muscle and region from which fatty tissue has been removed
  7 Medial rectus muscle, a millimeter strip and sclera
  8 Superomedial angle of the wall of the maxillary sinus and the conchal lamina
  9 Septal spur posteriorly on the right side
  10 Nasal septum with an anterior spur on the left side
  11 Palatine glands
  12 Maxillary sinus and the inferior concha
  13 Inferior rectus muscle and floor of the orbit

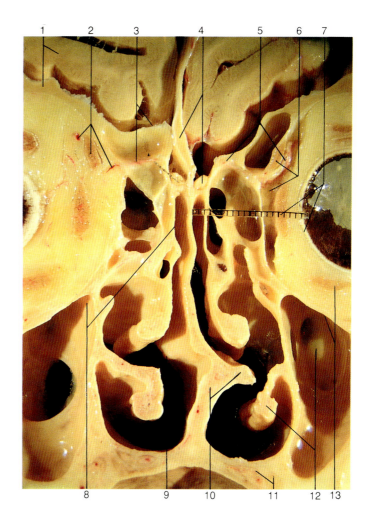

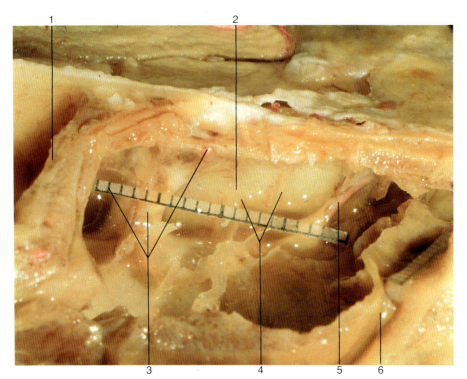

Fig. **121** Ethmoidal arteries after removal of
the superior ethmoidal cells (left side from
right and below in a 72-year-old woman)
1 Anterior wall of the sphenoidal sinus
2 Roof of the ethmoidal labyrinth
3 Posterior ethmoidal canal, posterior
  ethmoidal artery and a millimeter strip
4 Remnants of the walls of the ethmoidal
  cells
5 Anterior ethmoidal canal, dehiscence and
  anterior ethmoidal artery
6 Anterior wall of the ethmoidal bulla

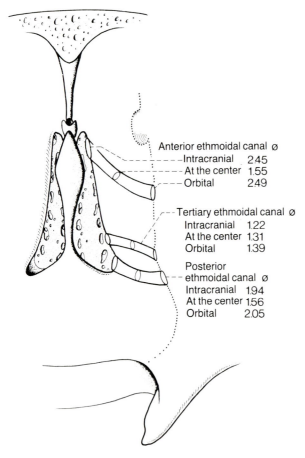

Anterior ethmoidal canal ø
---Intracranial   2.45
--- At the center 1.55
--- Orbital   2.49

Tertiary ethmoidal canal ø
Intracranial   1.22
At the center   1.31
Orbital   1.39

Posterior
ethmoidal canal ø
Intracranial   1.94
At the center 1.56
Orbital   2.05

Fig. **122** Ethmoidal canals showing widths at its intracranial and
orbital openings, and in the center of the canal (Lang et al., 1979)

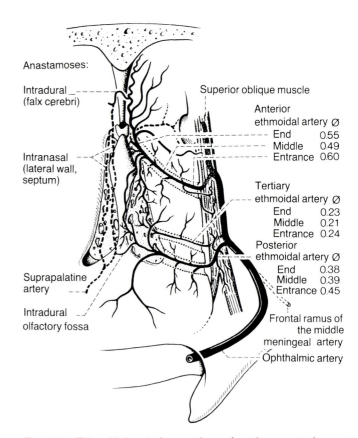

Anastamoses:

Intradural
(falx cerebri)

Intranasal
(lateral wall,
septum)

Suprapalatine
artery

Intradural
olfactory fossa

Superior oblique muscle

Anterior
ethmoidal artery ø
    End   0.55
    Middle   0.49
    Entrance 0.60

Tertiary
ethmoidal artery ø
    End   0.23
    Middle   0.21
    Entrance 0.24

Posterior
ethmoidal artery ø
    End   0.38
    Middle   0.39
    Entrance 0.45

Frontal ramus of
the middle
meningeal artery
Ophthalmic artery

Fig. **123** Ethmoidal arteries, values for the most frequent
course, anastamoses, origins and width (Lang and Schaefer,
1979)

Sphenoidal Sinus

A clearly developed sphenoethmoidal recess lay in front of the sphenoidal sinus in 48% of our material (Lang and Sakals, 1982). It was 10.5 (8–14.5) mm high, 5.5 (2–28.5) mm long and 4.3 (1.5–12) mm deep.

Ostium of the Sphenoidal Sinus

(Fig. **124**)

The ostium of the sphenoidal sinus in our material was round in 70% of cases with a mean diameter of 2.4 mm. Pinhead-sized openings were found in 15% of cases, whereas round openings up to 3.5 mm in size were unusual. The opening was elliptical in about 30% of cases, the greater diameter being more often vertical than oblique or horizontal. Inflammation of the mucosa of the sphenoid sinus is more common when the ostium is narrow than when it is wide. The ostium of the sphenoidal sinus most often lies in the superior quadrant, a few millimeters from the cribriform plate (Peele, 1957). More rarely it lies close to the floor of the sinus, or opens into a posterior ethmoidal cell. Onodi (1893, 1895, 1901, 1903) described one case in which the ostium lay in the posterior segment of the semilunar hiatus. Tunis (1912) described one ostium opening into a bony canal running between the posterior segment of the ethmoid bone and the sphenoidal bone. Van Gilse (1922, 1924, 1925) recorded ducts of the sphenoidal sinus in the root of the pterygoid process, and vary rarely in the orbital process of the palatine bone. The ostium lies 4.8 (0.6–9.0) mm from the midline (Lang et al., in press) (Figs. **124–128**).

Size of the Sphenoidal Sinus

(Fig. **124**)

The sphenoidal sinus of adult elderly subjects was 13.5 (5–20.5) mm wide in its superior segment, 16.9 (8.5–24) mm in the center and 18.7 (6.5–26.5) mm in its lower segment. The sphenoid was 19.4 (6.5–32) mm long in its upper part, 4.8 (9–36) mm long in the center and 18.5 (7–31) mm long in the lower part. Small sphenoidal sinuses were termed conchal, and medium-sized sellar, in type. Hammer and Radberg (1961) found conchal sphenoidal sinuses in 2.5% of cases; the posterior border of the sinus lay between the sphenoidal concha and the body of the sphenoidal bone. They found presellar types in 11%, sellar types in 59% and mixed types in 27%. Elwany et al. (1983) found presellar sphenoidal sinuses in 27% of male and in 31% of female specimens. Postsellar sphenoidal sinuses were found in 73% of men and 79% of women. The transverse diameter of presellar sinuses was 12 (7–14) mm, that of postsellar 19 (14–24) mm. In the sellar type, in the material described by Fujii et al. (1979), the anterior wall of the pituitary fossa was 0.4 (0.1–0.7) mm thick. In 6 of the presellar type of sphenoidal sinus investigated by these authors, the anterior wall of the sella was 0.7 mm thick. Dixon (1937) measured the length of the sphenoidal sinus parallel to the roof on 1600 skulls, findings values between 20 and 23.2 mm. The vertical height between the floor and roof measured 16.4–20.4 mm, and the greatest width lay between 15.3 and 17.1 mm in men. The dimensions in women were somewhat less. Schaeffer (1912) estimated the mean volume of the sphenoid sinus as 7.4 cm^3, whereas Dixon gave values between 0 and 14 cm^3.

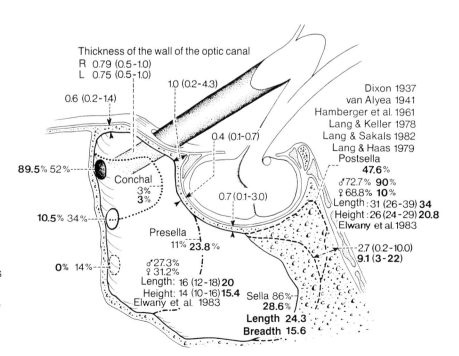

Fig. **124** Height of the ostium of the sphenoidal sinus, shape of the sphenoidal sinus, thickness of the neighboring bone (Fujii et al., 1979). Types of sphenoidal sinus according to various authors (Dixon, 1937; van Alyea, 1941; Hamberger et al., 1961; Lang and Keller, 1978; Lang and Haas, 1979; Lang and Sakals, 1982; Elwany et al., 1983; Lang et al., 1988 [thick numbers])

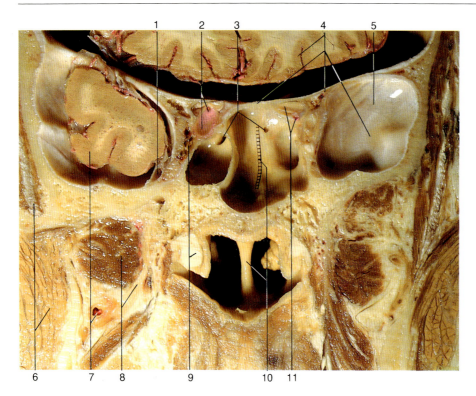

Fig. **125**   Differences in the ostia of the sphenoidal sinus between the two sides. Frontal section 8 mm behind the anterior wall of the sphenoidal sinus, showing a view from behind

1 Superficial middle cerebral vein draining into the cavernous sinus
2 Anterior genu of the internal carotid artery, and origin of the ophthalmic artery
3 Ostia of the sphenoidal sinus. The difference between the two sides, and the septum lying on the left side should be noted in particular
4 Frontal lobe of the brain, sphenoidal plane, lesser wing of the sphenoid bone and depression for the temporal pole
5 Inferior edge of the superior orbital fissure
6 Temporal muscle and parotid gland
7 Temporal lobe and maxillary artery
8 Lateral pterygoid muscle and mandibular nerve
9 Anterior segment of the cavernous sinus and tubal cartilage
10 Millimeter strip on the anterior wall of the sphenoidal sinus, and medial wall of the choana
11 Optic nerve and ophthalmic artery at the entrance to the canal

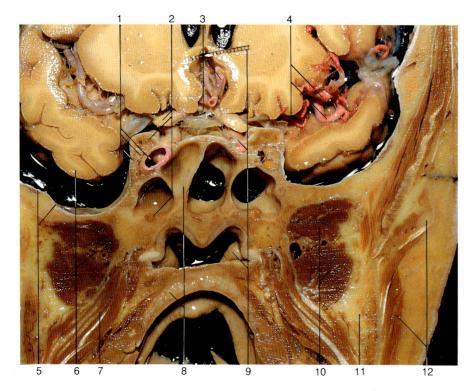

Fig. **126**   Variations of the septa of the sphenoidal sinus: frontal section viewed from in front.

1 Lateral wall of the cavernous sinus, anterior genu of the internal carotid artery and oculomotor nerve
2 Anterior clinoid process, optic nerve and pterygoid canal
3 Optic chiasma and pericallosal part of the left anterior cerebral artery distal to the anterior communicating artery
4 Vallecula and branches of the middle cerebral artery
5 Frontal ramus of the middle meningeal artery and floor of the middle cranial fossa
6 Lateral pterygoid muscle and pole of the temporal lobe elevated
7 Medial pterygoid muscle
8 Soft palate and vertical septum in the sphenoid sinus
9 Millimeter strip, internal carotid artery leaving the cavernous sinus, and torus tubalis
10 Lateral pterygoid muscle, infratemporal and pterygoid heads
11 Mandible
12 Zygomatic arch and masseter muscle

Fig. **127** Relation of the central part of the ostium of the sphenoid sinus to the median sagittal plane, and width of the sphenoidal sinus 4 mm posteriorly in the plane of the ostium. The structures are drawn in a transverse section seen from below. On the right hand side the roof of the sphenoidal sinus has been removed revealing the optic nerve, the internal carotid artery and the position of the anterior lobe of the pituitary gland. Sex differences are also given (Lang et al., 1988)

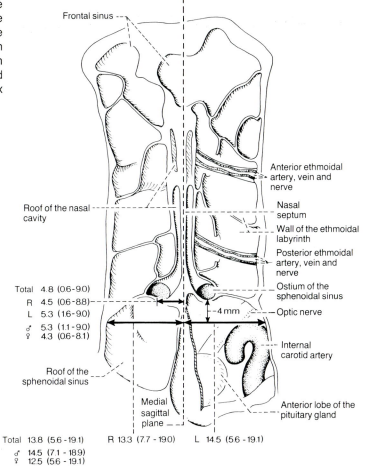

Frontal sinus

Anterior ethmoidal artery, vein and nerve

Roof of the nasal cavity

Nasal septum

Wall of the ethmoidal labyrinth

Posterior ethmoidal artery, vein and nerve

Ostium of the sphenoidal sinus

Optic nerve

Internal carotid artery

Anterior lobe of the pituitary gland

Total 4.8 (0.6–9.0)
R 4.5 (0.6–8.8)
L 5.3 (1.6–9.0)
♂ 5.3 (1.1–9.0)
♀ 4.3 (0.6–8.1)

Roof of the sphenoidal sinus

Medial sagittal plane

Total 13.8 (5.6 – 19.1)   R 13.3 (7.7 – 19.0)   L 14.5 (5.6 – 19.1)
♂ 14.5 (7.1 – 18.9)
♀ 12.5 (5.6 – 19.1)

Fig. **128** Transverse section through the roof of the nose seen from below
1 Anterior and posterior ethmoidal arteries
2 Trochlea, superior oblique muscle and sclera
3 Orbital fat removed
4 Frontozygomatic suture and temporalis muscle
5 Lateral rectus muscle and temporal lobe
6 Section through the optic nerve, and ophthalmic artery
7 Section through the frontal sinus, and roof of the labyrinthine paries; millimeter strip
8 Sphenoidal sinus, roof and ostium
9 Roof of the nasal cavity, and septum
10 Optic nerve, anterior lobe of the pituitary gland and internal carotid artery exposed

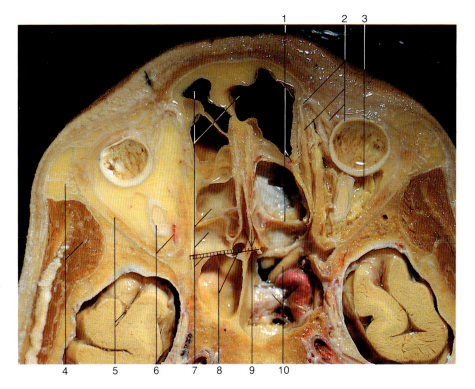

Septum of the Sphenoidal Sinus
(Figs. **125–128**)

The septum of the sphenoidal sinus often deviates from the midline. It may be oblique or transverse, as described many years ago by Morgagni (1682–1771), and is vertical in only 25% of cases (Hammer and Radberg, 1961). Accessory septa, arising from synchondroses of the sphenoid, are often found within the sinus. The septum of the sphenoidal sinus lies in the midline in 27% of cases. In 43% of cases only the anterior part lies in the midline, whereas in the rest the septum is S-shaped, C-shaped or has other shapes. Accessory septa are found in 76% of cases, of which 48% are unilateral and 28% bilateral (Elwany et al., 1983).

Accessory Septa and Lateral Craniopharyngeal Canal

Toldt (1883) was the first to point out that accessory, oblique and transverse septa in the sphenoid sinus occur most often in the area of the former synchondroses of the sphenoid bone. Cope (1917) investigated 300 sphenoid sinuses, and Congdon (1920) 212 specimens, looking for these additional septa (Fig. **129**). A large number of the septa were found in the area of the former synchondroses and of the lateral craniopharyngeal canal. The latter canal was first described by Sternberg (1890): it runs from the posteroinferior root of the lesser sphenoid wing, between the inner and outer surfaces of the skull base. The canal is a remnant lying between the ossification centers of the three synchondroses of the sphenoid bone. The canal runs within the synchondroses (Congdon, 1920) which only disappear completely in the thirteenth year of life (Koelliker, 1879; Toldt, 1882). The walls of the canal are formed of a thin layer of compact bone, and lie in the region of the anterior transverse septum. Usually the canal is curved, convex anteriorly. The lower part of the canal is often visible from the sphenoid sinus. A septum in the plane between the presphenoid and the basi-sphenoid usually lies transversely, but is occasionally also longitudinal. It lies below the tuberculum sellae and extends as far as the anterior third of the pituitary fossa. Congdon (1920) demonstrated septa or grooves in this area in about 30% of specimens, most often in the roof of the sphenoid sinus. Cope (1917) found these septa in 20% of cases.

Onodi Cells (Posterosuperior Ethmoidal Cells Lying Within the Sphenoid Bone)

Developmental origin (Figs. **130, 131**): An anterior and a posterior ossification center can be recognized in the midline of the head of an eight-month-old fetus. These chondral ossification centers are destined to form the sphenoid bone. Parts of the sphenoidal conchae on each side arise in the fifth fetal month from the perichondrium of the still thick nasal septum, a little above the anlage of the vomer. In the seventh to eighth fetal month desmal ossification centers arise close by; they unite in the perinatal period with the ossification centers arising within the cartilage (Told, 1882).

Other connective tissue ossification centers lying close to the inferior wall of the developing sphenoid cavity take part in the formation of the sphenoidal conchae during the perinatal period. The triangular, approximately sagittal, bony plates (concha) lie on each side of the primary rostrum. Normally the concha grows during the first year of life, increasing more in height than in breadth, remaining independent until the fourth and occasionally the sixth year of life. Subsphenoidal ossicles are also present (Zuckerkandl, 1896). At birth the mucosal bud of the sphenoidal cavity is bounded above, behind and laterally by cartilage. The upper part of the wall of the sphenoid sinus ossifies during the first year of life followed by the posterior. A

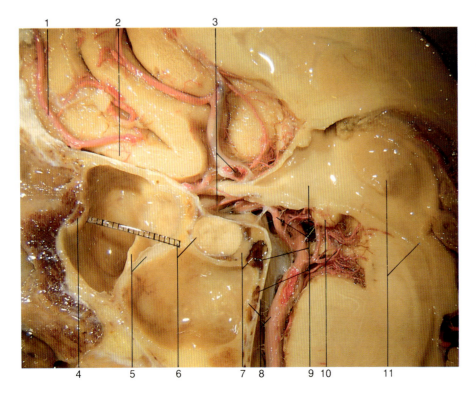

Fig. **129** Median sagittal section through the sphenoidal sinus with additional septa, and surrounding area. The sphenoidal sinus is very large
1 Frontopolar ramus of the anterior cerebral artery
2 Gyrus rectus
3 Internal carotid and anterior cerebral arteries
4 Millimeter strip in the ostium of the sphenoid sinus
5 Oblique septa
6 18-mm-long millimeter strip extending to the end of the posterior oblique septum, and the pituitary gland
7 Neurohypophysis and rarefaction of the dorsum sellae
8 Thin posterior wall of the sphenoidal sinus, dura mater and basilar artery
9 Third ventricle, posterior communicating artery and basilar venous plexus
10 Mamillary body and interpeduncular rami
11 Interthalamic adhesion and cerebral aqueduct

small part of the lateral wall of the sphenoidal sinus can be formed by a part of the perpendicular plate of the palatine bone. The lateral wall of the sphenoidal concha is often supplemented by the orbital process of the palatine bone or by a sutural bone.

In one six-year-old boy the sphenoid cavity was 11 mm long, 10 mm wide and 6 mm high (Toldt, 1882). At this age only the anterior and medial segments of the wall are formed by the sphenoidal concha. The ethmoid bone projects anterolaterally, so that the aperture of the

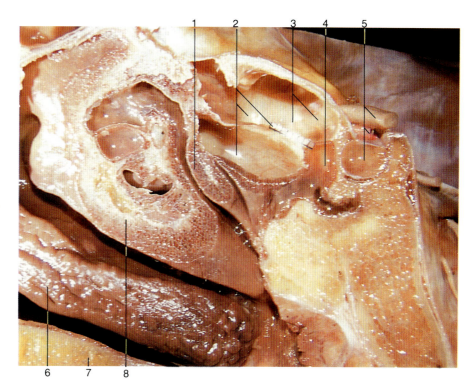

Fig. **130** Onodi's cell in a paramedian sagittal section seen from the medial surface
1 Superior nasal concha
2 Two Onodi cells with a millimeter strip
3 Medial wall of the optic canal
4 Sphenoidal sinus; the ostium is shown in section anteriorly
5 Optic nerve, internal carotid artery and pituitary gland
6 Inferior nasal concha
7 Hard palate
8 Middle nasal concha with a conchal sinus

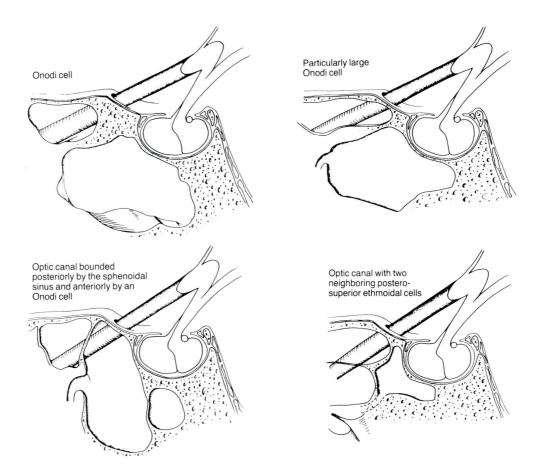

Onodi cell

Particularly large Onodi cell

Optic canal bounded posteriorly by the sphenoidal sinus and anteriorly by an Onodi cell

Optic canal with two neighboring postero-superior ethmoidal cells

Fig. **131** Various types of Onodi (Grünwald) cells, which occur in 11.7% of our material. We describe only those cells as Onodi cells which surround the medial optic canal both above and below (after Lang, 1988)

sphenoidal sinus is displaced medially. The concha fuses with the ethmoid bone at the age of four. The sphenoidal conchae fuse partially or completely with the body of the sphenoid bone in the second year of life, inhibiting the growth of the conchae, particularly in their transverse and vertical diameter. The sphenoidal sinus then develops solely in the lower half of the body of the sphenoid bone, whereas the upper part of the body of the sphenoid bone unites with the ethmoidal labyrinth. In these cases posterosuperior ethmoidal cells can grow into the body of the sphenoid bone. Pit-like recesses appear over the actual sphenoidal sinuses, succeeded by two superimposed cavities with an intervening horizontal septum. The lower cavity represents the sphenoidal sinus proper. Ethmoidal cells had migrated in 9–12% of the material described by ourselves, and of that by von Alyea (1939) (see also Figs. **130–131**, and **177**). These cells demonstrated varying degrees of development; they surrounded the optic canal and reached the anterior wall of the sella turcica. Von Alyea found a similar cell which had completely overgrown a small sphenoidal sinus, and ended a little behind it. The upper wall of the optic canal is surrounded by ethmoidal cells in 25% of cases (Habal et al., 1976). In our material the bone lying between these posterior and postremal ethmoidal cells as well as that between the Onodi cells and the optic canal was 0.8 (0.5–1.5) mm thick on the right side, and 1 (0.5–1.5) mm on the left (Lang and Haas, 1979).

Rudimentary Development of the Sphenoidal Sinus

The sphenoidal sinus is absent in 1–1.5% of cases (Gruenwald, 1925; Wertheim, 1901). Small, lateral sphenoidal sinuses can be easily overlooked (Stupka, 1938). In our material, too, a very thick sinus septum had to be removed when the sphenoidal sinus was small (Lang and Kley, 1981). Peele (1957) described a particularly small sphenoidal sinus, complete agenesis of the sphenoidal sinus, and differences between the two sides.

Recesses of the Sphenoidal Sinus
(Figs. **132, 133**)

Septal recess – sphenovomerine bulla: If the sphenoidal sinus grows inferolaterally the rostrum of the sphenoid bone is completely pneumatized and projects downwards between the alae of the vomer into the nasal septum.

Ethmoidal recess: The sphenoidal sinus rarely extends into the posterior part of the ethmoid bone, most commonly extending into its posteroinferior angle (Peele, 1957). Extensions into the ethmoidal bulla, the orbit, the maxilla and the supraorbital region have also been described.

Superior and inferior lateral recess: A diverticulum of the sphenoidal sinus can encompass the optic canal laterally and above as far as the lesser sphenoid wing. The sphenoi-

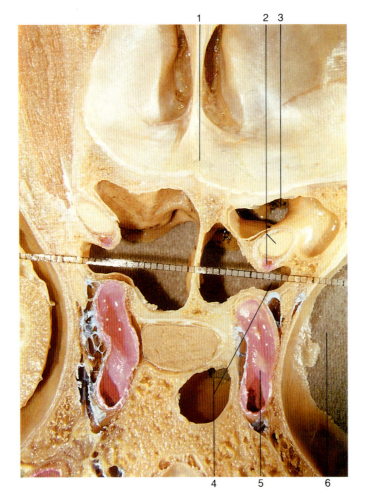

Fig. **132** Optic canal, sphenoidal sinus and pituitary region in an orbitomeatal plane from above
1 Sphenoidal plane
2 Optic nerve and ophthalmic artery
3 Posterosuperior ethmoidal cell embracing the optic canal above
4 Right sphenoidal sinus embracing the optic canal from the medial side and below
5 Internal carotid artery
6 Middle cranial fossa

dal sinus can also extend laterally, below the optic canal (Lang, 1981).

Palatine recess: The orbital process of the palatine bone may be pneumatized not only from the maxillary sinus but also from the sphenoidal sinus. Posterior ethmoidal cells, too, extended into the orbital process of the palatine bone in our material. According to Cope (1917) the recess of the sphenoidal sinus (termed by him the anterior recess) abuts on cells of the orbital process of the palatine bone, but never communicates with them. In his material an anterior recess was found in 5%, contacting the posterosuperior wall of the maxillary sinus in 2–3% of cases. Figs. **134** and **138** illustrate the relation of the pterygoid canal to the sphenoidal sinus and its floor, as well as dehiscences of the latter.

Inferolateral recess: The lower part of the sphenoidal sinus can extend laterally into the orbital face of the greater wing of the sphenoid, and pneumatize the posterolateral segment of the orbital wall. Rarely the sphenoidal sinus reaches the foramina rotundum and ovale. Peele described a sphenoidal sinus extending as far as the mandibular nerve, the trigeminal ganglion and the apex of the petrous bone. We also found this type of sinus in our material. Peele described a sphenoidal sinus whose lateral recess extended into the greater wing of the sphenoid bone.

Pterygoid recess: A sphenoidal sinus which has developed inferiorly and laterally quite often extends into the pterygoid process. The sinus can then reach the Eustachian tube (Mayer, 1841; Sluder, 1916).

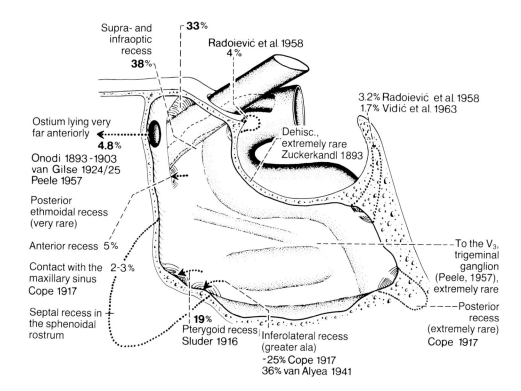

Fig. **133** Sphenoidal sinus and recess. The incidence of occurrence of the recess in our material is given in thick type, and of that of other workers in thin type. Zuckerkandl (1893) reported very unusual dehiscences of the floor of the sella (Lang et al., 1988)

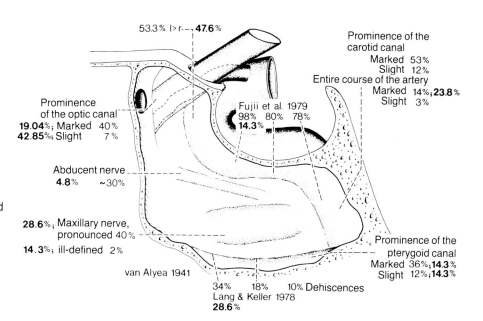

Fig. **134** Prominences in the lateral wall and the floor of the sphenoidal sinus. The data from our own material and from that of previous workers are given in thin type, and the percentages found in our more recent material in thick type (van Alyea, 1941; Land and Tisch-Rottensteiner, 1977; Lang and Keller, 1978; Fujii et al., 1979; Lang et al., 1988)

Posterior and posterosuperior recess: Very rarely does the sphenoidal sinus extend so far backwards and downwards into the occipital part of the clivus that it ends at the basion. We did not find an example of this in our material.

The posterior clinoid process is often pneumatized by upper and lower recesses from the sphenoidal sinus. Peele (1957) described the relation of the lateral wall of the sphenoidal sinus to the internal carotid artery and the neighboring nerves, as well as dehiscences related to these structures and in the floor of the sella turcica. In one case the superior wall of the sphenoidal sinus was completely absent in the region of the sella turcica (Zuckerkandl, 1893). Lang (1981, 1983) described prominences in the lateral wall of the cavernous sinus.

Median craniopharyngeal canal: Klinkosch (1764) reported an open craniopharyngeal canal in a 4-year-old girl, Suchannek (1887) observed an open canal extending through the nasopharynx to the dura of the sella turcica: the sac contained an ectopic pituitary gland. Wilson and Gehweiler (1970) described a midline facial teratoma connecting with Rathke's pouch in a 3-week-old girl. The canal contained meninges and remnants of the pituitary gland.

Prominences within the Sphenoidal Sinus caused by the Internal Carotid Artery and the Cranial Nerves

(Figs. **134–136**)

Adjacent structures project into the sinus, particularly if it is unusually long and wide (van Alyea, 1941; Lang and Tisch-Rottensteiner, 1977; Lang and Keller, 1978; Fujii et

al., 1979). Fig. **134** shows how often these prominences were observed by the above authors. Dehiscences, for example in the course of the internal carotid artery, were never found in our material, although they have occasionally been described by others (Fujii et al., 1979). It is of no practical significance whether a bony lamina less than 0.1 mm thick is present or whether it is completely absent. The surgical significance of these prominences lies in the vulnerability of the neighboring structures.

Pterygoid Canal

(Figs. **137–139**)

In our material (Lang and Keller, 1977) the pterygoid canal ran below the level of the floor of the sphenoidal sinus in 38% of cases, at the same level in 34% and within the sphenoidal sinus in 18%. The bony roof of the canal was dehiscent in 10%. The pterygoid canal was 16.2 (11.5–23) mm long. In 44% of cases it ran directly anteriorly and medially, in 52% it demonstrated lateral kinks in the center, and in 24% of cases it ran in a paramedian sagittal plane, particularly when the sphenoidal sinus was large. The posterior opening of the canal lay 15.3 (12.4–19.2) mm from the midline and the anterior opening 12.3 (5.5–17.5) mm from this point.

Spreading Inflammation of the Sphenoidal Sinus

Inflammation of the mucosa of the sphenoidal sinus was first described by Lieutaud in 1735 (Teed, 1938). A literature search shows that the sphenoidal sinus is implicated in

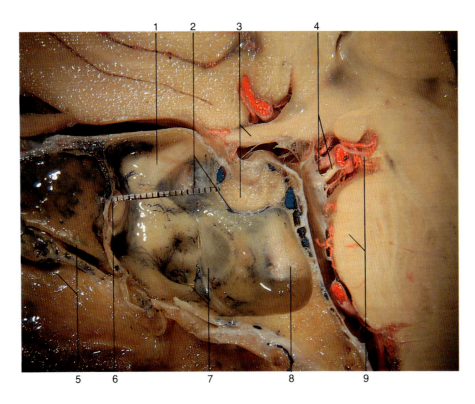

Fig. **135** Sphenoidal sinus showing prominences in the lateral wall
1 Prominence of the optic canal
2 Anterior carotid prominence and floor of the pituitary fossa
3 Intracranial course of the optic nerve and the anterior lobe of the pituitary gland
4 Liliequist's membrane and the oculomotor nerve
5 Posterior process of the uncinate process, and superior nasal concha
6 Millimeter strip in the ostium of the sphenoidal sinus
7 Prominence of the pterygoid canal, and an oblique septum
8 Posterior carotid prominence
9 Interpeduncular fossa and pons

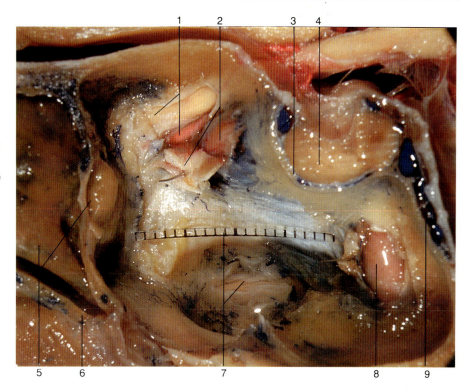

Fig. **136** Structures in the lateral wall of the sphenoidal sinus (dissected)
1 Optic nerve and ophthalmic artery exposed
2 Dural-periosteal layer of the optic canal retracted inferiorly, and anterior genu of the internal carotid artery
3 Anterior intercavernous sinus in the floor of the pituitary fossa
4 Anterior lobe of the pituitary gland
5 Superior nasal concha and ostium of the sphenoidal sinus
6 Cut edge of the middle nasal concha
7 Millimeter strip indicating the course of the abducens nerve, and the maxillary nerve exposed
8 Internal carotid artery, and posterior segment of the sinus
9 Basilar venous plexus

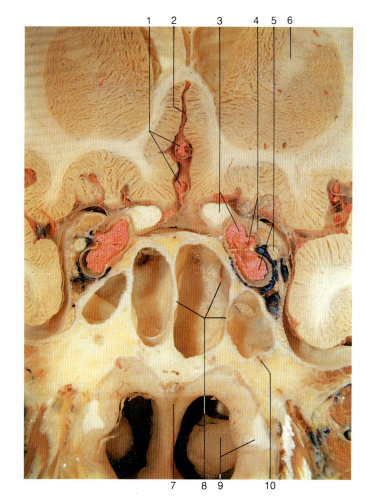

Fig. **137** Frontal section through the sphenoidal sinus, the anterior segment of the cavernous sinus, and the pterygoid canal
1 Anterior cerebral arteries
2 Interhemispheric fissure
3 Subarachnoidal part of the optic nerve and internal carotid artery
4 Origin of the ophthalmic artery, and the anterior clinoid process
5 Anterior cavernous curvature and oculomotor nerve
6 Internal capsule
7 Nasal septum seen from behind
8 Septum of the sphenoidal sinus and accessory septum
9 Inferior nasal concha and tubal cartilage
10 Pterygoid canal

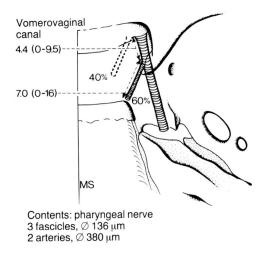

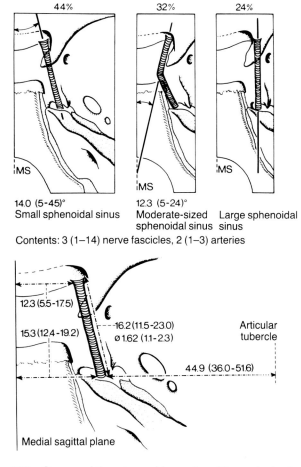

Contents: 3 (1–14) nerve fascicles, 2 (1–3) arteries

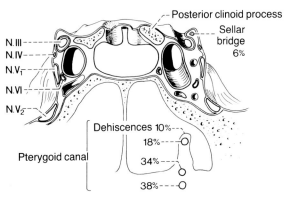

Fig. **138** Opening of the pterygoid and vomerovaginal canals. In our material the pharyngeal nerve usually consisted of three fascicles and was accompanied by two arteries. The lower view shows the prominences of the pterygoid canal and the dehiscences in its superior wall (Lang and Keller, 1978)

Fig. **139** Course of the pterygoid canal and its contents, length and diameter of the pterygoid canal and the distance from the anterior and posterior foramina to the median sagittal plane and to the articular tubercle (Lang and Keller, 1978)

16% of all cases of sinusitis, proceeding to meningitis in about 13% of these cases. Extradural abscesses, cerebral and occasionally cerebellar abscesses are also described. Sphenoidal sinusitis is often combined with otitis media. The inflammation can also extend to the cavernous sinus (causing sinus thrombosis), to the superior sagittal sinus and to the internal carotid artery.

Mucoceles and Trauma, Headaches and Other Sequelae

Mucoceles: A mucocele of the sphenoidal sinus was first described by John Berg in 1889: until 1971 only 69 mucoceles had been reported (Blum and Larson, 1973). The latter authors described a 24-year-old man who suddenly went blind in the right eye; he had suffered occipital headache for 5 days, right-sided photophobia, proptosis and subjective diplopia for 1 day. In previous cases the symptoms always extended over very long periods of time, as much as 20 years (Lundgrin and Olin, 1961). The pain of disease of the sphenoidal sinus also radiates within the skull to the occipital region; frontal and retro-orbital pain is also frequent. The optic, oculomotor and trigeminal nerves also may be compromised by extension of a mucocele or a pneumosinus dilatans anteriorly and laterally. Lesions of

the orbit, the cavernous sinus and the upper cranial nerves still occur, despite the introduction of antibiotics (Dale and Mackenzie, 1983). Mucoceles may be caused by trauma or tumors blocking the drainage of the sinus: the accumulation of mucus thins and erodes the bony walls of the sinus.

Pyoceles: Suppuration of the contents of a mucocele is termed a pyocele. Partial or complete obstruction of the ostium of a sinus by an osteoma is rare. Cystic dilatation of one or more mucous glands can close the ostium (Benjamins, 1910). We have not seen a specimen with an absent ostium, but primary constriction or absence of the ostium of the sphenoidal sinus, or a deviation of the nasal septum, can contribute to the development of a mucocele or pyocele (van der Hoeve, 1920). The latter author also described atrophy of the optic nerve due to a mucocele of the sphenoidal sinus and the posterior ethmoidal cells. The optic nerve or the chiasma could also be damaged by pressure from a mucocele leading to loss of vision or acute blindness.

The cavernous segment of the internal carotid artery can be displaced laterally, causing temporary or permanent damage to the optic nerve; this condition may be confused with a pituitary adenoma or an aneurysm. Mucoceles or pyoceles of the sphenoidal sinus or posterior ethmoidal

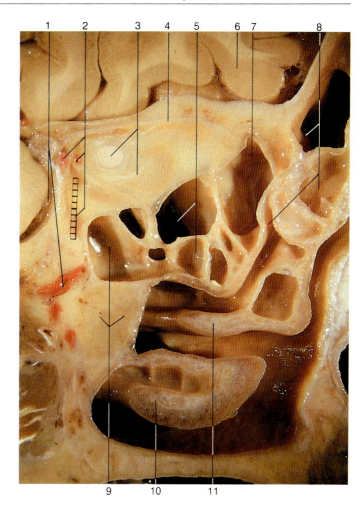

Fig. **140** Section from anteromedial to posterolateral through the ethmoidal labyrinth seen from the lateral side
1 Temporal pole and pterygopalatine part of the maxillary artery
2 Middle meningeal artery and the ophthalmic artery, orbitalis muscle and a millimeter strip
3 Optic nerve and medial rectus muscle with the muscular ramus
4 Superior oblique muscle and trochlear nerve
5 Ethmoidal cells
6 Orbital part of the frontal lobe
7 Anterior ethmoidal cell and roof of the orbit
8 Frontal sinus and nasal cell
9 Posterosuperior ethmoidal cell abutting on the sphenoidal sinus, and the medial segment of the wall of the maxillary sinus
10 Inferior nasal concha
11 Middle nasal concha

cells can cause the same effects at the orbital apex, often leading to exophthalmos due to strangulation of the ophthalmic vein (Lundgrin and Olin, 1961). They can also affect the sense of smell. Lateral displacement of the pituitary gland by a mucocele has been described. In 8 of 10 cases of paralysis of the oculomotor nerve by mucoceles, the reaction of the pupil to light was unchanged. The possible explanation is that the pupillary fibers run in the superior periphery of the oculomotor nerve, so that a lesion of these fibers is more probably due to increased intracranial pressure than to an extracranial lesion (Sunderland and Hughes, 1946). Lesions of the third cranial nerve due to mucoceles may be caused by strangulation of the vasa nervorum (Friedmann and Harrison, 1970).

Intra- and extracranial extension of mucoceles: Diaz et al. (1978) reported an exceedingly large mucocele with intra- and extra-cranial extension, but were unable to confirm its exact origin. An 11-year-old patient demonstrated an intra-orbital lesion 4 cm in size, and a lesion in the ptery-gopalatine fossa 6 cm in size. They also observed a calcified mass in the right olfactory fossa of a 15-year-old girl extending beyond the lesser wing of the sphenoid. An osteoma also lay deep within the ethmoidal labyrinth. Both children were operated on in two stages.

Large mucoceles may be drained into the nasal cavity by ethmoidal, transmaxillary, transseptal, or intranasal approaches (Fig. **140**).

A 15-year-old boy with a mucocele of a large sphenoidal sinus suffered occlusion of both internal carotid arteries 3 years after the first onset of symptoms which include a disorder of vision. The right internal carotid artery was completely occluded 2 cm above the bifurcation, whereas the left was narrowed and stretched over a round mass in the suprasellar region. The vertebrobasilar system appeared to be dilated, and irrigated the anterior part of the cerebral arterial circle (of Willis) including the anterior cerebral arteries (Doyle and Simeone, 1972).

Fractures of the Sphenoid Bone

A bleeding aneurysm within the sphenoidal sinus is common after fracture (Denecke and Hartert, 1954; Schloss-hauer and Vosteen, 1954). These authors injected thrombin into the aneurysmal sac, and also packed it with muscle. Blood can track through the ostium of the sphenoidal sinus or through a tear in its inferior wall into the pharynx. Drake (1965) recommended surgery. The optic nerve, followed by the third cranial nerve, the olfactory tract and then the fifth and sixth cranial nerves are those most often injured by this type of trauma. Petersen et al. (1981) reported a caroticocavernous fistula after an external sphenoethmoidectomy for purulent sinusitis in a 57-year-old woman. The capsular arteries to the floor of the pituitary fossa, as well as numerous branches to the dura mater arise from the caroticocavernous trunk. Trauma can tear these structures leading to bleeding or caroticocavernous fistula.

Cerebrospinal Leak

A CSF leak through the sphenoidal sinus is due to frontal trauma in 68% of cases (Robinson et al., 1967); the prognosis is poor. Occasional CSF rhinorrhea has been reported after hypophysectomy via the frontal approach (Campbell et al., 1966; Gutsche, 1895; Friedmann, 1932).

Chordomas and chondromas also occasionally develop in the sphenoid sinus.

Bleeding during Operations on the Sphenoidal Sinuses

(Fig. **141**)

Forschner (1950) reported that bleeding from the nasopalatine artery (which we term the posterior septal rami) and adjacent vessels can occur during exposure of the sphenoid bone. He preferred the term artery of the sphenopalatine recess for this vessel. Damage to this vessel is the cause of late hemorrhage after surgery.

Meningoceles and Encepheloceles

Virchow (1863) was the first to describe an encephalocele: it presented in the pharynx of a neonate (Danoff et al., 1966). In 1882 Heinecke distinguished three types of basal encephelocele:

1) *Sphenopharyngeal,* projecting between the ethmoidal and sphenoidal bones or through a cleft between these two structures into the nasal cavity or into the nasopharynx.
2) *Speno-orbital,* passing through the superior orbital fissure into the orbit.
3) *Sphenomaxillary,* projecting through the superior and inferior orbital fissures into the pterygopalatine fossa.

Fenger (1895) stated that these celes arise solely in nonviable monsters, but 13 years later he reported a successful intranasal operation in a 29-year-old man. Of 546 children with meningoceles and 84 with encephelocele only 6 had an intranasal cerebral mass. One had a defect of the cribriform plate (Ingraham and Mattson, 1943).

Transphenoidal encepheloceles: These rare types of encephalocele are due to a congenital malformation (Gisselsson, 1947). Defects during closure of the neural tube, a temporary rise of the intraventricular pressure during embryonal development, developmental anomalies arising during the ossification of the sphenoidal sinus or persistence of the craniopharyngeal canal may all be important causes (Pollock and Newton, 1971). Meningoceles may be found in the sphenoidal sinus. A 40-year-old woman demonstrated a thin-walled mucocele 5×1 cm in size; it had penetrated through a dehiscence of the lateral wall of the sphenoidal sinus, causing CSF rhinorrhea (McCoy, 1963). Absence of the corpus callosum is also occasionally found in encephelocoeles (Manelfe et al. 1978). Hypertelorism, marked widening of the temporal region of the skull and an abnormally broad nasal root may also be found in transsphenoidal encepheloceles (Pollock et al., 1968; Pollock and Newton, 1971).

A cystic mass may also be found in the superomedial part of the nasopharynx (Manelfe et al., 1978). Pressure on the jugular veins causes it to enlarge. Symptoms arising

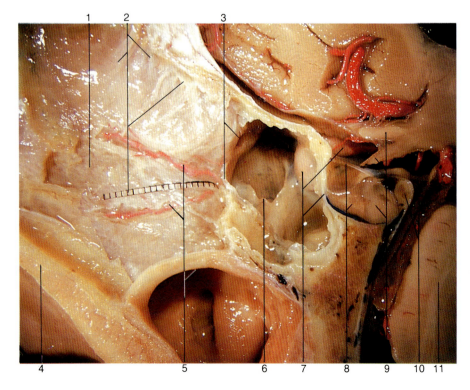

Fig. **141**   Posterior septal rami arising from the sphenopalatine artery on the right side. The view is from the left side, and the vomer has been removed
1 Mucoperiostium of the septal mucosa (the bony septum has been removed)
2 Olfactory filaments to the septal mucosa with a millimeter strip
3 Ostium of the sphenoidal sinus and the anterior wall of the sinus. The position relative to the septal rami should be noted
4 Hard palate and nasal crest of the maxilla
5 Posterior septal rami and choana, and mucosa of the medial wall
6 Partial oblique septum of the sphenoidal sinus
7 Anterior carotid prominence in the sphenoidal sinus, internal carotid artery and floor of the sella
8 Diaphragma sellae and anterior lobe of the pituitary gland
9 Optic chiasma, stalk and posterior lobe of the pituitary gland
10 Dorsum sellae and basilar artery
11 Pons

from the chiasma or the hypophalamus are also described, as is blindness due to herniation of the optic chiasma and adjacent parts of the hypopthalamus through the defect in the sphenoidal bone.

Surgical Access to the Sphenoidal Sinus

Transnasal access to the pituitary gland: In 1853 the outstanding anatomist Josef Hyrtl summarized the contemporary feeling when he stated that the sphenoidal sinus was entirely beyond the reach of surgery. Horsley was the first to describe 10 transfrontal and transtemporal excisions of the pituitary in 1906 (Schloffer, 1907). Schloffer himself carried out the first extracranial partial hypophysectomy on a 30-year-old man, for a tumor that had extended downwards into the sphenoidal cavity. After reflecting the nose to the right side, all the turbinates, the nasal septum, the orbital plate of the ethmoid bone, the medial wall of the maxillary sinus and part of the maxillary bone were excised. The method was attended by numerous complications, but was eventually reintroduced by Guiot in 1958 after many preliminary experiments. Hardy (1971) devoted great attention to this method of access. Further particulars and more recent developments are described by Lang (1985), Kageyama et al. (1985), Fukushima (1985), Fahlbusch and Buchfelder (1985) and Pia et al. (1985).

Position of the ostium of the sphenoidal sinus: The ostium of the sphenoidal sinus is first looked for on one side of the septum during transnasal (subperiostial-subperichondrial) access. Its blood supply is shown in Figs. **141** and **142**.

The distance between the *ostium of the sphenoidal sinus and the floor of the sella* (Fig. **143**) was given by Fujii (1979) as 17.1 (12–23) mm; in our material it was 14.6 (9–23) mm. The ostium lay 4.8 (0.6–9.0) mm from the

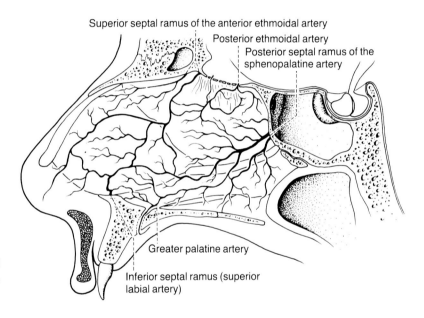

Fig. **142** Arterial supply of the nasal septum showing the commonest arrangement in our material (Lang, 1985)

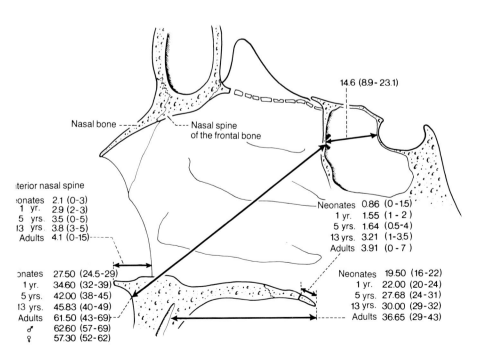

Fig. **143** Distance between the subnasale and the ostium of the sphenoidal sinus during the postnatal period and in adults. Sex differences in adults are also indicated (Krauss, 1986). The length of the anterior and posterior nasal spines and the distance between the ostium of the sphenoidal sinus and the anterior edge of the sella turcica are shown (Lang and Baumeister, 1982; Krauss, 1987)

midline. The distance was greater on the left side than on the right, and in men than in women. The distance between landmarks at the *piriform aperture* and the *ostium* of the sphenoidal sinus is important in trans-sphenoidal (transnasal) access to the pituitary gland. In our neonatal material the distance between the subspinale and the aperture of the sphenoidal sinus was 27.5 (24.5–29) mm. In the five-year-old it measured 42.0 (38–45) mm, in the 13-year-old 45.8 (40–49) mm, and in adults 61.5 (43–69) mm. (Lang and Baumeister, 1982; Krauss, 1987) (see Fig. **143**).

Transmaxillary access to the pituitary gland (see Fig. **140**): Jansen, in 1894, was the first to describe transmaxillary access to the sphenoidal sinus. Later Turnbull (1929) and Hamberger et al. (1961) gave a more accurate description of this approach. Hoyt et al. (1983) emphasized that the transeptal access can be difficult in the presence of congenital anomalies; they developed the transantral approach to the pituitary gland further. They did not destroy the nasal conchae, but dissected the ethmoidal bulla and the anterior ethmoidal cells lateral and parallel to the middle nasal concha. They divided the anterior wall of the sphenoidal sinus down to the floor, and removed its septum, exposing the posterior wall of the sinus. The posterior part of the inferior turbinate, the mucoperiosteum of the posterior part of the perpendicular plate and of the vomer together with the posterior septal rami of the sphenopalatine artery, were displaced medially and downwards. After resection of the posterior part of the perpendicular plate and the vomer, bleeding from the sphenopalatine artery and its branches was dealt with by cautery, and the floor of the sella was exposed. The angle of access measured 25° to the median sagittal plane. After the operation fat, muscle or fascia were placed into the sella, and the wound was drained.

Inferior Nasal Meatus (Anatomy of the Routes of Access)

Measurements

The height between the floor of the nasal cavity and the attachment of the inferior nasal concha is 19.5 (12–23) mm (Hajnis et al., 1967). We measured the breadth of the nasal cavity at the level of the inferior meatus, and the distance of the conchae from the floor of the nasal cavity (Figs. **69** and **70**) (Lang and Baumeister, 1982).

Ostium of the Nasolacrimal Duct

The anterior limb of the attachment of the inferior nasal concha to the lateral wall of the nasal cavity forms an angle of 30°–45° with the floor of the nasal cavity, whereas the posterior limb lies at an angle of 15°–30° (see Fig. **144**) (Lang and Sakals, 1981).

The *nasolacrimal duct* in the newborn is 7.5 mm long, and stands more vertically than in later life (Peter, 1938). According to Peter the opening into the inferior nasal meatus is present in the neonate, whereas Schaeffer considered that the duct only breaks through into the nasal cavity during or after maturation of the child. Exact data about the postnatal elongation of the canal, and its relation to the growth of the maxillary segment are not available (Peter, 1938). Gundobin (1921) distinguished two growth periods: the first between the age of seven months and three years during which the duct elongates from 8 to 12 mm, and a further period between the ages of twelve and fourteen years during which the canal increases in length from 14 to 20 mm. The axis of the canal in the newborn points to the anterior edge of the future first deciduous molar, in the seventh month of life it points more posteriorly, in the ninth month it points to the center of the tooth, and in the fourth year of life through its posterior edge. In the fifth and sixth year of life it points towards the anterior edge of the second deciduous molar, in the seventh year through its center, and after the age of fifteen through the posterior edge of the second premolar (Peter, 1938). Fig. **145** illustrates the axis of the canal in adults.

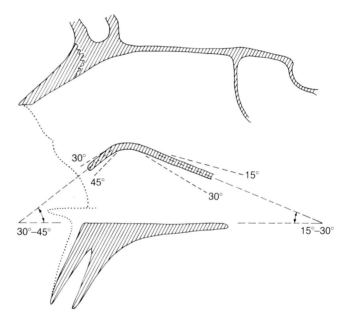

Fig. **144** Angle between the anterior and posterior insertion of the inferior nasal concha (Lang and Sakals, 1982)

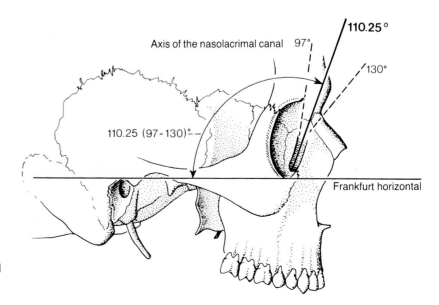

Fig. **145** Angle formed by the nasolacrimal canal with the Frankfurt horizontal

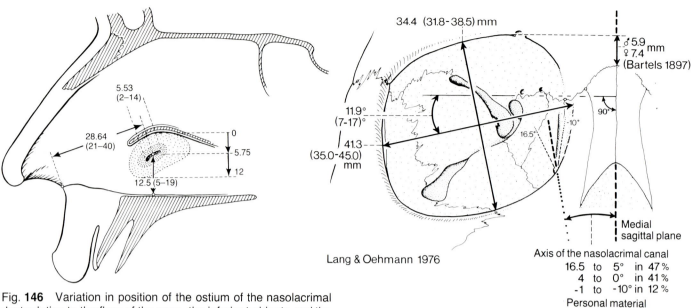

Lang & Oehmann 1976

Fig. **146** Variation in position of the ostium of the nasolacrimal duct relative to the floor of the nose, the inferior turbinate and the nares. The frequencies are indicated by varying shades of grey (Lang and Sakals, 1981)

Fig. **147** Angle formed by the nasolacrimal duct with the median sagittal plane (personal material). Measurements of the height and width of the orbit are adapted from Lang and Oehmann (1976), and of the distance between the nasion and the upper edge of the orbit in men and women from Bartels (1897)

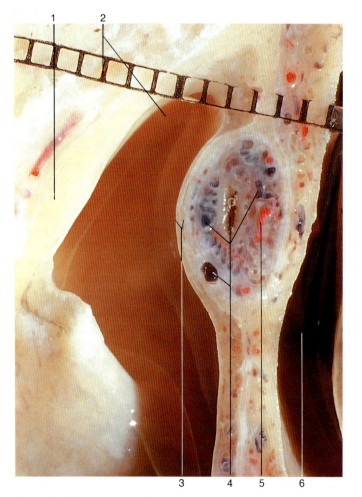

Fig. **148** Transverse section through the nasolacrimal duct from below.
1 Anterior wall of the maxillary sinus
2 Prelacrimal recess and millimeter strip
3 Mucosa and the nasolacrimal canal. The lateral wall is 0.1 millimeters thick
4 Nasolacrimal duct and venous plexus
5 Arteria comitans
6 Nasal cavity

The ostium of the nasolacrimal duct moves upwards on the lateral wall of the inferior meatus in the postnatal period, and is increasingly arched over by the inferior turbinate. In the fourth year of life the initially cleft-shaped opening has become a horizontal ellipse (Peter, 1938). The ostium in adults lies 22 to 25 mm behind the edge of the nares either close to the vault of the turbinate, or passing from there downwards about as far as the center of the inferior nasal meatus (Mihalkovics, 1896). In our material the ostium lay 5.8 (0–12) mm from the superior edge of the inferior nasal meatus (Fig. **146**). The distance to the anterior zone of attachment of the inferior nasal concha was 7.7 (0–14) mm, and to the floor of the nasal cavity 12.5 (5–19) mm. In our material of 95 half-heads the distance to the anterior nasal spine from the superior extent of the lateral ostium was 23.8 (11–47) mm, and from its inferior extent 21.83 (11–32) mm. The distance to the lateral wall of the piriform aperture was about 14 (9–30) mm, and that to the posterior edge of the nares was 31 (12.5–45.5) mm. The shortest distance in a straight line to the nares was 28.6 (21–40.5) mm (Lang and Sakals, 1982).

Nasolacrimal Canal and Angle with the Frontal Plane
(Fig. **147**)

In 47% of our cases the nasolacrimal canal ran from superolateral to inferomedial, at angles varying between 5° and 16.5°. 41% of the canals ran inferiorly, and 12% inferolaterally.

Nasolacrimal Duct

The maximal width of the nasolacrimal duct in its superior part was 2.6 (0.9–4.9) mm, and its greatest breadth 1.4 (0.6–3.4) mm (Lang and Papke, 1984). In this region, the canal possessed an anterioposterior length of 6.4 (4.1–10.1) mm, and a width of 4.9 (3.0–7.4) mm. A loose, highly vascular, connective tissue lay between the mucosa of the duct and the internal surface of the nasolacrimal canal, and these vessels have connections to the orbit and to the nasal cavity (Fig. **148**). Fig. **149** illustrates the course of the nasolacrimal duct from the medial side.

The distance between the nasal ostium of the nasolacrimal duct and the greater palatine canal is 32.3 (23–44) mm on the right side, and 36.4 (30–45) mm on the left side (Lang and Vaeth, 1989). Further details are shown in Figs. **150–152.**

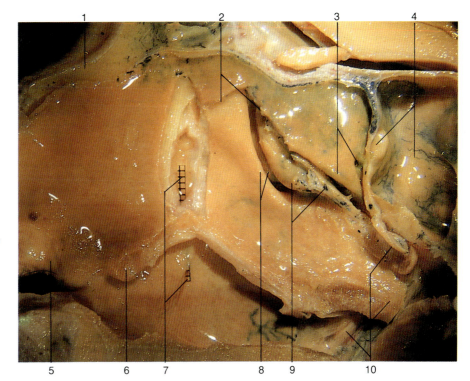

Fig. **149** Nasolacrimal duct opened, and displayed by a probe. The relation of the conchae to the pterygopalatine canal are also shown.
1 Nasal bone
2 Cut edge of the middle nasal concha, lateral wall of the nasofrontal duct
3 Superior nasal concha and sphenoethmoidal recess
4 Sphenoidal sinus and ostium
5 Limen nasi
6 Anterior part of the cut edge of the inferior nasal concha
7 Millimeter strip in the opened nasofrontal duct
8 Uncinate process and semilunar hiatus
9 Ethmoidal bulla and area of fusion with the middle concha
10 Posterior end of the middle and inferior nasal conchae, and the greater palatine nerve

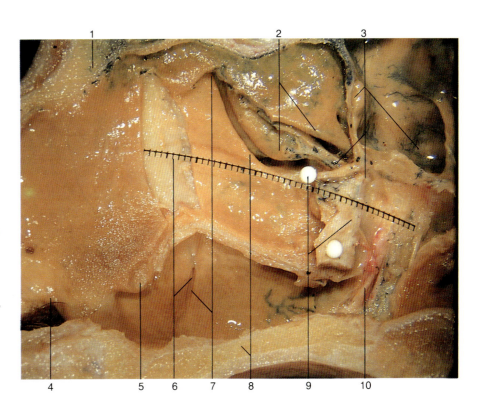

Fig. **150** Nasolacrimal and palatine canals
1 Nasal spine of the frontal bone
2 Ethmoidal bulla and superior nasal concha
3 Cut edge of the posterior attachment of the middle nasal concha, the sphenoidal sinus and its ostium
4 Nares
5 Section through the inferior nasal concha anteriorly
6 Central part of the nasolacrimal canal, millimeter strip and nasal ostium of the nasolacrimal duct
7 Section through the middle nasal concha, and lacrimal sulcus
8 Uncinate process and hard palate
9 Nasal mucosa retracted anteriorly and fixed with drawing pins
10 Greater palatine nerve with its canal opened

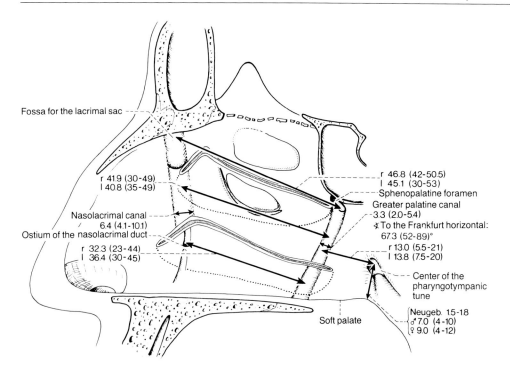

Fossa for the lacrimal sac

r 41.9 (30-49)
l 40.8 (35-49)

Nasolacrimal canal
6.4 (4.1-10.1)
Ostium of the nasolacrimal duct
r 32.3 (23-44)
l 36.4 (30-45)

r 46.8 (42-50.5)
l 45.1 (30-53)
Sphenopalatine foramen
Greater palatine canal
3.3 (2.0-5.4)
To the Frankfurt horizontal:
67.3 (52-89)°
r 13.0 (5.5-21)
l 13.8 (7.5-20)

Center of the
pharyngotympanic
tune

Soft palate

Neugeb. 1.5-1.8
♂ 7.0 (4-10)
♀ 9.0 (4-12)

Fig. **151**   Distances between the lacrimal ducts and the sphenopalatine foramen, the inferior part of the pterygopalatine fossa and the greater palatine canal. The distance between the pharyngeal ostium of the pharyngotympanic tube and the greater palatine canal and the superior surface of the soft palate are also given. The measurements were taken from Hassmann (1975), Lang and Sakals (1982), Lang and Papke (1985) and Vaeth (1989) and Haas (1987)

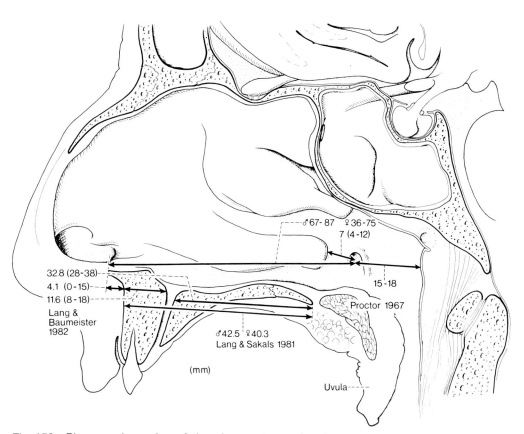

♂ 67- 87   ♀ 36-75
7 (4-12)

32.8 (28-38)
4.1 (0-15)
11.6 (8-18)

15-18

Lang &
Baumeister
1982

Proctor 1967

♂ 42.5 ♀ 40.3
Lang & Sakals 1981

(mm)

Uvula

Fig. **152**   Pharyngeal opening of the pharyngotympanic tube. Distances and dimensions in the hard palate

Choanae

Measurements

Alginate impressions showed that the mean height of the choanae was 10.9 mm in 3- to 6-year-olds, 13.6 mm in 7- to 9-year-olds, 15.9 mm in 14- to 16-year-olds and 17.5 mm in 20- to 25-year-olds. In our adult material the height of the bony choanae was 25.4 (21–33) mm. This value was clearly lower than those previously reported (Figs. **153, 154**).

The distance between the two tubal openings was 17.8 mm in 3- to 6-year-olds and 21 mm in 10-year-olds; the latter distance was also found in 56- to 90-year-old subjects. The distance between the tubal elevations was 16.2 mm in 3- to 6-year-olds, 18.2 mm in 10-year-olds, and 18.8 mm in 56- to 90-year-old subjects. The maximal width of the pharyngeal recess was 32.1 mm in 3- to 6-year-olds, 34.6 mm in 10-year-olds, and 33.9 mm in 56- to 90-year-old subjects (Hildmann et al., 1982).

The medial boundary of the choanae is formed by the posterior edge of the vomer, and its posteroinferior boundary by the horizontal plate of the palatine bone with the nasal crest of the palatine bone. Lateral to the ala of the vomer the choanae are bounded by the vaginal process of the pterygoid process above, and by the perpendicular plate of the palatine bone laterally. The posterior part of the medial pterygoid plate usually deviates laterally and thus does not form part of the boundary of the choanae. Fig. **153** shows the height and breadth of the choanae during postnatal development in our material (Lang and Baumeister, 1982).

Zuckerkandl (1893) gives far and away the greatest measurements for the choanae; Hopmann (1895) reported that in man the choana has a mean height of 27 mm, and a mean width of 13 mm (Merkel, 1896); in women it measures 25 × 12 mm. These values agree closely with our findings.

Since the soft tissues at the choanae are 2–3 mm thick (Luschka, 1867), the mean values during life are 24 × 11 mm for men, and 22 × 10 mm for women.

Choanal Asymmetry

The choana is not usually affected by deviations of the nasal septum. The difference in width between the choanae is not more than 3 mm (Zuckerkandl, 1893). The choanae are symmetrical in 84.3% of cases; they point obliquely to the right side in 1.2% of cases and to the left in 1.7%, in 4.7% the right choana is wider than the left, and in 8.1% the left is wider than the right (Stier, 1895).

Asymmetries arise most frequently if one pterygoid process inclines more horizontally in an inferolateral direc-

tion than the other. This is more frequent on the right side than the left (Bergeat, 1896).

Choanal Atresia

Choanal atresia was first described by Roederer in 1755, and was first operated on successfully by Emmert in 1851 (Jung, 1977). Luschka (1867) was the first to describe the anatomy of choanal atresia, in a girl who died immediately after birth. The bony membrane was formed by processes of the palatine bone on both sides, arising from the horizontal plate and running as thin compact laminae upwards and backwards towards the lower surface of the sphenoid

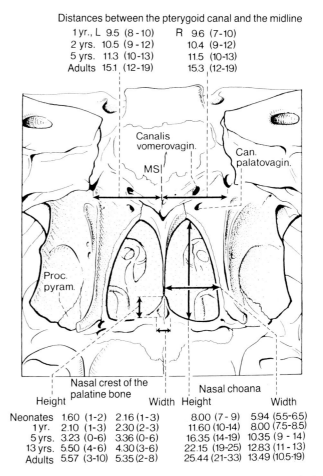

Distances between the pterygoid canal and the midline

1 yr., L	9.5 (8 - 10)	R 9.6 (7-10)
2 yrs.	10.5 (9 - 12)	10.4 (9-12)
5 yrs.	11.3 (10-13)	11.5 (10-13)
Adults	15.1 (12-19)	15.3 (12-19)

	Nasal crest of the palatine bone		Nasal choana	
	Height	Width	Height	Width
Neonates	1.60 (1-2)	2.16 (1-3)	8.00 (7-9)	5.94 (5.5-6.5)
1 yr.	2.10 (1-3)	2.30 (2-3)	11.60 (10-14)	8.00 (7.5-8.5)
5 yrs.	3.23 (0-6)	3.36 (0-6)	16.35 (14-19)	10.35 (9 - 14)
13 yrs.	5.50 (4-6)	4.30 (3-6)	22.15 (19-25)	12.83 (11 - 13)
Adults	5.57 (3-10)	5.35 (2-8)	25.44 (21-33)	13.49 (10.5-19)

Fig. **153** Postnatal growth of the height and width of the choanae, the nasal crest of the palatine bone and the distance of the posterior aperture of the pterygoid canal from the median, sagittal plane (Lang and Baumeister, 1982)

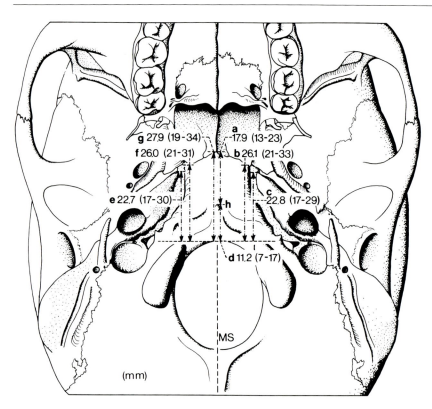

Fig. **154** Posterosuperior border of the vomer, the distance to the basion and the pharyngeal tubercle. Longitudinal measurements of the clivus lateral to it are also given

a Distance between the posterior edge of the vomer and the pharyngeal tubercle

b Length of the clivus between a plane transverse to the basion and the medial pterygoid plate

c Length between a transverse line to the basion and the petrosal apex

d Length between the basion and the pharyngeal tubercle

e Length between a line transverse to the basion and the petrous apex on the right side

f Length between a line transverse to the basion and the medial plate of the pterygoid process on the right side

g Length of the clivus between the basion and the vomer (central region)

h Pharyngeal tubercle

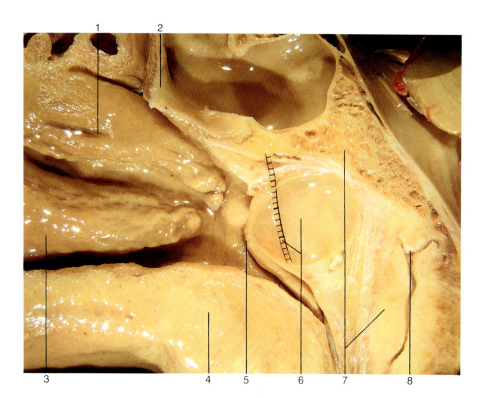

Fig. **155** Large cyst in the roof of the pharynx in a 77-year-old man

1 Middle nasal concha (notch)
2 Anterior wall of the sphenoidal sinus
3 Inferior nasal concha
4 Soft palate with section through the palatine glands
5 Pharyngeal ostium of the pharyngotympanic tube
6 Cyst in the nasopharynx, and a millimeter strip
7 Clivus and the anterior arch of the atlas
8 Bony process on the basion (tertiary condyle) articulating with the anterior arch of the atlas and the apex of the dens (a rare variant)

bone. At that point they joined each other with a notched edge. Laterally the bony plate bounds the medial aspect of the medial pterygoid plate with a sharp edge. Atresia may be membranous, bony, complete or incomplete, unilateral or bilateral (Beinfield, 1853). Choanal atresia probably has a complex origin, although failure of the superior segment of the buccopharyngeal membrane to atrophy may be the cause (Soeprapto and Surjono, 1977).

Pharyngeal Hypophysis and Cysts of the Roof of the Pharynx

Hinrichsen et al. (1986) described the development of the epipharynx and of the pharyngeal hypophysis. A swelling can be clearly recognized in their Figs. 8–11 in the area of the pharyngeal hypophysis in 17.5 and 26.0 mm embryos. They state that the pharyngeal bursa was recognized by Tourneux and Tourneux (1912), Corning (1925) and Christ et al. (1988) but lying inferior to the pharyngeal tonsil. The pharyngeal hypophysis had been described by Haberfeld (1909), Frazer (1911), Cristeller (1914), Atwell (1926), Mueller (1955), Boyd (1956) and Romeis (1940).

Cysts of the Nasopharynx Constricting the Choanae

Cysts filled with mucus were quite often found in our material arising from the roof of the pharynx and narrowing the choanae. One example is shown in Fig. **155**. These are probably Tornwaldt cysts (Tornwaldt, 1885). Guggenheim (1967) gave a fuller description of these midline cysts of the nasopharynx, and described their relation to the nasopharyngeal fascia. He felt that they could arise from the pharyngeal bursa (Tourtual, 1846; Ganghofner, 1879; Killian, 1888).

Posterosuperior Border of the Vomer

The distance between the posterior edge of the vomer and the pharyngeal tubercle is roughly equal in children and adults (Merkel, 1890; Piersol, 1930). The posterior edge of the nasal septum moves backwards during postnatal growth to the base of the sphenoid bone (appositional growth) (Takagi, 1964). The posterior wall of the pharynx arises at the posterior edge of the sphenoid bone (Takagi et al., 1962). As a result of posterior migration of the vomer the lower surface of the sphenoid bone forms less and less of the roof of the pharynx, since the posterior edge of the adult vomer reaches almost as far as the previous sphenooccipital synchondrosis. We confirmed this finding on our material (Issing, 1987) and carried out further measurements on the external base of the skull. The pharyngeal tubercle lies 17.9 (13–23) mm from the posterior edge of the vomer, whereas it lies at a distance of 27.9 (19–34) mm from the anterior edge of the foramen magnum (Lang and Issing, 1989).

Vessels of the Nasal Cavity and Paranasal Sinuses

Arteries of the Lateral Nasal Wall

(Fig. **156**)

The sphenopalatine artery is the main vessel supplying the nasal mucosa (Zuckerkandl, 1884, 1893). It gives off the posterior lateral nasal and septal artery of the nose. The sphenopalatine artery arises in the pterygopalatine fossa from the maxillary artery, and divides either proximal to, or within, the sphenopalatine foramen. In 97% of cases the posterior lateral nasal and septal artery arises from the bifurcation of the sphenopalatine artery, in 1.7% cases from the maxillary artery, and in 1.7% from a trunk formed by the artery of the pterygoid canal and the descending palatine artery (trifurcation) (Navarro et al., 1982). The larger branch is usually destined for the lateral wall of the nasal cavity, and the other for the medial wall. The sphenopalatine foramen is often split into two by a band, in which case the nasopalatine artery runs above the band, and the descending palatine artery intended for the lateral nasal wall runs below it. The main branch of the descending palatine artery runs on the lateral wall of the nose, lateral to the posterior end of the middle and inferior nasal conchae and divides into three sagittal branches, after giving off a branch for the middle nasal meatus at the inferior turbinate. A vessel running to the inferior nasal concha can be shown in 21.6% of cases arising from the descending palatine, the greater palatine or the lesser palatine artery (Navarro et al., 1982). The most robust of these branches then runs forwards, between the upper and lower edge of the turbinate to reach the cartilaginous segment of the nasal cavity where it anastamoses with branches of the superior labial artery. The next largest branch runs along the free edge of the turbinate, gives off a branch in the anterior segment of the inferior nasal meatus, and, like the middle artery, reaches the nasal vestibule at the anterior anastamotic area. One branch, usually the smallest, runs forwards along the insertion of the inferior nasal concha and then on the wall of the middle nasal meatus. On the conchae the vessels are partly embedded in deep grooves, and also are sometimes bridged by a bony bar. The largest vessel for the middle nasal concha runs forwards partly along the edge of the concha and partly under it. The superior and supreme nasal conchae receive a direct blood supply from the nasopalatine artery. Branches for these conchae run downwards from the lower surface of the body of the sphenoid bone towards the lateral wall of the nose. The septum, the lateral wall of the nose and the

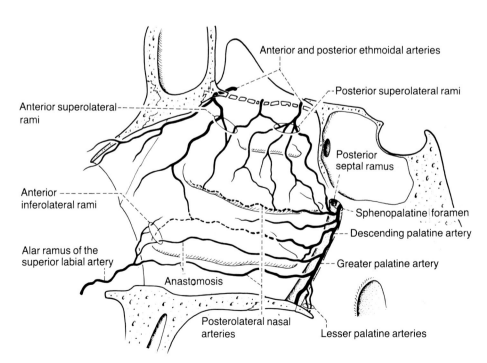

Fig. **156** Arteries of the lateral wall of the nose

upper part of the nasal cavity are supplied by branches of the anterior and posterior ethmoidal arteries (Lang and Schaefer, 1979). The descending palatine artery also takes part in the supply of the nasal cavity; it too arises from the maxillary artery in the pterygopalatine fossa. Fine branches from this vessel pass through the medial wall of the greater palatine canal, mainly into the middle nasal meatus, to anastamose with the posterolateral nasal artery arising from the sphenopalatine artery.

Arteries of the Nasal Septum

(Fig. **157**)

Zuckerkandl showed that the sphenopalatine artery usually gives off an upper and a lower posterior septal ramus at the nasal septum. The lower, larger branch, runs inferiorly and anteriorly along the vomer. One of its branches runs towards the incisive canal and anastamoses with the penetrating branch of the greater palatine artery. In our material this area was supplied more from the greater palatine artery than from the sphenopalatine artery.

Anastomoses and Variations

(Fig. **142**, page 97)

The angular and ophthalmic arteries anastomose via the ethmoidal arteries, although these anastomoses may be absent (Zuckerkandl, 1893). Shaheen (1975) infused dye in the living subject into the external carotid artery, and into the internal carotid artery after ligation of the external carotid artery. After injection of the internal carotid artery a dramatic suffusion of the upper half of the face, of the area between the cribriform plate and the upper third of the nasal septum and of the lateral wall of the nose was noticable. Injection of the external carotid artery showed that the facial artery was patent in 8 of 13 patients. In 3 of these patients the entire septum and lateral nasal wall were perfused, perfusion of the lateral nasal wall being less intense above the middle nasal concha. In the remaining 5 subjects the lower two-thirds of the nasal cavity was perfused intensively. In 5 patients subjected to injection of the external carotid artery in whom the facial artery was not patent, the entire septum and lateral nasal wall were perfused, although less intensively above the middle nasal concha.

The anterior ethmoidal artery is absent on one side in 14% of cases, and on both sides in 2% of cases (Shaheen, 1976). The anterior ethmoidal artery can arise from a common stem with the posterior ethmoidal artery, and share in the supply of the orbital contents, including the superior oblique and medial rectus muscles and the orbital fat. If the anterior ethmoidal artery is absent it is replaced by a branch from the posterior ethmoidal artery that runs forwards upon the dura along the lateral edge of the olfactory fossa, and then enters the nasal cavity (Lang and Schaefer, 1979). In this case the anterior ethmoidal nerve traverses the ethmoidal canal without an arteria comitans. Also the posterior ethmoidal artery may be rudimentary on one side, being replaced by a posterior ramus of the anterior ethmoidal artery, by the contralateral posterior ethmoidal artery or by branches of the sphenopalatine artery (Lang and Schaefer, 1979). The ethmoidal arteries can also arise from the middle meningeal arteries. The ethmoidal arteries give off branches to the ethmoidal cells during their further course (Fig. **123**, page 84).

Further anastomoses exist with the branch of the ophthalmic artery that penetrates the nasolacrimal canal to anastomose with the infraorbital artery (Zuckerkandl, 1893).

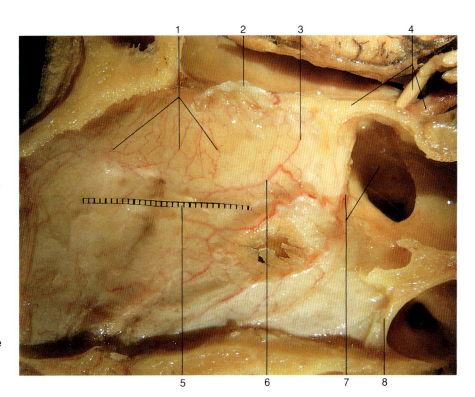

Fig. **157** Arteries of the posterosuperior segment of the nasal septum after removal of the skeletal part of the septum
1 Branches of the ethmoidal artery
2 Dura mater of the olfactory fossa
3 Branches of the posterior ethmoidal artery
4 Sphenoidal plane, optic nerve retracted upwards and the internal carotid artery
5 Millimeter strip
6 Anastomoses of the septal rami of the sphenopalatine artery
7 Branches of the sphenopalatine artery for the nasal septum on the anterior wall of the sphenoid sinus
8 Posterior edge of the vomer

Cavernous Plexus

Cavernous conchal plexuses are found in the lamina propria of the mucosa in the region of the erectile tissue. The veins of the plexus are between 0.1 and 0.5 mm wide; they anastomose with each other, and with veins from the neighboring bone (Baison, 1954). Narrow capillaries and veins arise within the submucosal layer, as in the superficial layers. The capillaries are surrounded by an incomplete layer of flat pericytes. The endothelium is fenestrated between the processes of the pericytes, usually on the side nearest the surface (Cauna et al., 1969). The entire plexus is permeated by smooth muscle fibers. The cushion veins are thought to control the blood flow through the arteries and the post-capillary veins (Temesrecasi, 1969).

Capillaries of the nasal mucosa: 52% of the capillaries of the anterior end of the inferior turbinate are not fenestrated, whereas 31% can be regarded as fenestrated (Watanabe and Watanabe, 1980). Numerous microvilli project from the endothelium into the lumen of the capillary, and others into the interstitium. On the dorsal part of the inferior turbinate, about 67% of capillaries were fenestrated, 25% were nonfenestrated and 8% were open capillaries lying between the neighboring endothelial cells. The fenestrated capillaries possessed a smooth-walled lumen, and few pericytes in the basal lamina.

Arteriovenous Anastomoses

Numerous arteriovenous anastomoses are present in the deep layer of the mucosa and around the mucosal glands (Cauna, 1970). These often resemble simple glomeruli, and are enclosed by a connective tissue capsule. The neighboring arterial walls contain long muscle bundles. The transition from thick-walled arteries to thin-walled veins is abrupt. The walls of the vein are thinner than those of similar veins elsewhere, and they may be almost completely without muscles. Electron microscopy showed non-myelinated nerve fibers with agranular vesicles in the region of the arteries, but never in the tunica media, and it is likely that these are cholinergic nerves (Cauna, 1970) (see also the section on nerves, page 115).

Blood Supply of the Paranasal Sinuses

Maxillary Sinus

The maxillary sinus is supplied by branches from the sphenopalatine and infraorbital arteries. The branches of the sphenopalatine artery enter the sinus through the semilunar hiatus or the nasal fontanelle. The posterosuperior alveolar rami also take part in the supply of the bone and mucosa of the maxillary sinus. In our material 2–3 posterior alveolar rami usually penetrated the posterior wall of the maxillary sinus. The foramina for nerves, arteries and veins lay 20 (11–36) mm from the superior wall of the maxillary sinus (Lang and Papke, 1984). During childhood the arterial and venous connections between the maxillary sinus and the orbit are relatively wide, facilitating spread of infection between these two structures.

Frontal Sinus

Branches of the anterior artery of the falx, and of the supraorbital and supratrochlear arteries penetrate the frontal sinus; branches from the medial posterior lateral nasal artery also enter it through the ostium. The venous drainage, too, follows several different pathways (Fig. **158**).

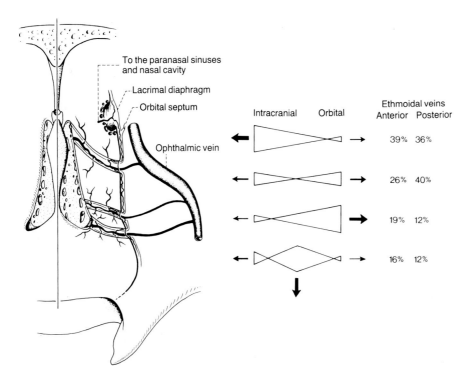

Fig. **158** Course, width and direction of flow of the ethmoidal veins of the anterior and posterior ethmoidal canals. Several tributaries to the ethmoidal veins and connections with the orbital periostium and the venous network around the lacrimal sac and the nasolacrimal duct are also shown (Lang et al., 1979)

Ethmoidal Cells

The ethmoidal cells receive their blood supply from the ethmoidal arteries and from branches of the arteries of the nasal cavity via their ostia.

Sphenoidal Sinus

One branch of the sphenopalatine artery enters the sphenoidal sinus from in front and below to supply the mucosa of the sinus (Mosher, 1903). In our material the inferior hypophyseal artery took part in the supply of the mucosa of the sphenoidal sinus and of the neighboring bone. This sinus is also irrigated by numerous neighboring vessels.

Veins of the Nasal Cavity

Veins arise from the dense venous network of the nasal mucosa to run in different directions accompanying the arteries. The main drainage from the nasal septum runs backwards accompanying the sphenopalatine artery. The ethmoidal arteries are usually acommpanied by veins that anastomose with veins of the dura mater of the anterior cranial fossa, and with the superior sagittal sinus through the foramen caecum which is occasionally open (Kiesselbach, 1884). In our material the ethmoidal veins drained mainly to the orbit, to the anterior cranial fossa or to the veins of the ethmoidal cells (Lang et al., 1980). These veins act as pathways of spread of inflammation from the paranasal sinuses to the orbit (Fig. **158**). An external nasal plexus drains towards the external nasal opening, destined for the facial vein and its tributaries (Zuckerkandl, 1893).

One vein runs in a posteroinferior direction towards the soft palate and the pharynx. Venous drainage in a posterosuperior direction is through the sphenopalatine foramen to the pterygopalatine fossa.

Small venae comitantes of the end branches of the greater palatine artery penetrate the incisive canal, to end in the veins of the hard palate and its overlying mucosa.

Zuckerkandl distinguished a superficial and a deep venous system in the nasal cavity. The superficial system lies at the posterior ends of the turbinates, and drains into the pharyngeal venous plexus and the palatal veins. Veins from the posterosuperior ethmoidal turbinates penetrate the sphenopalatine foramen to reach the pterygopalatine fossa as venae comitantes of the posterior lateral nasal artery. Further drainage passes via the pterygoid venous plexus. Fine veins from the nasal mucosa run through the pterygopalatine canal to reach the palatal veins.

Lymphatics

(Fig. **159**)

Lymphatic drainage from the nasal cavity passes both anteriorly and posteriorly; the number and caliber of the lymph vessels is dictated by the thickness and tension of the mucosa (Most, 1901).

Posterior Drainage

The posterior lymphatics of the nose collect on the lateral pharyngeal wall, just behind the hard palate and close to the pharyngeal ostium of the pharyngotympanic tube. The lymphatic pathway from the nasal septum runs along the floor of the nose to the upper surface of the soft palate. The lymphatic pathway divides into two on the lateral pharyngeal wall; one of these consists of three or four trunks which run in a straight line externally and down-

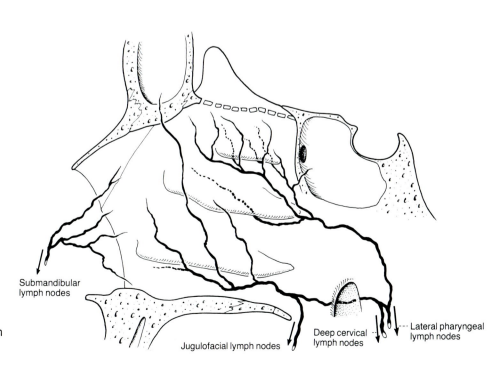

Fig. **159** Main lymphatic drainage from the lateral wall of the nose

Submandibular lymph nodes

Jugulofacial lymph nodes

Deep cervical lymph nodes

Lateral pharyngeal lymph nodes

wards to join the lymph vessels of the palatine arch and tonsil. The deep cervical chain of lymph nodes is strung along this pathway behind the submandibular gland and the digastric muscles, at the level of the bifurcation of the common carotid artery. The most important node of this group is the *jugulofacial lymph node.* The other drainage pathway, consisting of two to four vessels, runs directly backwards from the pharyngeal ostium of the pharyngotympanic tube in a posterior direction to the *lateral pharyngeal lymph nodes,* and thence to the deep cervical lymph nodes. A lateral pharyngeal lymph node always fills during injection experiments (Most, 1901). The same lymphatic drainage area was perfused after injection into the mucosa of the paranasal sinuses as after injection into the nasal mucosa. Lymphatic vessels arising from the sphenoethmoidal recess immediately turn deeply behind the mucosa of the roof of the pharynx. They run backwards and downwards between this structure and the pericranium to the lateral pharyngeal lymph nodes.

Anterior Lymphatic Drainage and Lymphatics of the External Nose

(Fig. **31**, page 21)

Lymph from the most anterior part of the nasal cavity in front of the piriform aperture drains towards the external nose, and thereafter in the subcutaneous fatty tissue, occasionally under or between the facial muscles, towards the facial vein and the submandibular lymph nodes. Three groups of lymphatic vessels drain the external nose. The upper arises at the root of the nose, and runs through the upper eyelid close to the supraorbital margin to reach the

parotid lymph nodes. The central stream also arises from the root and superolateral parts of the nose; it runs horizontally along the inferior orbital rim to the anterior border of the parotid gland where it turns downwards to reach the lymph nodes lying in the tail of the parotid gland. The third group, consisting of six to ten vessels, arises from all parts of the external nose and joins the facial vein. The buccal lymph nodes may be incorporated into this pathway. The main drainage may pass from one group of lymphatics to another.

Lymphatic Drainage of the Maxillary Sinus

It has been known since ancient times that otitis media and sinusitis are common in children: between 82% and 92% of middle ear effusions resolve after treatment of the sinusitis. Lymphangiography has shown that the lymph drains not only via the ostia and fontanelles, but also via transverse connections to the pharyngotympanic tube and to the nasopharynx (Mann, 1980). Those running in the area of the pharyngeal recess and the torus tubarius and thence to the posterior wall of the pharynx and to the opposite side have been confirmed by dye studies. Nasendoscopy was unable to demonstrate lymphatic vessels in the middle and inferior nasal conchae after injection of the posterior wall of the maxillary sinus. In contrast, injection of the medial wall of the maxillary sinus showed staining of the middle and inferior nasal concha. Mann (1980) therefore concluded that the lymphatic vessels follow the blood vessels (the superior alveolar vessels). The inferior part of the maxillary sinus possesses lymphatic vessels that penetrate the semilunar hiatus to reach the nasal lymphatics, and also the bone to reach the lymphatics of the face (Andre, 1905).

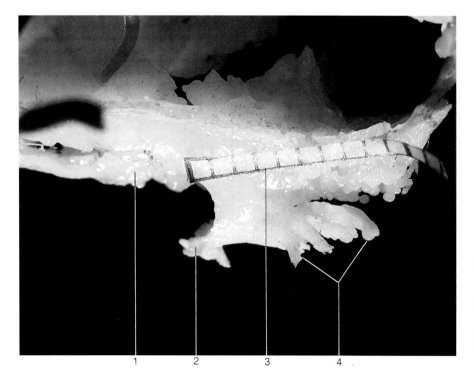

Fig. **160** Arachnoid sheaths and olfactory filaments of the olfactory fossa and of the cisterns of the olfactory filaments after plastic injection
1 Region of the sphenoidal plane
2 Arachnoidal sheaths of the posterior filaments filled with plastic
3 Millimeter strip
4 Arachnoid sheaths of the anterior olfactory filaments

The Lymph and the Cerebrospinal Fluid

(Fig. **160**)

Lymph vessels were first demonstrated by Rudbek in 1659 in the presence of Queen Christina of Sweden (Hartz, 1911). The cerebrospinal fluid communicates with the lymphatics of the nasal mucosa via the subarachnoid space along the perineural clefts of the olfactory filaments. Thus it can reach the deep cervical lymph nodes (Key and Retzius, 1875; Weed, 1914; Woollard, 1924; Naumann and Naumann, 1977). There are connections between the right and left side of the nose, and with the lower airway (Hartz, 1911). We came to the same conclusions as Key and Retzius (1875) about the connections through the cribriform plate. The nasomeningeal tract is confined mainly to the olfactory region. In the discussion of Hartz's paper, Stucky stated that he had recently observed three cases in which infection had passed from the nasal mucosa through the cribriform plate to the frontal lobe. Connections have also been shown between the subarachnoid cavity and the lymphatics of the nasal cavity of cats and apes (Yoffey and Drinker, 1940). On several occasions we have demonstrated small cisterns along the olfactory filaments passing through the cribriform plate. If they are torn by trauma or surgery a CSF leak may result.

Innervation of the Nasal Cavity

Sensory Nerves

(Fig. **161a, b**)

The nasal septum derives its sensory nerve supply from branches of the ophthalmic and maxillary nerves. The *anterior ethmoidal nerve* runs with the anterior ethmoidal artery through the cribroethmoidal foramen, and then passes forwards and downwards along the border between the nasal septum and the lateral wall of the nose.

The main stem then emerges on the external surface of the nose between the nasal bone and the lateral cartilage. Within the nasal cavity numerous branches of the nerve pass to the anterior segment of the nasal septum, from the cribriform plate down to an area lying above the premaxilla. The fibers of the posterior ethmoidal nerve are mainly autonomic. The *nasopalatine* (Scarpa's) nerve arises from the maxillary nerve, and passes through the sphenopalatine foramen to reach the nasal septum. It runs in an anteroinferior direction towards the incisive canal, embedded in grooves in the vomer. Its end-branch penetrates the canal and supplies the superior gingiva as far as the canine tooth. During its course within the nasal cavity it gives off numerous branches to the septal mucosa. The sensory branches of the maxillary nerve run with the autonomic nerves (v.i.).

The *nervus terminalis* probably supplies a small segment of the nasal septum (Lederer and Dinolt, 1943). It is also said to carry autonomic fibers (Brookover, 1917; Pearson, 1941).

Autonomic Nerves

(Fig. **161a, b**)

The nasopalatine nerve, too, carries autonomic fibers, and it supplies part of the nasal vestibule. It usually anastomoses with nasal rami arising from the anterior superior alveolar branch of the infaorbital nerve. The medial superior posterior nasal branches of the greater palatine nerve share in the supply of the posterior segment of the septum and of the body of the sphenoid bone. The lateral posterior nasal rami pass through the sphenopalatine foramen to the superior and medial nasal concha and the neighboring meatus. They give branches to the nasal cavity, the roof of the pharynx, the mucosa of the nasopharynx, the sphenoidal sinus and the pharyngeal ostium of the pharyngotympanic tube. Lateral inferior posterior nasal rami run downwards with the greater palatine nerve in its canal, and leave it at the level of the inferior nasal concha. They supply the mucosa of the concha, and of the medial and inferior nasal meatus.

Pterygopalatine Ganglion

(Fig. **164**)

The pterygopalatine ganglion lies in the pterygopalatine fossa (Table 14). Fig. **162** shows the complex anatomy of its posterior wall. All the aforementioned nerves are branches of the pterygopalatine ganglion. The ganglion is 3.3

Table **14**   Pterygopalatine fossa, orifices

Orifices		Contents	Course
Lateral orifice	Pterygomaxillary fissure	Maxillary artery, superior and posterior alveolar arteries, veins, and nerves	Infratemporal fossa
Posterior orifice	a) Foramen rotundum superior and lateral	Maxillary nerve and artery	Middle cranial fossa
	b) Pterygoid canal, superior and medial	Pterygoid nerve, artery of the pterygoid canal	Lower surface of the base of the skull
	c) Vomerovaginal canal, more medial	Small arteries and nerves	Pharyngeal fornix
	d) Palatovaginal canal, medial	Pharyngeal branches of the sphenopalatine ganglion and artery	Roof of the pharynx
Medial orifice	Sphenopalatine foramen, above and medial	Nasal branches of the posterior sphenopalatine artery	Nasal cavity
Anterior orifice	Orbital fissure, below and infront	Infraorbital arteries and nerves, zygomatic nerve	Orbit, facial region
Lower orifice	Greater palatine canal	Greater and lesser palatine arteries, veins, and nerves	Hard and soft palate, nasal cavity

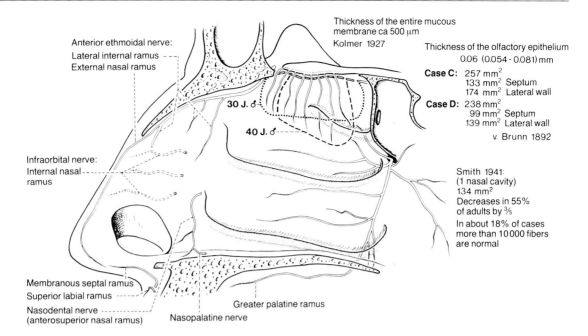

Fig. **161a** Nerves of the lateral wall of the nasal cavity. Data for the area of the olfactory region (v. Brunn, 1882; Smith, 1941), and for mucosal thickness (Kolmer, 1927) are also given

Anterior ethmoidal nerve:
Lateral internal ramus
External nasal ramus

Infraorbital nerve:
Internal nasal ramus

Membranous septal ramus
Superior labial ramus
Nasodental nerve
(anterosuperior nasal ramus)

Nasopalatine nerve

Greater palatine ramus

30 J. ♂
40 J. ♂

Thickness of the entire mucous membrane ca 500 μm
Kolmer 1927

Thickness of the olfactory epithelium
0.06 (0.054 - 0.081) mm

Case C: 257 mm²
133 mm² Septum
174 mm² Lateral wall
Case D: 238 mm²
99 mm² Septum
139 mm² Lateral wall
v. Brunn 1892

Smith 1941:
(1 nasal cavity)
134 mm²
Decreases in 55% of adults by ⅗
In about 18% of cases more than 10 000 fibers are normal

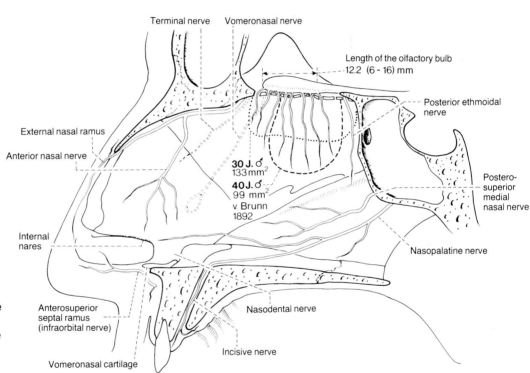

Fig. **161b** Innervation of the nasal septum. The extent of the olfactory region, the course of the nervus terminalis and of the vomeronasal nerve are also given

Terminal nerve   Vomeronasal nerve

Length of the olfactory bulb
12.2 (6 - 16) mm

Posterior ethmoidal nerve

External nasal ramus

Anterior nasal nerve

30 J. ♂
133 mm²
40 J. ♂
99 mm²
v. Brunn 1892

Internal nares

Anterosuperior septal ramus (infraorbital nerve)

Vomeronasal cartilage

Incisive nerve

Nasodental nerve

Nasopalatine nerve

Posterosuperior medial nasal nerve

(2–6) mm high and 1.8 (1–3) mm wide (Tanaka, 1932), and is sometimes split into two or more parts. It lies behind the pterygopalatine artery, and between the maxillary nerve and the sphenopalatine foramen. Fig. **163** shows the distance from various landmarks.

The ganglion contains the following structures:

1) Two or three ganglionic (pterygopalatine) rami arising from the maxillary nerve (Fig. **164**).
2) The greater petrosal nerve as its parasympathetic root.
3) The deep petrosal nerve as the sympathetic root.

The deep petrosal nerve arises from the internal carotid plexus, runs through the inferior sphenopetrosal ligament and then penetrates from behind into the pterygoid canal. It unites with the greater petrosal nerve proximal to or within the canal to form the nerve of the pterygoid canal. The sympathetic fibers pass through the pterygopalatine ganglion without interruption, whereas most of the sensory fibers synapse. Its ganglionic cells are mainly parasympathetic fibers. It also probably transmits motor fibers for the levator palati muscle. The greater petrosal nerve probably contains vasodilator and secretory fibers which it transmits to the pterygopalatine ganglion. The sympathetic fibers are vasoconstrictor.

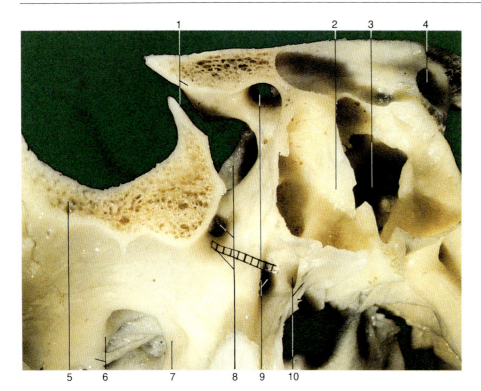

Fig. **162**   Pterygopalatine fossa with posterior foramina and surrounding area in frontal section seen from in front
1   Superior orbital fissure
2   Oblique septum of the sphenoidal sinus
3   Left sphenoidal sinus
4   Left optic canal
5   Floor of the middle cranial fossa
6   Sphenoidal lamina
7   Lateral plate of the pterygoid process
8   Dorsum sellae and foramen rotundum; millimeter strip
9   Optic canal and anterior aperture of the pterygoid canal
10 Palatovaginal canal and palatine bone (sphenoidal process)

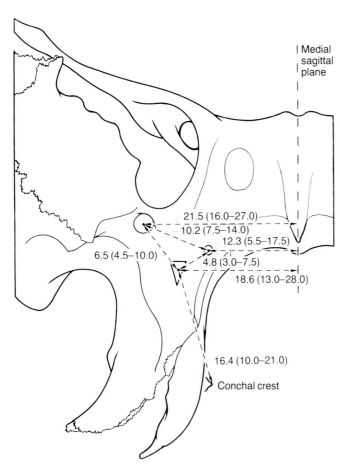

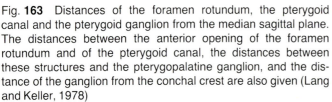

Fig. **163**   Distances of the foramen rotundum, the pterygoid canal and the pterygoid ganglion from the median sagittal plane. The distances between the anterior opening of the foramen rotundum and of the pterygoid canal, the distances between these structures and the pterygopalatine ganglion, and the distance of the ganglion from the conchal crest are also given (Lang and Keller, 1978)

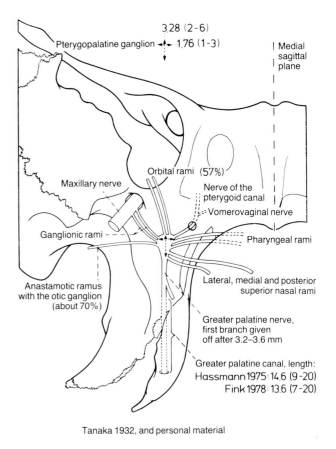

Fig. **164**   Size of the pterygopalatine ganglion when it is fully developed, and branches of the pterygopalatine ganglion (Tanaka, 1932; Hassmann, 1975; Lang and Keller, 1978; Fink, 1978)

Nerve of the Pterygoid Canal, and Vidian Neurectomy

Good results have been reported to follow division of the greater petrosal nerve or the nerve of the pterygoid canal in chronic vasomotor rhinopathy with recurrent polyposis (Golding-Wood, 1961, 1962, 1973). This procedure eliminates the parasympathetic innervation of the nasal mucosa. We investigated the junction between the greater petrosal nerve and the deep petrosal nerve, the course within the pterygoid canal and the position of the pterygopalatine canal (Lang and Keller, 1978). A parasympathetic ganglion has been found at the junction between the greater petrosal nerve and the deep petrosal nerve (Chorobwski and Penfield, 1932).

Golding-Wood (1961, 1970) prefers transantral access for destruction of the pterygopalatine ganglion or the nerve of the pterygoid canal. A permeatal approach through the middle nasal meatus to the pterygopalatine ganglion was described by Takahashi and Tsutsumi (1970).

Sewall recommended a transantral approach to the pterygopalatine and infratemporal fossae (1926, 1937). Golding-Wood (1973) reported the results of Vidian neurectomy via the transantral route on 242 patients with vasomotor rhinopathy. The immediate result was good in 94% of cases and excellent in 57%; 2% of patients suffered an ophthalmoplegia. Good results have also been reported for senile epiphora, crocodile tears and chronic epiphora (Chandra, 1967). Lesions of the oculomotor muscles occurred with the use of a 2 mm thick diathermy probe; Golding-Wood now insulates the needle more securely.

Specific Function of the Pterygopalatine Ganglion

Burger (1927) showed that the pterygopalatine ganglion can inhibit vasoconstriction. Swelling, redness, increased secretion from the nasal mucosa and hyperemia of the orbital contents could all be explained by stimulation of the ganglion. The pterygopalatine ganglion is thus a peripheral regulatory center for the innervation of the vessels of the nasal mucosa. Operations on the nasolacrimal duct, removal of the lacrimal gland and division of the nerve of the pterygoid canal may all be considered for chronic epiphora. The accessory glands and the goblet cells of the conjunctiva also contribute to the excessive secretion of tears (Golding-Wood, 1973), because the lacrimal glands are supplied by branches of the pterygopalatine ganglion.

Sluder's syndrome: Sluder (1908, 1909) described neuralgia of the pterygopalatine ganglion. He found that the ganglion lay 1–9 mm from the mucosa of the nasal cavity. Also he investigated the relationship of the ganglion to the sphenoidal sinus, to the maxillary sinus (lying at a distance of 3–4 mm), to the optic nerve and to the posterior ethmoidal cells. Inflammation of the nasal sinuses could affect the ganglion producing neuralgia after resolution of the inflammation. The pain irradiates from the root of the nose downwards over the maxilla, backwards towards the mastoid process, to the occiput, to the neck, to the scapula, to the shoulder, and occasionally to the maxilla. It irradiates to the parietal bone after inflammation of the posterior ethmoidal cells, and to the occiput after inflammation of the sphenoidal sinus. Dysart (1944) applied cocaine to the pterygopalatine ganglion and observed an improvement in Sluder's neuralgia and corneal ulceration.

Sympathetic Fibers for the Nasal Cavity

The sympathetic fibers to the nasal mucosa arise from the superior cervical ganglion (Blier, 1930; Malcolmson, 1959; Larsell and Fenton, 1936). If the sympathetic and parasympathetic fibers are stimulated at the same time the vasoconstrictor effect is more powerful than the vasodilator effect. The sympathetic innervation of the nasal mucosa is abnormal after paralysis of the nerve of the pterygoid canal.

Stimulation of the hypothalamus causes vasoconstriction (Fowler, 1943; quoted by Malcolmson, 1959). The nasal mucosa does not respond to stimulation if the nerve of the pterygoid canal or the pterygopalatine ganglion have been divided (Malcolmson). The autonomic nerves, both cholinergic (parasympathetic) and adrenergic (sympathetic), regulate the flow of blood through the nasal vessels, the secretion from the seromucinous glands and the activity of the cilia of the nasal and sinus mucosa. Burnstock (1972) has reported the presence of purinergic nerves. The transmitter substance *neuropeptide Y* can be shown both in the central and in the peripheral nervous system (Ekblad et al., 1984). Neuropeptide Y fibers are found in the smooth vascular muscles and also in other smooth muscles, around the acini of exocrine glands as well as beneath the epithelial surface. Surgical or chemical sympathectomy leads to suppression of adrenergic and neuropeptide Y fibers. It is assumed that the neuropeptide Y fibers complement the vasoconstrictor function of the noradrenergic sympathetic fibers. The nasal mucosa has a generous supply of neuropeptide Y fibers, particularly in the inferior turbinates (Uddman and Sundler, 1986).

Substance-P was discovered by Euler and Gaddum in 1931. It contains 11 amino acids (Chang and Leeman, 1970), and has been found in central and peripheral nervous systems, particularly in the posterior horn of the spinal cord. Peripherally, substance-P produces contraction of smooth muscle fibers, vasodilatation and increased glandular and pancreatic secretion. Substance-P probably induces vasodilatation and increased fluid production from capillaries, and is probably a transmitter substance of the primary sensory neurons at the periphery (Lembeck, 1953). Substance-P fibers have been found in the nasal mucosa, particularly around blood vessels and seromucinous glands, and in the respiratory epithelium (Lundblad et al., 1983). Numerous substance-P immunoreactive perikarya and nerve fibers are also observed within the trigeminal ganglion. Division of the maxillary nerve leads to a loss of substance-P fibers in the nasal mucosa. Therefore it is likely that the substance-P fibers are sensory, and that their cells lie in the trigeminal ganglion. Electrical stimulation of the maxillary nerve or local application of substance-P causes increased vascular permeability and interstitial edema of the nasal mucosa in animal experiments (Lundblad et al., 1983). The *calcitonin-gene-related peptide fibers* probably run with the fibers carrying substance-P (Rosenfeld et al., 1983), sharing in the regulation of the local bloodflow, the tone of the smooth muscle fibers, and the glandular secretion.

Gastrin-releasing peptide has also been found around small blood vessels and nasal glands in animal experiments.

Acetylcholinergic fibers have been demonstrated by the acetylecholinesterase reaction lying around the glandular cells and blood vessels of the nasal mucosa (Ishii and Toriyama, 1972). Most of these fibers for the lower part of the nasal cavity arise from the pterygopalatine ganglion, whereas a smaller upper segment possibly arises from the ciliary ganglion (Grothe et al., 1975). We feel that these are orbital rami of the pterygopalatine ganglion.

Electrical stimulation of the pterygopalatine ganglion causes an atropine-sensitive secretion of the nasal glands, and an atropine-resistant vasodilatation (Angard, 1974). This finding indicates that the postganglionic parasympathetic mediators for the secretion of the nasal glands have a cholinergic innervation, whereas vasodilatation is achieved by non-cholinergic transmitter substances. The latter is probably a neurotransmitter, called *vasoactive intestinal polypeptide* (VIP) a peptide containing 28 amino acids. Many VIP fibers have been found in the nasal mucosa.

Other reflexes: A slight *apnea* as well as a *sneezing reflex* are produced by application of water to the face or nose. The sneezing reflex can also be induced by the administration of histamine or substance-P, by cooling of the body, irritation of the scalp or the external ear, shining light into the eyes or psychogenic factors (Widdicombe, 1986).

The *sniffing reflex* leads the airstream to the olfactory region; it is provoked by various scents. Sniffing can reach a frequency of 12–15 times a second in small experimental animals, and is probably important in sexual identification. The nose is cleared of mucus and obstruction by voluntary sniffing in man.

Irritation of the nasal mucosa causes *bronchoconstriction or dilatation,* and constriction of the larynx. Negative pressure in the nasal cavity, the pharynx or larynx, leads to reflex contraction of the *laryngeal abductor muscles*. The sensory nerves of the nasal mucosa are said to be responsible for the protective reflex: smoke and acid fumes etc. causes breath holding and averting movements of the head.

Mucosa of the Nasal Cavity and Paranasal Sinuses

Koelliker in 1896 named the connective tissue layer beneath the mucosa of the nose and nasopharynx the Schneiderian membrane, in honor of Schneider (1614–1680). The thickness of the nasal mucosa varies between 0.3 and 5 mm, depending on the development of the cavernous plexus and the mucosal glands. The mucosa over the medial surface of the middle and inferior nasal conchae is thicker than elsewhere. At this point the conchal cavernous plexus is embedded in the lamina propria. A similar plexus is also found on the nasal septum, as discovered by Morgagni (1682–1771). This area is now termed the corpus cavernosum of the septum, the anterior tubercle of the septum or Kiesselbach's ridge. This swelling lies at the connection between the vomer and the septal cartilage, and is present even in the newborn. Its level depends on the shape of the lateral nasal wall: posteriorly it extends between the middle and inferior nasal conchae.

Kiesselbach's Plexus

At the anterior end of the swelling the mucosa is thin, rich in vessels and loosely bound to the underlying perichondrium. This is Kiesselbach's plexus. Epistaxis is usually due to venous or arterial bleeding from this area. The arrangement of the vessels of Kiesselbach's plexus may represent rudimentary erectile tissue that is possibly connected with the vomeronasal organ (Heiss, 1936). This blind-ending duct lies about 2 cm behind the nares: immediately in front of it lies the remnant of the incisive duct which in man does not open into the oral cavity. The lamina propria of the epithelium of the nasal cavity possesses no papillae, although it does in Kiesselbach's plexus.

Respiratory Region

A capillary network lies beneath the epithelium of the respiratory region; its matrix is about 0.025 mm wide (see Fig. 20 in Lang, 1977). Delicate connective tissue with a few lymphocytes, neutrophils, plasma cells and macrophages may be found in this area (Cauna, 1982). In the deeper layers may be found tubuloalveolar glands, and also a venous network with the cavernous plexus both in this zone and under it. Some of the glands extend to the periostium or the perichondrium. The basal membrane is visible under light microscopy, and is between 1.6 and 10 microns thick (Heiss, 1936). Under light microscopy it is homogeneous, but electron microscopy shows fine collagen fibers lying parallel to the surface but running in differing directions. This collagen layer must be distinguished from the basal lamina which is about 1 micron thick. The basal lamina is covered by the epithelium of the respiratory region. It is between 40 and 100 micron thick. The ciliated cells are 15 micron wide and between 15 and 20 micron high (Busuttil et al., 1977). There is a wide variation in the total number of cilia per cell. More cilia are present at the central segment of the cell than at the edges. These zones often demonstrate microvillae. The cilia are about 6 micron long and 0.3 micron wide, the microvillae have a length of 0.5 to 4 micron and a width of 0.1 micron. Towards the basal lamina the diameter of the cell, and the plasma-nucleus ratio become less. The cells here are smooth and their nuclei plumper. Neighboring epithelial cells are united by tight junctions or terminal bars.

Nasal Mucus, Glands and Capillaries

Development of the Nasal Glands

Nasal glands begin to appear in the nasal vestibule at the beginning of the fourth month of fetal life (Richter, 1952). Glandular anlages can be found in the septum and above the medial nasal concha in the middle of the fourth fetal month (13 cm length) (Fig. 5). At the end of the fourth month of fetal life glandular anlages may be found in the maxillary sinus; in the fifth month of fetal life they are better developed in the anterior than in the posterior part of the nasal cavity.

The secretion of the nasal glands humidifies the inhaled air, but increasing glandular secretion does not lead to increased humidification (Perwitzchky, 1927). The capillaries at the anterior end of the inferior nasal concha are not fenestrated in about 52% of cases, whereas 31% are (Watanabe and Watanabe, 1980). In the posterior part of the inferior turbinate 67% of the capillaries were fenestrated, 25% were non-fenestrated and 8% demonstrated openings between the neighboring endothelial cells. Cauna (1982) therefore concluded that the subepithelial network of the fenestrated capillaries was responsible for moistening the air. He stated that the feeling of dryness of the nose, and the development of crusts in disease could occur after emptying of the glands, and is more commonly due to atrophy of or damage to the fenestrated capillaries, or the presence of metaplastic squamous epithelium in the respiratory region than to dysfunction of the glands. The normal air is raised from a temperature of 4°C and a relative humidity of 40%, to a temperature of 32°C and 98% humidity, measured in the subglottic space (Ishii,

1980). If the mucous layer produced by the goblet cells cannot produce satisfactory humidification of the inspired air the subepithelial fenestrated capillaries dilate, producing more fluid from the nasal mucosa. The total amount of secretion from the nasal mucosal glands is less than 200 g per day; the mucosal area is about 123 cm² (Kortekangas, 1977). Mucus consists of about 96% water, and about 3% mucin (Malcolmson, 1959). The nasal secretion contains at least 12 proteins which are present in plasma, and six further proteins which are not (Reisman cited by Ishii, 1980). Antibody activity against a whole range of viruses including poliomyelitis, Coxsackie A9, ECHO 28 and para-influenza 3 may be found in the nasal secretion of healthy subjects. Antiviral antibodies of immunoglobin class A are also present in the secretions.

Control of Secretion

The hypothalamus possesses a reflex and integration center for the production of mucus in the nose; this center responds to emotional stimuli, endocrine changes and other factors, for example stimulation of the nasal mucosa (Golding-Wood, 1963). The superior salivatory nucleus, too, is responsible for mucus secretion: its impulses are conducted by the parasympathetic pathways to the ptery-gopalatine ganglion via the greater petrosal nerve.

Profound changes in volume of the cavernous nasal plexus can be induced by mechanical, thermal, psychogenic, sexual or chemical stimuli (Cauna, 1982). They change the airway as well as the speed of the air-stream through the nasal cavity (Mink, 1916).

Circular and subendothelial longitudinal muscle fibers were demonstrated long ago on the arteries supplying the blood to the conchal plexus. It is thought that these can control the blood supply to the plexus. Their activity is under the influence of both nerves and circulating blood

(Cauna, 1982). Furthermore cushion veins have been shown in the plexus that are also capable of controlling blood circulation through the plexus. The tubuloalveolar glands of the respiratory region are mainly seromucinous and demonstrate von Ebner's demi-lunes; they are surrounded by myoepithelial cells. The mast cells of the nasal mucosa which are responsible for the liberation of his-tamine are very important in hyperreflex rhinopathy whose symptoms include sneezing attacks, hypersecretion and nasal obstruction (Terrahe, 1985). Medical treatment may be achieved by:

1) Mast cell stabilization by corticosteroids, H_1 receptor blockers, etc.
2) Mediator antagonists.
3) Inhibition of the reflex.
4) Hydrotherapy.

Ciliary Beat and Mucus Transport

General Observations

Ciliary movement was discovered by Antonius de Heide in 1683. Valentin gave a full account of this phenomenon in 1842 (Erhard, 1910). Ciliary movement can continue even if the nucleus of the ciliated cell is removed (Englemann, 1868; Peter, 1899), and in the absence of basal bodies (Maier, 1903). Each cell possesses 20–30 kinocilia, that are 5–7 micron long and about 0.3 micron thick in man. The effective ciliary beat lasts about one-quarter of the time of the return beat (Tremble, 1951); 250–300 ciliary beats are accomplished per minute, and the cilia of the nasal cavity attain a frequency of 15 cycles per second (Guillerm et al., 1971). Each of these cycles can be divided into two phases: a rapid active phase and a slow recovery phase. Fig. **165** illustrates the direction of the ciliary beat in the nasal cavity.

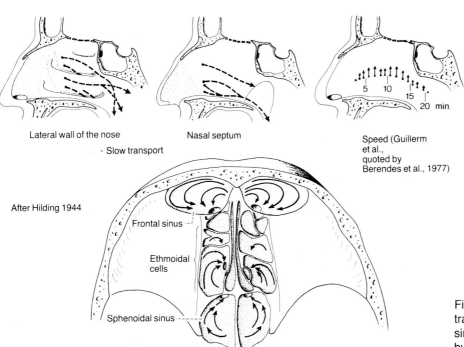

Lateral wall of the nose   Nasal septum

= Slow transport

Speed (Guillerm et al., quoted by Berendes et al., 1977)

After Hilding 1944

Frontal sinus

Ethmoidal cells

Sphenoidal sinus

Fig. **165** Airstream in the nasal cavity, and transport of secretion in the paranasal sinuses (Hilding, 1944; Guillerm et al., quoted by Berendes et al., 1977)

Ciliary Beat and Airstream in the Paranasal Sinuses
(Fig. 165)

A fluid introduced into the frontal sinus is usually subjected to a spiral movement. Similar movements are present in the ethmoidal cells. In two opened sphenoidal sinuses the fluid streamed towards the opening of the left sphenoidal sinus; spiral forward movements of the fluid was also seen (Hilding, 1944).

Frontal sinus: The mucus in the frontal sinus flows from the upper part of the frontonasal duct medially and upwards along the anterior and posterior walls of the sinus and its septum (Kortekangas, 1977). On reaching the roof of the frontal sinus the fluid stream arches laterally, and then runs downwards along the lateral side of the cavity towards the frontonasal duct. Variations of the frontal recess are clinically important in transport of secretion (Messerklinger, 1982). Only a part of the secretion of the frontal sinus reaches the middle nasal meatus; the rest forms a whirlpool, and then rejoins the circuit.

Disease of the frontal recess can be due to extension of a nasal infection. However diffuse or circumscribed mucosal swellings may be present, for example over the agger nasi. Variations of the anterior end of the middle nasal concha, or of the position of the uncinate process and the ethmoidal bulla can facilitate the development of infections. Paradoxically curved (lateral-convex) middle nasal conchae can also narrow the medial infundibular wall. The total secretion of the frontal sinus only reaches the nasal cavity completely in about one-third of cases (Vogt and Schrade, 1979; Prott, 1971, 1973, 1975). In the rest the drainage pathway divides as it passes through the ethmoidal bone to reach other ethmoidal cells or the maxillary sinus.

Maxillary sinus: The oxygen concentration in the maxillary sinus is about 19%, falling to 9% when the ostium is closed (Kortekangas, 1977). The secretory stream has a speed similar to that in the nasal cavity. A gel placed on the floor of the maxillary sinus radiates in all directions and finally reaches the ostium via the walls of the maxillary sinus. Mucous, tubuloalveolar and mixed glands may be found in the mucosa of the paranasal sinuses.

Temperature and air exchange: The mean temperature within the maxillary sinus is 31°C during inspiration, and 37°C during expiration (Muesebeck and Rosenberg, 1980). If the ostium is open the air within the maxillary sinus is completely exchanged by 15 breaths in one minute, with wide individual variations. The maximum variation of temperature is 4°C, but this is absent if the ostium is obliterated or closed.

Olfactory Region

The olfactory region comprises an area of only 134 mm² on each side. The olfactory region decreases in size during ageing in 55% of adults and is completely absent in 13% (Fig. 150a). The normal number of olfactory nerve fibers (10,000 or more) was found in only 29 of 169 adults (Smith, 1941).

Only substances soluble in water and lipid that reach the olfactory region can be smelt. The mucous film in this region is 20μ thick. A detection threshold (the weakest concentration of a stimulatory substance which provokes a sense of smell), a recognition threshold, and a distinction threshold are described. There is no clear boundary between the olfactory and respiratory regions in man (Kolmer, 1927). The mucosa of the olfactory region is 480–500μ thick, the epithelium 30–80μ thick. In newborns it is about 96μ thicker than in the adult. Older textbooks state that the yellowish color of the olfactory mucosa indicates the extent of the olfactory region, but Kolmer was unable to confirm this.

The olfactory region possesses supporting and olfactory cells. The *supporting cells* are of the same length as the thickness of the mucosa and are about 4μ wide. The nucleus has a width of 3μ. Each *sensory cell* possesses a uniform middle part about 7μ thick in which lies the nucleus. From here a process of varying length extends towards the surface. The central process serves to conduct the sense of smell. In adults the central processes of the olfactory cells possess 2–20 neurotubules, each of which is 20μ thick and possesses a central filament. These axons run initially between the basal processes of the supporting cells, and then several axons run together, being originally enclosed by processes of the supporting cells and then by dark basal cells, to form thick bundles. Thereafter Schwann cells provide their covering at the base of the epithelium. One Schwann cell usually contains 5–10 fibers, some up to 30 and a few more than 100 axones. The axones become more tightly packed towards the cribriform plate to form olfactory filaments (Seifert, 1970). Further details are given by Lang (1985).

Anomalies of the Sense of Smell

About 0.2% of humans suffer from anomalies of the sense of smell (Herberhold, 1978). Testing with well-known odors suffices for screening, if the patient will co-operate. Quantitative and qualitative, respiratory and sensorhinoneural disorders of smell must be distinguished. In the latter group, lesions of the central nervous olfactory pathways (the olfactory epithelium, the olfactory nerves, the olfactory bulb, the olfactory tract, or the pathways of the olfactory cortex) must be distinguished from each other. Qualitative dysosmia can cause spontaneous hallucinations of smell in the absence of an olfactory substance.

Parosmia, that is the incorrect identification of olfactory substances, indicates organic cerebral disease.

Hyperosmia is rare, but can occur, for example, in cystic fibrosis.

Carriage of odors may be abnormal due to disorders of nasal ventilation, particularly polypi and inflammation due to foreign bodies.

Hyposmia, anosmia, and olfactory hallucinations – reversible or irreversible, acute or chronic – may be caused by single or repeated contact with certain noxious agents.

10% cases of hyposmia, anosmia or parosmia are due to injury to the skull. Concussion usually leads to hyposmia whereas contusion causes anosmia, in about 20% of cases. About 30% of olfactory disorders resolve spontaneously, with the exception of anosmia. The latter is now recognized as a cause of reduced earning capacity, of about 10%, or even as much as 20%, in some occupations.

Nasal Cavity

Airstream

Bidder (1844) showed that the air passes for preference along the floor of the nose and the inferior meatus during quiet respiration, whereas in deep breathing it passes along the medial wall more superiorly and posteriorly (Rethi, 1900). If the agger nasi is well developed a groove lies between it and the dorsum of the nose through which part of the air is conducted into the olfactory region (Fick, 1864). Further investigations were carried out by Paulsen (1882, 1885), Zuckerkandl (1893) etc. In the normal nose during quiet respiration the air initially passes in a superior direction; then it turns backwards at the anterior end of the middle turbinate (see Fig. 17 in Naumann, 1966). Next it flows medial to the middle nasal concha, and passes downwards at the posterior end of the concha towards the nasopharynx. There is little air movement in the roof of the nose (Rethi, 1900). A whirlpool arises in the inferior nasal meatus. The airstream is deflected by mucosal thickenings or cartilaginous or bony projections. Stoksted (1952) and others have investigated the airstream in the nasal cavity and reported similar findings. The shape of the external nose is said to affect the airstream (Fig. 18 and 19 in Naumann, 1966). During inspiration and expiration the airstream in 80% of humans amounts to about 200 ml/s and at the beginning and end of the respiratory phase, to about 150 ml/s (Jost et al., 1973; Wegener, 1983; Lenz et al., 1985).

Intranasal Investigations and Operations

Ethmoidal Labyrinth, Intranasal Procedures on the Sphenoidal and Frontal Sinuses

(Figs. **166**, **167**)

General Remarks

This method was used many years ago by Mikulicz (1886), Halle (1906) and Dahmer (1909). In 1912 Stenger reported his experiences with clearance of the ethmoid cells and the neighboring paranasal sinuses. He used his own modification of Heymann's forceps to identify the ethmoidal bulla as the first step. He showed that the multilocular system of the ethmoidal cells is divided from the neighboring structures by smooth, even, bony surfaces, and that the walls of the ethmoidal cells are usually perpendicular to these party walls. After wide opening of the ethmoidal bulla he used Hartmann's conchotome to remove the thin bony laminae of the anterior and posterior ethmoidal labyrinth, without tearing or breaking them.

The frontal sinus too can be exposed and its duct widened via this endonasal approach.

Opening of the sphenoidal sinus is the simplest procedure of all. Anatomical conditions determine whether the medial nasal concha should be removed (Kastenbauer, 1975). The lateral part of the anterior wall of the sphenoidal sinus is thinner than the medial part, so that this area provides ready access. Earlier authors as well as Kasten-

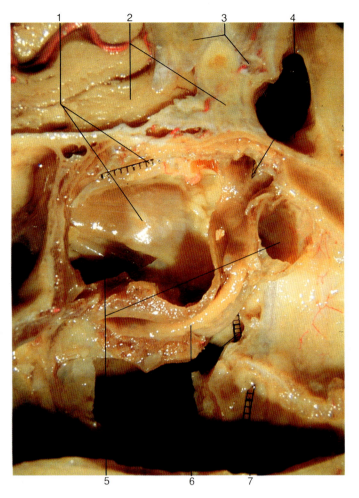

Fig. **166** Ethmoidal arteries after the removal of the superior ethmoidal cells and the orbital plate (view from the right side in a 72-year-old woman)
1 Medial rectus muscle and a millimeter strip
2 Gyrus rectus and crista galli
3 Falx cerebri and anterior falceal artery
4 Frontal sinus and a millimeter strip in the frontal ostium
5 Inferior rectus muscle and agger cells
6 Uncinate process and a millimeter strip in the maxillary ostium (far anterior)
7 Millimeter strip in the nasal lacrimal duct

bauer (1975) have demonstrated the dangers of operations on the ethmoid bone and sphenoidal cavity, and draw attention particularly to the fact that the cribriform plate can sometimes lie very low; in 70% of cases it lies 4–7 mm below the level of the immediately lateral ethmoidal cell, and in 18% of cases 8–16 mm below this plane (Keros, 1962) (Fig. **168**). Kastenbauer also emphasizes the close relationship of the sphenoidal sinus to the neighboring nerves and the cavernous sinus. Intranasal ethmoidal operations are carried out in a relatively narrow field. Rarefaction due to pressure by polyps or secondary inflammation may have destroyed the orbital plate of the ethmoid bone already. Furthermore the inflamed mucosa may be adherent to the periorbital fascia which tears allowing the orbital contents to be grasped. If the orbital wall is pierced, the medial rectus and superior oblique muscles are usually injured (see Fig. **166**). Sometimes the inferior ramus of the

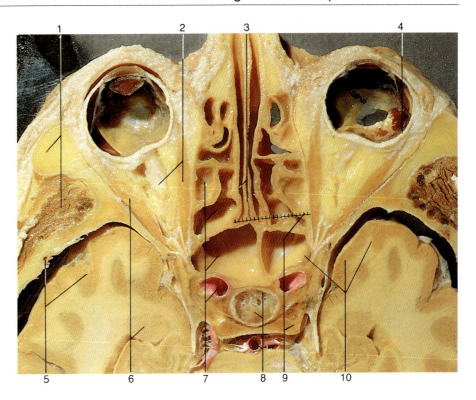

Fig. **167** The ethmoidal labyrinth and neighboring structures in transverse section from below

1 Zygomatic bone and temporal muscle
2 Optic nerve and medial rectus muscle
3 Superior segment of the nasal cavity, and the nasal septum
4 Sclera of the bulb
5 Middle meningeal artery, frontal ramus and temporal lobe
6 Lateral rectus muscle and amygdaloid body
7 Ethmoidal cells, sphenoidal sinus and anterior genu of the internal carotid artery
8 Hypophyseal cistern, stalk of the hypophysis and basilar artery
9 Millimeter strip and dorsum sellae
10 Prominence of the optic canal and temporal pole

oculomotor nerve, and more rarely its superior ramus, may also be damaged.

During the last ten years, Wigand and his team have paid particular attention to refinements of intranasal surgery. An attempt is made to clear the diseased mucosa in chronic sinusitis, and in diffuse polypoid-hypoplastic mucosal disease of the sinus, preserving apparently healthy tissue. The aim is to create a wide opening of the nasal cavity lined with mucosa and communicating with the sinus. Polypi and diseased mucosa are removed. Wigand emphasises that the secretion of the nasal sinuses, except for that of the frontal sinus, drains through a superiorly placed ostium in the upright posture. The isthmus (or sphincter) must be enlarged if it is swollen (Fig. **169**).

Inlet Sphincter

A circular or lip-shaped vascular plexus is present at the entrance of the nasal sinuses that possibly provides a sphincter mechanism (Zange, 1940).

Foci of sinusitis often lie in hidden cells and niches of the sinus, for example in the prelacrimal recess of the maxillary sinus, the maxilloethmoidal junctional area and in the anterolateral ethmoidal segment. The bullous conchae as well as the septal recesses of the buccal and sphenoidal cavities also require attention. *Accurate knowledge of topographic anatomy* and modern instruments are *absolute prerequisites* for surgery of the sinuses. This operation is one of the most dangerous of ear, nose and throat surgery (Wigand, 1981).

Dangers. The operation often begins with a septal correction to improve the airflow and the view of the superior ethmoidal region. The middle nasal concha is removed with the exception of the part of the turbinate bordering anteriorly and laterally on the cribriform plate. The olfactory filaments with their CSF sheaths run in this area,

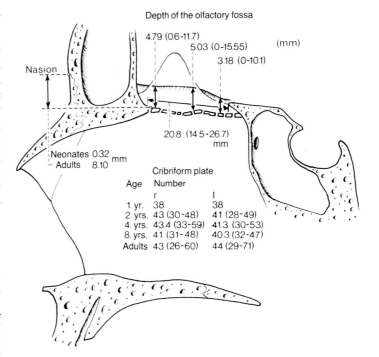

Fig. **168** Relation of the cribriform plate to the nasion, number of cribriform foramina (Schmidt, 1974, 1975) and depth of the anterior, middle and posterior segments of the olfactory fossa (Lang and Haas, 1988). The length of the upper surface of the cribriform plate is also given

carrying the *danger of CSF leak*. The posterior ethmoidal cells are splayed apart exposing the entrance to the *sphenoidal cavity*. In our material the ostium of the sphenoid sinus lay 4.8 (0.6–9.0) mm from the midline (Pahnke, 1986). The internal carotid artery lying in the cavernous sinus may on occasion lie only 4 mm away.

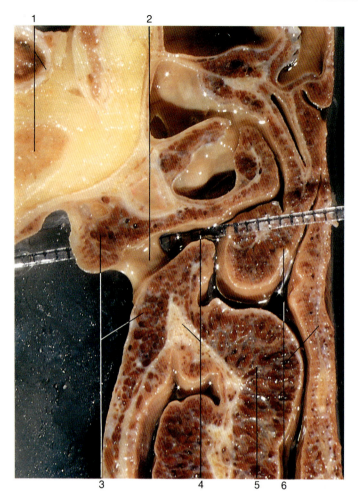

Fig. **169**   Thickened mucosa in the ostium of the sinus
1 Dura of the optic nerve and the inferior rectus muscle
2 Maxillary ostium
3 Thickened mucosa at the maxillary ostium (inlet sphincter)
4 Millimeter strip in the accessory ostium, and uncinate process
5 Thickened mucosa of the inferior concha
6 Middle nasal concha and nasal septum

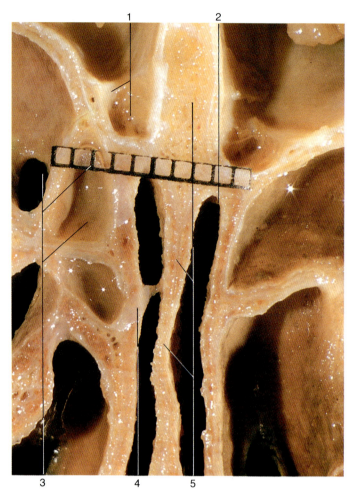

Fig. **170**   Cribriform plates lying at different levels, and anterior tentorium of the olfactory fossa in frontal section from behind
1 Anterior olfactory tentorium, and anterior wall of the olfactory fossa
2 Narrow roof of the nasal cavities lying at different levels
3 Ethmoidal cells and millimeter strip
4 Conchal lamina, and mucosa
5 Crista galli and perpendicular plate of the ethmoidal bone

Bleeding from branches of the posterior septal rami is dealt with by biopolar coagulation forceps. The anterior wall of the sphenoidal sinus is then removed.

The cell walls of the *ethmoidal labyrinth* are not removed completely. The course of the *ethmoidal artery, vein and nerves* is usually visible: they are preserved. Fig. **118** demonstrates the level of their canals relative to the cribriform plate. The left and right cribriform plates do not lie in the same transverse plane in 80% of cases (Fig. **170**). Figs. **127** and **128** show the paramedian distances of the ostia of the sphenoidal sinus from the midline, their breadth and their relationship to the wall of the ethmoidal labyrinth. Fig. **167** is a transverse section through this region. The agger nasi must usually be resected in order to reach the anterior ethmoidal cells. Then the ethmoidal infundibulum and the frontonasal duct as far as the frontal infundibulum are widened by Killian's method (Fig. **171**).

Fig. **92** shows the distance between the posterior surface of the anterior wall of the frontal sinus and the anterior edge of the cribriform plate. The sphenoidal plane grows during the postnatal period and projects over the upper surface of the cribriform plate. Fig. **168** also shows the number of the cribriform foramina. The height of the nasion above the cribriform plate, its position relative to the lowest point of the saddle at the root of the nose, the depth of the olfactory fossa and the height of the superior wall of the ethmoidal labyrinth are indicated.

Maxillary Sinus

Antroscopy

Onodi in 1906 was amongst the first to recommend opening of the maxillary antrum from the middle meatus. According to his data, the medial wall of the antrum between the middle and inferior concha is 30–40 mm long and 15 mm high. The first attempt at direct observation of the maxillary antrum using an optical instrument was made by Hirschmann in 1901 (Draf, 1978). Valentin (1903) carried out endoscopy of the nasopharynx; he was followed by

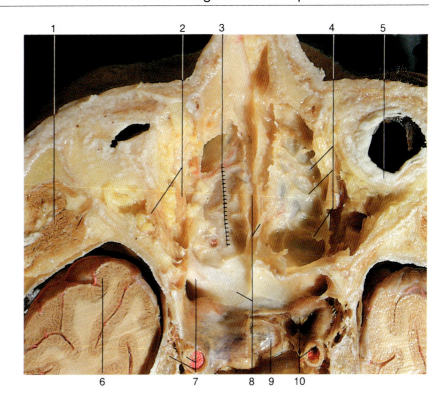

Fig. **171**   Roof of the ethmoidal labyrinth and surrounding area from below
1 Temporalis muscle
2 Section through inferior and medial rectus muscles
3 Anterior ethmoidal artery, nerve and canal, and millimeter strip
4 Walls of the ethmoidal cells forming the upper part of the ethmoidal labyrinth
5 Sclera of the bulb
6 Temporal pole
7 Prominence of the optic canal, internal carotid artery and trigeminal ganglion
8 Roof of the nasal cavity, nasal septum and roof of the sphenoidal sinus
9 Diaphragma sellae with the pituitary gland removed on this side
10 Internal carotid artery showing its course within the cavernous sinus

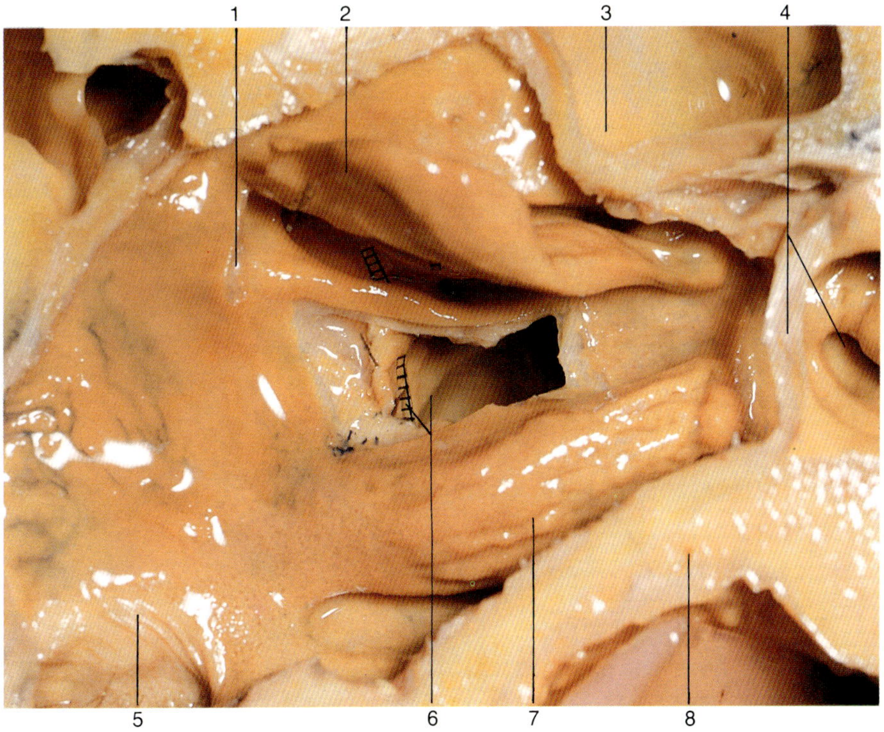

Fig. **172**   Maxillary sinus opened widely in the middle meatus
1 Area of the middle nasal concha which has been removed
2 Middle nasal concha retracted superiorly
3 Sphenoidal sinus
4 Remnants of mucosa of the medial wall of the choane and the ostium of the pharyngotympanic tube
5 System of folds at the limen nasi
6 Large opening of the maxillary sinus with a millimeter strip
7 Inferior nasal concha
8 Palatine glands

Spielberg (1922), Maltz (1925), Portmann (1926) and others. According to Zarniko (1940) this type of endoscopy "gives more the impression of being an interesting toy than an essential method of investigation".

Transmaxillary ethmoidectomy is also carried out if the maxillary sinus needs to be cleared for a patient with ethmoidal sinusitis. In this case a contact surface with the posterior ethmoidal labyrinth of sufficient size is present in only 70% of cases (Rudez, 1966; cited by Terrahe and Muendnich, 1974). If the medial wall of the antrum is displaced laterally, and part of the orbital floor borders directly on the nasal cavity, the orbit may be opened. If the maxillo-ethmoidal party wall is then punched out with forceps the sphenopalatine artery may be damaged. In Wigand's hands the last step of radical clearance is to create a wide antrostomy in the middle meatus.

Fig. **172** shows the maxillary sinus opened medially. The upper part of the antrum is the commonest site for recurrence of polypi, so that the maxillary sinus should be opened from the middle meatus (Wigand, 1986). At the moment Wigand regards ethmoidal procedures with clearance of the sphenoid sinus as indicated only for diffuse polyposis. For circumscribed inflammatory disease he chooses access via the middle meatus, opens the semilunar hiatus and then the neighboring ethmoid cells. The distance between the fossa for the lacrimal sac and the nasolacrimal canal anteriorly, and the sphenopalatine foramen and pterygomaxillary canal or the greater palatine canal with its nerves and vessels is very important in all intranasal operations on the walls of the ethmoidal labyrinth. These distances are shown in Fig. **151** which also records the distances to the center of the pharyngotympanic tube, and to the soft palate, as well as the width of the canal.

Draf (1986) described clearance of the ethmoidal labyrinth and the sphenoidal cavity, and widening of the frontonasal ostium (or duct). After displacing, and possibly removing, the middle nasal concha he first widens the frontonasal duct and then clears the ethmoidal labyrinth in whose superior wall the ethmoidal canals, particularly those of the ethmoidal arteries, serve as landmarks. The anterior ethmoidal canal runs 2 (4–11) mm above the cribriform plate (Fig. **118**), the tertiary ethmoidal canal 1 (1.1–3.25) mm above it and the posterior ethmoidal canal 1.5 (0.84–3.1) mm above it (Lang and Haas, 1988). Dehiscences of varying lengths were found in the course of the anterior ethmoidal canal in 93% of cases, in the tertiary ethmoidal canal in 39% and in the posterior ethmoidal canal in 59% of cases. The contents of the ethmoidal canal should be preserved. Differences in the height of the cribriform plate between the two sides must be looked for carefully. The sphenoidal sinus is opened from in front after clearance of the ethmoidal labyrinth. The posterior end of the middle nasal concha should be preserved as a landmark for possible future surgery. Knowledge of the relationship of the neighboring internal carotid artery and the cranial nerves is very important during clearance of the

sphenoidal sinus (further details are described in the section on prominences within the sphenoid sinus on pages 91 and 92). The nasolacrimal canal and the position of the sphenopalatine foramen and the greater palatine canal must be carefully respected during all these procedures. Access is wider above through the posteroinferior course of the nasolacrimal canal and the anteroinferior course of the greater palatine canal than in the lower segment. Further details are given in Fig. **151**. Figs. **94** and **95** show the anteroposterior extent of the frontal sinus, the thickness of its anterior and posterior walls, and the height of the nasion and the paranasion relative to the cribriform plate. Fig. **122** records the diameter of the ethmoidal canals. The mean diameter was measured in the orbital area, in the central area and at the intracranial foramina. The course of the septal branches on the anterior wall of the sphenoid sinus must be respected during the approach to the sphenoid sinus. These arteries can be up to 1.5 mm thick (see Fig. **157**).

Antral Irrigation

The antrum is usually irrigated through either the inferior nasal meatus (sharp irrigation) or the semilunar hiatus of the maxillary infundibulum (blunt irrigation). In sharp irrigation the lateral nasal wall in the inferior nasal meatus is pierced, the contents of the maxillary sinus are sucked out, irrigated, or a drug instilled.

For blunt irrigation local anesthesia of the middle nasal meatus is first induced; then the ostium of the maxillary sinus is found, and a blunt, curved irrigation cannula is passed into the maxillary sinus. Fig. **100** shows the relation of the maxillary infundibulum to various landmarks such as the limen nasi, the apex of the nose, the base of the nose and the posterior edge of the nares (subnasale). In our most recent material the entrance to the antral cavity most commonly lay in the posterior half (see Fig. **116**, page 80).

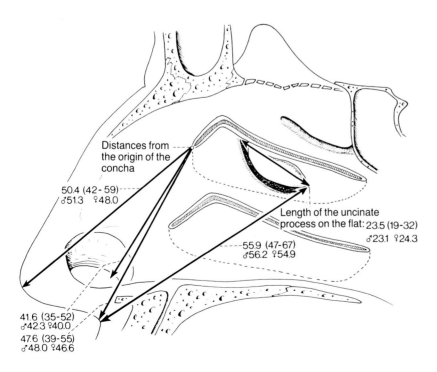

Distances from the origin of the concha

50.4 (42- 59)
♂51.3 ♀48.0

Length of the uncinate process on the flat: 23.5 (19-32)
♂23.1 ♀24.3

55.9 (47-67)
♂56.2 ♀54.9

41.6 (35-52)
♂42.3 ♀40.0
47.6 (39-55)
♂48.0 ♀46.6

Fig. **173** Distances between the anterior attachment of the middle nasal concha and the tip of the nose, the posterior part of the lower edge of the nares (laterally) and the cutaneous subnasale. The distance between the cutaneous subnasale and the posterior edge of the uncinate process, and this length measured in a straight line are also given (Lang and Bressel, 1988)

Diagnostic and Surgical Landmarks

Fig. **173** records the distance between the most anterior point of attachment of the middle nasal concha, and the nasal apex, the lower edge of the nares and the subspinale. The distance between the subnasale and the posterior edge of the uncinate process is also shown. An area of attachment of the middle nasal concha can often be found immediately above the posterior edge of the ethmoidal bulla. The conchal lamina, that is the area of attachment of the middle nasal concha to the lateral edge of the cribriform plate, therefore extends as far as this area.

Anterior edge of the uncinate process: Fig. **174** shows the distances between the anterior edge of the uncinate process and the tip of the nose, the limen nasi, the base of the nose and the subnasale. The distance between the limen nasi and the anterior attachment of the middle nasal concha can also be seen.

Olfactory fossa and olfactory filaments: The anterior part of the bony olfactory fossa is 5.9 (1–16) mm deep, and its posterior third 4.8 (1–10) mm deep. The distances between the cribriform plate and the highest point of the ethmoidal labyrinth are 6.9 (2–18) mm in the anterior third, and 5.8 (2–18) mm in the posterior third. A shallow fossa (1–3 mm deep) is found in about 12% of cases, a fossa of modest depth (2–4 mm) in 17% and a deep fossa (8–16 mm) in about 18% of cases (Keros, 1962). In our material there was usually a posterior step between the anterior edge of the sphenoidal plane and the cribriform plate, measuring about 2 mm (Schmidt, 1974). The deepest intracranial point of the cribriform plate in our material on both the right and left sides lay 7.9 (0.2–17) mm below the nasion. During the postnatal period the olfactory fossa usually deepens by accretion and enlargement of the frontal sinus and the ethmoidal cells. The roof and medial wall of these paranasal sinuses is usually provided by the frontal bone, but sometimes the ethmoidal bone also shares in the provision of the roof of the ethmoidal cells. The deepest point of the cribriform plate lies 13.5 mm above the Frankfurt horizontal in the newborn, and 21.1 mm above it in the adult. In the two-year-old the medial endofrontal fovea for the gyrus rectus of the frontal lobe of the brain lies 20 mm above the Frankfurt horizontal, and in adults 27.2 mm above it (see Lang et al., 1976).

The *olfactory bulb* (Fig. **175**) in our material was 12.2 (6–16) mm long. Its anterior pole lay 8.9 (0–24) mm from the rounded transition to the anterior wall of the anterior cranial fossa (Lang and Reiter, 1985). The central processes of the olfactory cells consist of non-myelinated fibers 0.2 micron thick (Seifert, 1970) that unite with other similar olfactory cells to form the olfactory filaments. Ten, to more than 100, axones are thus ensheathed, initially by supporting cells, then by Schwann cells and by processes of the dura mater of the olfactory fossa. We also found *arachnoid sheaths* of the olfactory filaments penetrating the cribriform plate. The olfactory filaments then penetrate the anterior, inferior and posterior surface of the olfactory bulb (Lang, 1983; Lang, 1985). We also observed thin veins of the frontal lobe of the brain connecting with the veins of the nasal cavity through the cribriform plate (Fig. **175**).

Optic Canal: Medial Approach

(Fig. **176**)

Neighboring Paranasal Sinuses

In 1952 Hooper described 58 patients with orbital complications after cranial trauma. Decompression of the optic nerve is unsuccessful for sudden and complete blindness, but often achieves partial recovery for progressive loss of vision. He decompressed the optic canal from above using a neurosurgical approach (Fukado, 1981). In adults, Fukado first induces local anesthesia and then makes a skin incision 40 mm long between the medial end of the eyebrow and the lacrimal sac; then he removes a 10×15 mm piece of

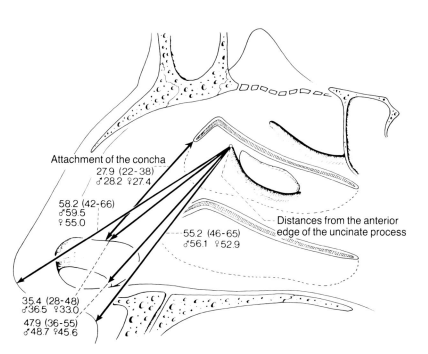

Fig. **174** Distances between the anterior edge of the attachment of the uncinate process and the tip of the nose, the limen nasi, the posterior edge of the nares and the subnasale. The distance between the most anterior point of attachment of the medial nasal concha and the limen nasi is also shown (Lang and Bressel, 1988)

Attachment of the concha
27.9 (22-38)
♂28.2 ♀27.4

58.2 (42-66)
♂59.5
♀55.0

55.2 (46-65)
♂56.1 ♀52.9

Distances from the anterior edge of the uncinate process

35.4 (28-48)
♂36.5 ♀33.0

47.9 (36-55)
♂48.7 ♀45.6

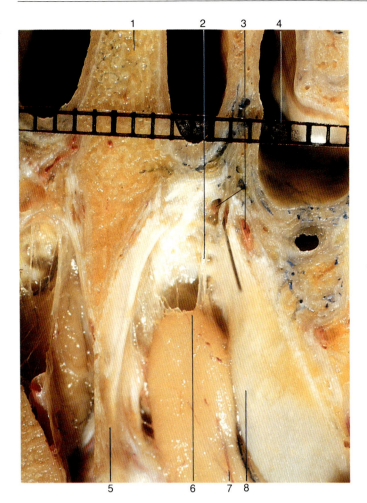

Fig. **175** Olfactory filaments with pial sheath, from above, in an 89-year-old subject
1 Perpendicular plate of the ethmoidal bone
2 Olfactory filament in its pial sheath
3 Anterior ethmoidal artery running to the cribroethmoidal foramen
4 Nasofrontal duct (millimeter strip)
5 Falx cerebri
6 Apex of the olfactory bulb
7 Olfactory tract with a branch of the anterior cerebral artery
8 Lateral wall of the olfactory fossa

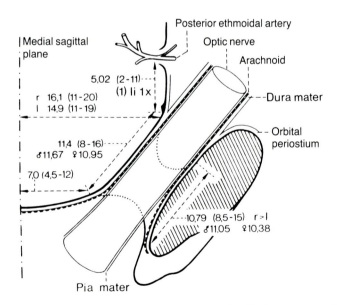

Fig. **176** Distances of the intracranial and orbital apertures of the optic canal from the midline, and from the posterior ethmoidal foramen. The lengths of the medial and lateral wall of the optic canal, and sex differences are also shown (Lang and Oehmann, 1976; Lang and Roth, 1984; Lang and Schlehahn, 1978; Lang and Reiter, 1985)

bone from the junction between the frontal process of the maxilla, the frontal bone and the ethmoidal bone. Next he anesthetizes the mucosa of the ethmoidal cells, and removes the labyrinthine septa. The medial wall of the orbit must *not* be removed initially to avoid damage to the optic nerve. The posterior ethmoidal cells lie at a depth of 40–45 mm, and the optic canal produces a prominence in these cells. Then he proceeds from the deepest segment of this ethmoidal cell to the medial wall of the orbit, and removes a piece of bone about 10 mm in size. This opening provides a view of the medial wall of the optic canal, and it is widened as far as possible. Fukado (1981) stresses the occasional anatomical variations: for example the optic canal may run deeply, at the superior end of the ethmoidal labyrinth, or may produce a prominence within the ethmoidal labyrinth. For these cases he recommends removing the roof of the ethmoidal labyrinth after perforating the medial wall of the orbit; the white optic nerve with its sheath of dura then comes into view. He controls bleeding from the neighboring bone and mucosa with adrenalin solution. The operation ends with closure of the periosteum of the maxilla and the frontal bone, and then of the skin. Data about the relative position of the medial wall of the optic canal to the paranasal sinuses are therefore clinically very important. In the material described by van Alyea (1941) there was a marked projection of the optic canal into the sphenoidal sinus in 40% of cases, and a slight protrusion in 7% (Fig. **134**). The optic canal is usually visible from the

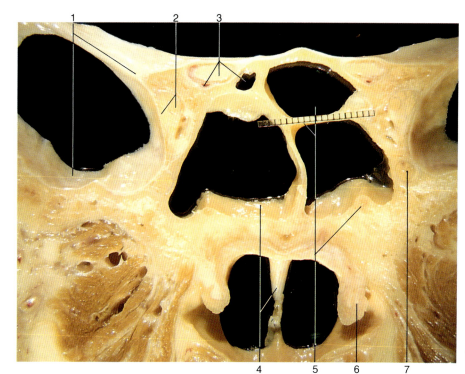

Fig. **177** Onodi cell in frontal section, seen from behind

1 Floor of the middle cranial fossa and lesser wing of the sphenoid bone
2 Ophthalmic and oculomotor nerves
3 Ophthalmic artery, optic nerve and Onodi cell
4 Floor of the sphenoidal sinus and medial boundary of the choanae
5 Large Onodi cell, millimeter strip and pterygoid canal
6 Tubal cartilage
7 Maxillary nerve

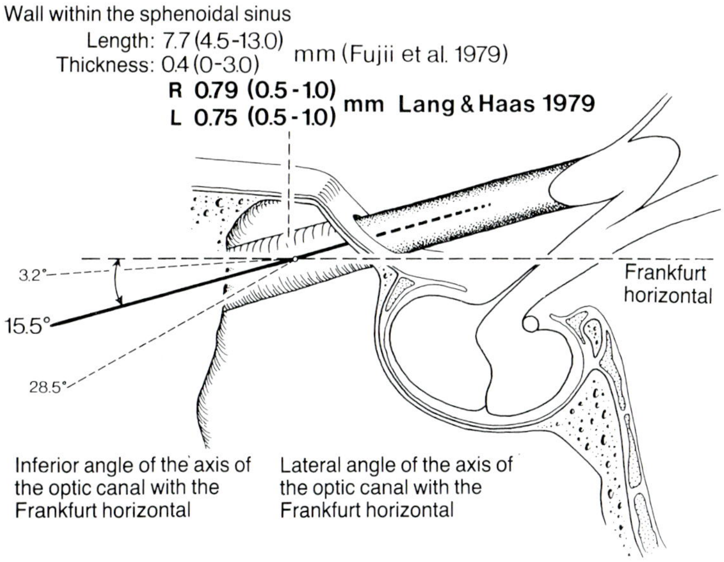

Fig. **178** Axis of the optic canal, and the thickness of the medial wall of the canal (Fujii et al., 1979; Lang and Oehmann, 1976). The axis of the optic canal in our material ran anteroinferiorly at an angle of 15.5° (3.2°–28.5°). Furthermore it ran at an angle of 39.1° (33°–44.5°) in a lateral direction. The thickness of the optic canal relative to the posterosuperior ethmoidal cells was also measured by Lang and Haas (1979)

Wall within the sphenoidal sinus
Length: 7.7 (4.5-13.0)
Thickness: 0.4 (0-3.0)   mm (Fujii et al. 1979)
R 0.79 (0.5 - 1.0)
L 0.75 (0.5 - 1.0)   mm Lang & Haas 1979

3.2°
15.5°
28.5°

Frankfurt horizontal

Inferior angle of the axis of the optic canal with the Frankfurt horizontal

Lateral angle of the axis of the optic canal with the Frankfurt horizontal

sphenoid sinus (Fujii et al., 1979). In our material the medial wall of the optic canal bordered the sphenoid sinus in 80% of cases. Depending on the size of the sphenoid sinus, this segment of the wall is therefore of varying thickness and length. The wall is 0.1–0.4 mm thick in 70% of cases, 0.5–0.9 mm in 14%, less than 0.1 mm in 4% and more than 8 mm in 8%: in some cases no bony wall can be found (Fujii et al., 1979). The prominence of the optic canal is 7.7 (4.5–13) mm long. The axis of the optic canal relative to the Frankfurt horizontal declines anteroinferiorly at an angle of 15.5° (3.2°–28.5°) (Lang and Oehmann, 1976) (Fig. **178**). Furthermore the canal runs from posteromedially in an anterolateral direction at an angle of 39.1° (33°–44.4°) with the midline sagittal plane in adults. Lang (1979) provides details about the postnatal

change in this angle. In our material, the medial wall of the optic canal was 11.4 (8–16) mm long. The intracranial foramen of the canal lay 7.0 (4.5–12) mm from the midline, the intraorbital foramen lay 16.1 (11–20) mm from the midline on the right side and 14.9 (11–19) mm from the midline on the left side (Lang and Oehmann, 1976; Lang and Reiter, 1985). The entrance to the canal for the posterior ethmoidal artery lay 5 (1–11) mm in front of the orbital aperture of the optic canal (Lang and Schlehahn, 1978) (Fig. **176**). Opening of the medial wall of the optic canal demonstrates a dural – endocranial layer representing a transitional zone between the cerebral dura mater and the orbital periosteum and the dural sheath of the optic nerve. Beneath this dural layer lies the arachnoid of the optic nerve, then the subarachnoid space and finally the pia

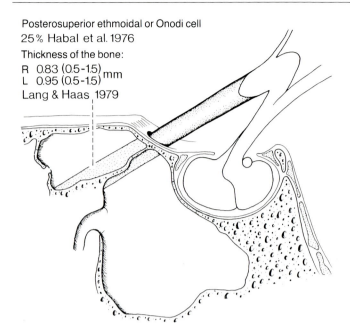

Posterosuperior ethmoidal or Onodi cell
25% Habal et al. 1976

Thickness of the bone:
R 0.83 (0.5-1.5)
L 0.95 (0.5-1.5) mm
Lang & Haas, 1979

Fig. **179**   Incidence of ocurrence of a posterosuperior ethmoidal cell in the upper wall of the optic canal; the thickness of the bone separating it from the optic canal is also shown

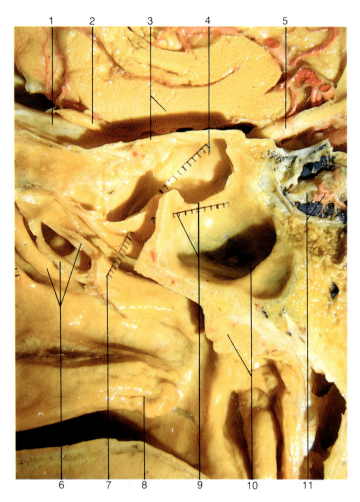

Fig. **180**   Onodi cell with deep position of the aperture and the sphenoidal sinus
1   Lateral wall of the olfactory fossa
2   Olfactory bulb displaced superiorly
3   Sphenoidal plane and gyrus rectus
4   Optic canal bordered by an Onodi cell
5   Intracranial segment of the optic nerve
6   Ethmoidal bulla and medial nasal concha, cut edges
7   Millimeter strip in the ostium of the Onodi cell
8   Inferior nasal concha
9   Boundary zone between the sphenoidal sinus and Onodi cell, and a millimeter strip in the mucosal ostium of the sphenoidal sinus
10 Sphenoidal sinus and pharyngeal tonsil
11 Internal carotid artery, anterior genu in the cavernous sinus and caroticocavernous branch

mater of the optic nerve. Below the optic nerve the ophthalmic artery lies embedded in this dural-endocranial sheath for a varying length. In the material reported by Habal et al. (1976) the upper wall of the optic canal was surrounded by a posterosuperior ethmoidal cell in 25% of cases. The bone in these cases was 0.8 (0.5–1.5) mm thick on the right side, and 0.9 (0.5–1.5) mm on the left side (Lang and Haas, 1979) (Fig. **178**). In our material the ophthalmic artery overlapped the medial side of the optic canal in the orbit in 16% of cases and therefore is in danger of injury (Engel, 1975). The optic canal itself demonstrates a narrow zone in the center of the canal that we termed the isthmus. In adults it is 4.6 (4–5.1) mm wide and 5.1 (1.1–6.2) mm high (Lang and Oehmann, 1976). A junctional zone of the arteries supplying the optic nerve lies within the optic canal. The intracranial part of the nerve is supplied by branches of the internal carotid, the ophthalmic and anterior cerebral arteries, whereas the intraorbital part is supplied by branches of the central retinal artery (Lang, 1983). The anterior origin of the superior oblique muscle can lie close to the posterior ethmoidal canal (Lang, 1983).

Injury to the ethmoidal arteries can usually be controlled by packing. Fracture of the cell walls of the ethmoidal bone can open up the anterior cranial fossa or lead to tearing of the dura, causing a CSF leak. Spontaneous CSF leak may follow opening of small meningocoeles which may be single or multiple congenital defects (Fig. **181**).

Infections Spreading from the Paranasal Sinuses to the Orbit

Inflammation of the orbit secondary to disease of the paranasal sinuses was reported by Beer in 1819, by Juengken in 1832 and by Berger and Tyrman in 1886 (Onodi, 1915). Two-thirds of orbital inflammations are said to be secondary to disease of the sphenoidal sinus (Berger and

Tyrman, 1886). 67% of all inflammations arise primarily in the nasal sinuses, 32% from the frontal sinus, 22% from the maxillary sinus, 20% from the ethmoidal cells, 6% from the sphenoidal sinus, and 15% from several sinuses (Birch-Hirschfeld; cited by Onodi, 1915). 16% of patients demonstrated permanent blindness, and 12% a temporary disorder of vision. Disease of the lacrimal drainage system spreads via the nasal route in 94% (Kuhnt; cited by Onodi, 1915).

Orbital complications of sinusitis have become much less common since the introduction of antibiotics. Bockmuehl (1963) reported a 4% incidence of orbital and eyelid complications, mostly in children. Probst (1973) observed a

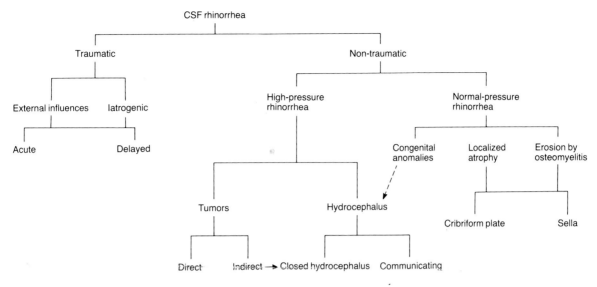

Fig. **181**   Diagram of traumatic and nontraumatic causes of CSF rhinorrhea (Freeland, 1973)

progressive paralysis of the oculomotor muscles lying at the supraorbital margin and the medial canthus following maxillary and ethmoidal sinusitis. Our studies show that the ethmoidal veins in particular are responsible for the spread of infection to the orbit. Their tributaries originate from the ethmoidal cells and the sphenoidal sinus. Fig. **158** records the width of these veins and the orbital foramina, in the centre of the ethmoidal canal and at the intracranial foramina. Dural veins also flow into the ethmoidal veins. The course of the nasolacrimal duct probably also represents a further danger zone. This area is surrounded by a dense venous network that communicates with the veins of the nasal cavity and of the fossa for the lacrimal sac (Fig. **148**).

Blindness after Intranasal Operations

Total blindness or restriction of the field of vision may follow pansinusitis (Gold et al., 1974; Plate and Asboe, 1981; Silberstein, 1906; Zahn, 1910; Rowe et al., 1967). Defects of the field of vision were observed in about 0.2% of cases after a nasal operation in one series (Plate and Asboe, 1981). These may be due to the following:

1) Vascular injury.
2) Direct mechanical trauma to the optic nerve.

The vascular damage can be propagated by intra-arterial injection of anesthetic agents into the ethmoidal and ophthalmic arteries. Injection of adrenaline or noradrenaline into the mucosa of the nasal septum was probably the cause of an arterial spasm or thromboembolus in two further patients. Blindness in one eye has been recorded after injection of cortisone into the anterior segment of the inferior nasal concha; the posterior ethmoidal artery is the probable pathway of spread to the central retinal artery (Heise, 1962). Sudden severe disturbances of vision have been reported after division of the posterior ethmoidal artery (Zange, 1950). The vascular stumps may retract into the orbital periostium and retrobulbar fatty tissue, and there cause a hematoma that strangulates the central retinal artery. The bones bounding the orbit in minimal poly-

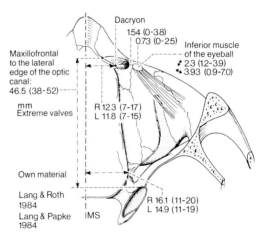

Fig. **182**   Breadth of the ethmoidal labyrinth in its anterior part (between the dacryon and median sagittal plane), as well as at the anterior (orbital) end of the optic canal. The distances between the maxillofrontale and the lateral edge of the optic canal, and the distance between the nasion and the frontozygomatic suture measured in the paramedian sagittal plane and the area of origin of the inferior oblique muscle as well as its relation to the nasolacrimal canal and the inferior orbital margin are also given (Lang and Roth, 1984)

poid lesions are usually robust, but in marked disease are soft and friable (Berendes, 1963). Every nasal surgeon must be completely familiar with the position of the optic nerve relative to the posterior ethmoidal cells (Figs. **176–182**).

Schroeder and Salzmann (1973) found 40 reports of damage to the optic nerve after operations on the nasal sinuses, and added a further five cases. Langnickel (1973) reported unilateral blindness after intranasal ethmoidectomy. He immediately opened the ethmoidal cells via an external incision, decompressed the orbital periostium and coagulated the posterior ethmoidal artery; the vision returned to normal. He thought that the compression or

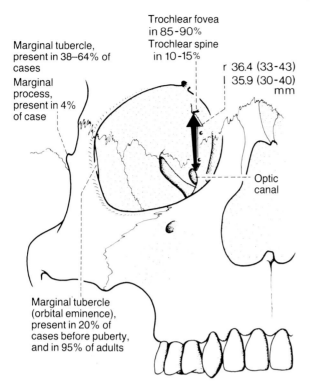

Marginal tubercle, present in 38–64% of cases

Marginal process, present in 4% of case

Trochlear fovea in 85-90%
Trochlear spine in 10-15%

r 36.4 (33-43)
l 35.9 (30-40) mm

Optic canal

Marginal tubercle (orbital eminence), present in 20% of cases before puberty, and in 95% of adults

Fig. **183**   Length between the fovea (trochlear spine) and medial edge of the optic canal. The marginal process (or tubercle) of the zygomatic bone, and the marginal tubercle on the internal side of the lateral orbital cavity are also shown

stretching of the optic nerve was caused by a retrobulbar hematoma.

In our material the medial wall of the optic canal bordered the posterosuperior ethmoidal cell (Onodi cell) in about 12% of cases (Figs. **177, 179**). Figs. **182** and **183** show some of the distances measured within the ethmoidal labyrinth and the optic canal.

Frontal Osteoma and Reversible Blindness

A 23-year-old patient with a large frontal osteoma leading to blindness has been reported: the vision recovered after its removal (Guettich and Mueller, 1967).

Malignant Disease of the Paranasal Sinuses

Macbeth (1965) provides a thorough review of malignant disease of the paranasal sinuses; metastatic carcinoma of the sphenoidal sinuses has been reported by McClatchey et al. (1985).

References

Abbate, L.: Considerazioni su di un anomalia del seno mascellare. Arch. Ital. Otol. 49 (1937) 431

Albinus, B. S.: Tabulae sceleti et musculorum corporis humani. Luydun, Batav. 1747 (cited after P. Eisler 1912)

Ambrus, P. S., R. D. Eavey, A. S. Baker, W. R. Wilson: Management of nasal septal abscess. Laryngoscope 91 (1981) 575–582

Andre, J. M.: Contribution à l'étude des lymphatiques du nez des fosses nasales. Thèsis, Paris 1905

Änggard, A.: The effects of parasympathic nerve stimulation on the microcirculation and secretion in the nasal mucosa of the cat. Acta Otolaryng. (Stockh.) 78 (1974) 98–105

Anton, W.: Zur Kenntnis der congenitalen Deformitäten der Nasenscheidewand. Arch. Ohrenheilk. 35 (1893) 304–308

Arnoldi, W.: Über die Genese der Nasenvorhofzysten. Z. Laryng. Rhinol. 18 (1929) 58

Augier, M.: Cartilage et osselet paraseptal chez le foetus humain. C. R. Ass. Anat. 26 (1931) 3–6

Aymard, J. L.: Some new points in the anatomy of the nasal septum, and their surgical significance. J. Anat. (Lond.) 51 (1917) 293–303

Bach, F.: cited after Martin, R., K. Saller 1957

Bachmann, W.: Die Nasenklappe, ein funktionell falsch verstandener Begriff. Arch. Klin. Exp. Ohr.-, Nas.- u. Kehlk.-Heilk. 194 (1969a) 451–454

Bachmann, W.: Die Topographie des anatomischen Ostium internum der Nase im Hinblick auf seine funktionelle Bedeutung. Z. Laryng. Rhinol. 48 (1969b) 263–270

Bartels, P.: Über Geschlechtsunterschiede am Schädel. Inaugural-Dissertation, Friedrich-Wilhelm-Universität, Berlin 1897

Basler, A.: Die Nasenform bei Chinesen. Z. Morph. Anthropol. 30 (1931) 559–563

Baud, C. A.: Harmonie der Gesichtszüge. Eine Studie über Schönheit, kosmetische Gesichtschirurgie und Mienenspiel. (German translation of the 4th French ed.) S. Karger, Basel, München 1982

Baum, S. J.: Introduction. Ear, Nose Thr. J. 61 (1982) 426–428

Becker, O. J.: Rhinoplasty: cultural, esthetic and psychological aspects. Chicago Med. 64 (1961) 15

Beckmann, G.: Zur Mitbeteiligung der Dura bei frontobasalen Frakturen. HNO 10 (1962) 239–241

Beer (1819): cited after A. Onodi 1915

Beinfield, H.: Treatment of complete unilateral bony atresia of the posterior nares: new technique and brief reference to asphyxia neonatorum. Arch. Otolaryng. 53 (1853) 530 (cited by H. Jung 1977)

Benjamins, C. E.: Mucocele des Sinus sphenoidalis. Arch. Laryng. Rhin. (Berl.) 24 (1910) 353–365

Berendes, J.: Grundsätzliches zur Begutachtung der iatrogenen Erblindung durch Siebbeinoperation. HNO 11 (1963) 25–28

Berendes, J.: Anwendung von Laser-Strahlen in der HNO-Heilkunde. Dtsch. Ärztebl. 74 (1977) 1528

Berg, J.: Bidrag till kännedom om sjukdomar i näsans bihalor samt till läran om cerebrospinalvätskas flytning ur näsan. Nord. Med. Ark. 21 (1889) 1–24

Bergeat, H.: Die Asymmetrien der knöchernen Choanen. Arch. Laryng. Rhin. (Berl.) 4 (1896) 409–420

Berger und Tyrman (1886): cited by A. Onodi 1915

Bidder, F. H.: Article on "Riechen" ("smell") in the Handwörterbuch der Physiologie. Braunschweig 1845 (cited after E. Zuckerkandl 1893)

Blier, Z.: Amer. J. Physiol. 93 (1930) 398 (cited by K. G. Malcolmson 1959)

Blind: Über Nasenbildung bei Neugeborenen. Diss., München 1890

Blum, M. E., A. Larson: Mucocele of the sphenoid sinus with sudden blindness. Laryngoscope (St. Louis) 83 (1973) 2042–2049

Bockmühl, F.: Orbitale Komplikation bei Nebenhöhlenentzündungen und ihre Behandlung. Z. Laryng. Rhinol. 42 (1963) 434–439

Boege, K.: Zur Anatomie der Stirnhöhlen (Sinus frontalis). Diss., Königsberg i. Pr.; Jber. Fortschr. Anat. Entw.-Gesch. 8/III (1903) 22

Boenninghaus, H.-G.: „Blow-out-fracture" des Orbitadaches. Z. Laryng. Rhinol. 48 (1969) 395–398

Bojsen-Møller, F.: Glandulae nasales anteriores in the human nose. Ann. Otol. (St. Louis) 74 (1965) 363

von Bonnsdroff, P.: Untersuchungen über Maßverhältnisse des Oberkiefers mit spezieller Berücksichtigung der Lagebeziehungen zwischen den Zahnwurzeln und der Kieferhöhle. Akademische Abhandlung, Helsingfors 1925

Boyden, G. L.: Etiology of non-traumatic nasal septal deviations. Trans. Pacific Coast Oto-ophthal. Soc. 29 (1948) 150–153

Boyer (1805): cited by E. Zuckerkandl 1893

Brandenburg, N. B.: Polypi of the nasal septum. Arch. Otolaryng. 22 (1935) 328–331

Broca, P.: Recherches sur l'indice nasale. Rev. Anthrop. (Paris) 1 (1872)

Broman, I.: Die knorpeligen Nasenwände. In: Normale und abnormale Entwicklung des Menschen. J. F. Bergmann, Wiesbaden 1911

Brookover, Ch.: The peripheral distribution of the nervus terminalis in an infant. J. Comp. Neurol. 28 (1917) 349–360

Bruck, H., G. Kittinger: Dermoide und Dermoidfisteln der Nase. HNO 11 (1963) 106–111

Brueggermann, A.: Arch. Laryng. Rhin. (Berl.) 33 (1920) 103 (cited by F. Montreuil 1949)

v. Brunn, A.: Beiträge zur mikroskopischen Anatomie der menschlichen Nasenhöhle. Arch. Mikr. Anat. 39 (1982) 632–651

Brusis, T.: Wie können neuralgische Beschwerden nach Kieferhöhlenoperationen vermieden werden? Laryng. Rhinol. Otol. 58 (1979) 54–65

Burger, H.: Das Ganglion spheno-palatinum. Acta Oto-laryng. (Stockh.) 11 (1927) 221–239

Burnstock, G.: Purinergic nerves. Pharmacol. Rev. 24 (1972) 509–580

Busuttil, A., I. A. R. More, D. Mcseveney: A reappraisal of the ultrastructure of the human respiratory nasal mucosa. J. Anat. (Lond.) 124 (1977) 445–458

Bynke, O., C. Radberg: Mucocele of the sphenoidal sinus. Neurochirurgia (Stuttg.) 28 (1985) 28–30

Caldwell, G. W.: Diseases of the accessory sinuses of the nose, and an improved method of treatment for suppuration of the maxillary antrum. N. Y. Med. J. 58 (1893) 526–528

Campbell, R. L., W. Zeman, J. Joyner: Spontaneous rhinorrhea due to pituicytoma. J. Neurosurg. 25 (1966) 208–210

Cauna, N.: The fine structure of the arteriovenous anastomosis and its nerve supply in the human nasal respiratory mucosa. Anat. Rec. 168 (1970a) 9–22

Cauna, N.: Electron microscopy of the nasal vascular bed and its nerve supply. Ann. Otol. (St. Louis) 79 (1970b) 443–450

Cauna, N.: Blood and nerve supply of the nasal lining. In: Proctor D. F., I. B. Andersen: The Nose: Upper Airway Physiology and the Atmospheric Environment. Elsevier, New York 1982

Cauna, N., K. H. Hinderer: Fine structure of blood vessels of the human nasal respiratory mucosa. Ann. Otol. (St. Louis) 78 (1969) 865–885

Chandra, R.: Treatment of a case of crocodile tears by vidian neurorectomy. J. Laryng. 81 (1967) 669–671

Chang, M. M., S. E. Leeman: Isolation of a sialogogic peptide from bovine hypothalamic tissue and its characterization as substance P. J. Biol. Chem. 245 (1970) 4784–4790

Chorobski, J., W. Penfield: Cerebral vasodilator nerves and their pathway from the medulla oblongata, with observations on the pial and intracerebral vascular plexus. Arch. Neurol. Psychiat. (Chic.) 28 (1932) 1257–1289

Christ, B., H. Jacob, R. Seifert: Über die Entwicklung der zerviko-okzipitalen Übergangsregion. In Hohmann, D., B. Kügelgen, K. Liebig: Neuroorthopädie 4. Springer, Berlin 1988 (S. 13–22)

Collignon: Etude anthropométrique élémentaire des principales races en France. Bull. Soc. Anthrop. (Paris) 3 (1883) 463–526 (cited by Martin, R., K. Saller 1957)

Congdon, E. D.: The distribution and mode of origin of septa and walls of the sphenoid sinus. Anat. Rec. 18 (1920) 97–123

Converse, J. M.: The cartilaginous structures of the nose. Ann. Otol. (St. Louis) 64 (1955) 220–229

Cope, V. Z.: The internal structure of the sphenoid sinus. J. Anat. (Lond.) 51 (1917) 127–136

Cottle, M. H.: The structure and function of the nasal vestibule. Arch. Otolaryng. 62 (1955) 173–181

Cottle, M. H., R. M. Loring, G. G. Fischer, I. E. Gaynon: The "maxilla-premaxilla" approach to extensive nasal septum surgery. Arch. Otolaryng. 68 (1958) 301–313

Czermak und Semmeleder: cited by E. Kallius 1905

Dahmer, R.: Die breite Eröffnung der Oberkieferhöhle von der Nase aus, mit Schleimhautplastik und persistierender Öffnung. Arch. Laryng. Rhin. (Berl.) 21 (1909) 325

Dale, B. A. B., I. J. Mackenzie: The complications of sphenoid sinusitis. J. Laryng. 97 (1983) 661–670

Daley, J.: Introduction of an artistic point of view in regard to rhinoplastic diagnosis. Arch. Otolaryng. 42 (1945) 33

Danoff, D., J. Serbu, L. A. French: Encephalocele extending into the sphenoid sinus: report of a case. J. Neurosurg. 24 (1966) 684–686

Davenport, C. B.: Postnatal development of the human outer nose. Proc. Amer. Phil. Soc. 80 (1939) 175–201

Dawes, J. D. K.: The management of frontal sinusitis and its complications. J. Laryngol. 75 (1961) 297–344

de Almeide, C. I. R.: Study of the adenovascular body of the posterior part of the nasal septum. Arch. Otolaryngol. 101 (1975) 344–347

Debakan, A.: Tables of cranial and orbital measurements, cranial volume, and derived indexes in males and females, from 7 days to 20 years of age. Ann. Neurol. 2 (1977) 485–491

Denecke, H. J., H. Hartert: Carotis interna-Verletzung mit unstillbarem Nasenbluten, geheilt durch intra-arterielle Thrombininjektion. Chirurg 25 (1954) 470

Denecke, H. J., R. Meyer: Plastische Operationen am Kopf und Hals. I. Nasenplastik. Springer, Berlin 1964

De Vries, E.: Note on the ganglion vomeronasale. K. Akad. van Wetenschappen te Amsterdam 7 (1905) 704

Diaz, F., R. Latchow, A. J. Duvall, C. A. Quick, D. L. Erickson: Mucoceles with intracranial and extracranial extensions. J. Neurosurg. 48 (1978) 284–288

Diewert, V. M.: A morphometric analysis of craniofacial growth and changes in spatial relations during secondary palatal development in human embryos and fetuses. Amer. J. Anat. 167 (1983) 495–522

Dion, M. C., B. W. Jafek, C. E. Tobin: The anatomy of the nose. Arch. Otolaryng. 104 (1978) 145–150

Dixon, A. D.: The early development of the maxilla. Dent. Pract. It. Dent. Rec. 3 (1952) 331–336 (cited by B. Vidić 1971)

Dixon, F. W.: A comparative study of the sphenoid sinus (a study of 1600 skulls). Ann. Otol. (St. Louis) 46 (1937) 687–698

Doyle, C. S., F. A. Simeone: Mucocele of the sphenoid sinus with bilateral internal carotid artery occlusion. J. Neurosurg. 36 (1972) 351–354

Draf, W.: Klinisch-experimentelle Untersuchungen zur Pathogenese, Diagnostik und Therapie der chronisch entzündlichen Kieferhöhlenerkrankungen unter Verwendung der direkten Beobachtung durch Sinuskopie. Habil.-Schrift, Mainz 1974

Draf, W.: Endoskopie der Nasennebenhöhlen. Technik, typische Befunde, therapeutische Möglichkeiten. Springer, Berlin 1978

Draf, W.: Die chirurgische Behandlung entzündlicher Erkrankungen der Nasennebenhöhlen. Arch. Oto-Rhino-Laryng. 235 (1982) 133–305

Draf, W.: Endoskopie der Nase und der Nasennebenhöhlen. Dtsch. Ärztebl. 80 (1983a) 23–30

Draf, W.: Endoscopy of the Paranasal Sinuses. Springer, Berlin 1983b

Draf, W.: personal communication, 1986

Drake, C. G.: Surgical treatment of ruptured aneurysms of the basilar artery: experience with 14 cases. J. Neurosurg. 23 (1965) 457–473

Drettner, B.: Measurements of the resistance of the maxillary ostium. Acta Oto-Laryng. (Stockh.) 60 (1965) 499–505

Dysart, B. R.: Modern view of neuralgia referable to Meckel's ganglion: report of cases showing relief of pain and sometimes arrest of develop-ment of ulcers of cornea by cocainization of ganglion. Arch. Otolaryngol. 40 (1944) 29–32

Edwards, W. C., R. W. Ridley: Blow-out fracture of medial orbital wall. Amer. J. Ophthal. 65 (1968) 248–249

Eisler, P.: Die Muskeln des Stammes. In: Bardelebens Handbuch des Menschen, Bd. II. Fischer, Jena 1912

Ekblad, E., L. Edvinsson, R. Uddman et al.: Neuropeptide Y coexists and co-operates with noradrenaline in perivascular nerve fibers. Regul. Pept. 8 (1984) 225–235

Eloff, F. C.: On the relations of the human vomer to the anterior paraseptal cartilages. J. Anat. (Lond.) 86 (1952) 16–19

Elwany, S., Y. M. Yacout, M. Talaat, M. El-Nahass, A. Gunied: Surgical anatomy of the sphenoid sinus. J. Laryng. 97 (1983) 227–241

Emmert, C.: Lehrbuch der Chirurgie. Dann, Stuttgart 1851

Engel, A.: Ursprungs- und Verlaufsvariationen der ersten Ophthalmica-Strecke. Diss., Würzburg 1975

Engelmann, T. W.: Über die Flimmerbewegung. Jena. Z. Med. Naturw. 4 (1868)

Erbs (1938): cited after Menger, W., V. Kocoglu 1969

Erhard, H.: Studien über die Flimmerzellen. Arch. Zellforsch. 4 (1910) 309–442

von Euler, U. S., J. H. Gaddum: An undentified depressor substance in certain tissue extracts. J. Physiol. (Lond.) 72 (1931) 74–87

Fahlbusch, R., M. Buchfelder: Present status of neurosurgery in the treatment of prolactinomas. Neurosurg. Rev. 8 (1985) 195–205

Farrior, R. T., M. E. Connolly: Septorhinoplasty in children. Otolaryng. Clin. N. Amer. 3 (1970) 345–364

Fawcett, E.: The development of the human maxilla, vomer and paraseptal cartilages. J. Anat. Physiol. 44 (1911) 378–405

Feingold, M., W. H. Bossert: Normal values for selected physical parameters: an aid to syndrome delineation. Birth Defects 10 (1974) 1

Fenger, C.: Basal hernias of the brain. Amer. J. med. Sci. 109 (1895) 1–17

Fenton, R. A.: Traumatism of the frontal sinuses. Arch. Otolaryng. 40 (1944) 157–159

Fick (1864) in Hermann, L.: Handbuch der Physiologie, Bd. III/2. (cited by E. Zuckerkandl 1893)

Finby, N., E. Kraft: The aging skull: comparative roentgen study, 25 to 34 year interval. Clin. Radiol. 23 (1972) 410–414

Fischer, A. J.: Nasal surgery in children. Arch. Otolaryng. 66 (1957) 497–502

Fleischer: S.-B. phys. med. Soc. Erlangen, 12. Nov. 1877 (cited by F. Merkel 1892)

Fleischmann, A.: Das Kopfskelett der Amnioten. Morphogenetische Studien. Gegenbaurs Morph. Jb. 31 (1903) 560–619

Flesch, M.: Varietäten-Beobachtungen aus dem Präpariersaale zu Würzburg in den Wintersemestern 1875/76 und 1876/77. Verh. Phys.-Med. Ges. Würzb. 13 (1879) 1–38

Fletcher, M. H.: Beobachtungen bei der Untersuchung von 500 Schädeln. Corresp.-Bl. Zahnärzte 25 (1896) 137–145

Fomon, S.: Cosmetic Surgery. Lippincott, Philadelphia 1960

Fomon, S., J. G. Gilbert, A. L. Caron, S. Segal, Jr.: Collapsed ala: pathologic physiology and management. Arch. Otolaryng. 51 (1950) 465–484

Forschner, L.: Über die Gefahr von Blutungen bei Eingriffen am Keilbein. Arch. Ohr.-, Nas.- u. Kehlk.-Heilk. 158 (1950) 271–275

Fowler, E. P., Jr. (1943): cited by Malcolmson, K. G. 1959

Freeland, A. P: Non-traumatic C. S. F. rhinorrhoea associated with congenitally malformed ears. J. Laryng. 87 (1973) 781–786

Friederich, H. C., K. D. Mörike: Über die Dehnbarkeit und Verschieblichkeit der Haut des Gesichtes beim Menschen unter klinischen und experimentellen Aspekten. Arch. Klin. Derm. 215 (1963) 496–512

Friedmann, A. P.: Sur le symptome de la liquorrhée nasale. Encéphale 27 (1932) 129–133

Friedmann, G., S. Harrison: Mucocele of the sphenoidal sinus as a cause of recurrent oculomotor nerve palsy. J. Neurol. Neurosurg. Psychiat. 33 (1970) 172–179

Fritz, K.: Funktionelle Methoden der ästhetischen Gesichtschirurgie einschließlich der Nasenscheidewandchirurgie. Urban & Schwarzenberg, München 1981

Fujii, K., S. M. Chambers, A. L. Rhoton, Jr.: Neurovascular relationships of the sphenoid sinus: a microsurgical study. J. Neurosurg. 50 (1979) 31–39

Fukado, Y.: Microsurgical transethmoidal optic nerve decompression: experience in 700 cases. In: Samii, M., P. J. Janetta: The Cranial Nerves. Springer, Berlin 1981 (pp. 125–128)

Fukushima, T.: Trans-sphenoidal microsurgical treatment of Nelson's syndrome. Neurosurg. Rev. 8 (1985) 185–194

Gherardi, F.: Contributo alla conoscenza della irrorazione sanguinea della mucosa del setto nasale. Otorinolaringol. Ital. 9 (1939) 132–148

Gilbert, J. G., R. Heights, S. Segal: Growth of the nose and the septorhinoplastic problem in youth. Arch. Otolaryng. 68 (1958) 673–682

Gisselsson, L.: Intranasal forms of encephalomeningocele. Acta Otolaryng. (Stockh.) 35 (1947) 519–531

Guiseppe (1942): cited after Salinger, S. 1948

Gold, R. S., L. Silver, E. Sager: Pansinusitis, orbital cellulitis, and blindness as sequelae of delayed treatment of dental abscess. J. Oral Surg. 32 (1974) 40–43

Golding-Wood, P. H.: Observation on petrosal and vidian neurectomy in chronic vasomotor rhinitis. J. Laryng. 75 (1961) 232–247

Golding-Wood, P. H.: Pathology and surgery of chronic vasomotor rhinitis. J. Laryng. 76 (1962) 969–977

Golding-Wood, P. H.: The surgery of nasal allergy. Int. Rhinol. 1 (1963) 188–193

Golding-Wood, P. H.: Vidian neurectomy and other transantral surgery. Laryngoscope 80 (1970) 1179–1189

Golding-Wood, P. H.: Vidian neurotectomy: its results and complications. Laryngoscope 83 (1973) 1673–1683

Goode, R. L.: Personal communications, 1983 (cited by Powell, N., B. Humphreys 1984)

Gray, L.: The deviated nasal septum, I: aetiology. J. Laryng. 79 (1965a) 567–575

Gray, L.: The deviated nasal septum, II: prevention and treatment. J. Laryng. 79 (1965b) 806–816

Grossehelleforth, A., J. Dücker: Sensibilitätsstörungen nach Kieferhöhlenoperationen. In: Schuchardt, K., G. Pfeifer: Fortschritte der Kiefer- und Gesichts-Chirurgie, Bd. XXI. Thieme, Stuttgart 1976 (S. 82–83)

Grote, J. J., W. Kuijpers, P. L. M. Huygen: Selective denervation of the autonomic nerve supply of the nasal mucosa. Acta Oto-Laryng. (Stockh.) 79 (1975) 124–132

Gruber, W.: Seltene Beobachtungen aus dem Gebiete der menschlichen Anatomie. Müllers Arch. (1848) 412–416

Gruber, W.: Über einen neuen Knochen im Antlitze des Menschen, mitgeteilt von Akademiker Baer. Bull. Cl. Physicomath. Acad. Sci. St. Petersbourg 8 (1850) 203–206

Grünwald, L.: Die Nasenmuscheln des Menschen. Dargestellt aufgrund der Entwicklung und des Vergleichs. Anat. H. 54 (1917)

Grünwald, L.: Deskriptive und topographische Anatomie der Nase und ihrer Nebenhöhlen. In Denker, A., O. Kahler: Die Krankheiten der Luftwege und der Mundhöhle. Springer, Berlin, Bergmann, München 1925 (S. 1–95)

Gudziol, H.: Funktionsdiagnostik des N. petrosus major mit Hilfe der Elektrogustometrie des weichen Gaumens und des Schirmer-Testes. Laryng. Rhinol. Otol. 61 (1982) 184–185

Guhrauer: Eine Resectio apicis intra sin. max. und andere Zahn-Nasenfälle. Diss., Berlin 1914 (cited after Schicketanz, H.-W., W. Schicketanz 1961)

Guillerm, R., R. Riu, R. Badré, R. LeDen, J. Hée: Pathophysiologische Aspekte der oberen Luftwege: Nase, Nasennebenhöhle, Ohrtrompete. Arch. Klin. Exp. Ohr.-, Nas.- u. Kehlk.-Heilk. 199 (1971) 1

Guillerm, R.: cited after J. Berendes 1977

Guiot, G.: La stimulation capsulaire chez l'homme: son intérêt dans la stéreotaxie pallidale pour syndromes parkinsoniens. Rev. Neurol. 98 (1958) 222–224

Gulisano, M., P. Pacini, G. E. Orlandini, G. Colosi: Considerazioni anatomo-radiologiche sui seni frontali: ricerca statistica su 520 casi umani. Arch. Ital. Anat. Embriol. 83 (1978) 9–32

Gülzow, J.: Notfall im Bereitschaftsdienst, Nasenbeinfraktur. Dtsch. Ärztebl. 76 (1979) 1690

Gundobin, N. P.: Die Besonderheiten des Kindesalters. Allgemeine Medizinische Verlagsanstalt, Berlin 1921

Gunter, J. P.: Anatomical observations of the lower lateral cartilages. Arch. Otolaryng. 89 (1969) 599–601

Gutsche, P.: Zur Pathogenese der Hypophysentumoren und über nasalen Abfluß sowie das Verhalten des Liquor cerebrospinalis bei einer Struma pituitomata. Int. Zbl. Laryng. 11 (1895) 460 (cited by Campbell, R. L., W. Zeman, J. Joyner 1966)

Güttich, H., E. S. Müller: Großes Stirnhöhlenosteom und reversible Blindheit. HNO 15 (1967) 155–158

Haas, A.: Wissenschaftliche Arbeit am Anatomischen Institut der Universität Würzburg, 1986

Habal, M. G., J. E. Maniscalco, W. C. Lineweaver, A. L. Rhoton: Microsurgical anatoma of the optic canal. Surg. Forum 27 (1976) 542–546

Hager, G., G. Heise: Über eine schwere Komplikation mit bleibender praktischer Erblindung eines Auges nach intranasaler Injektion. HNO 10 (1962) 325–328

Hajnis, K., T. Kustra, L. G. Farkas, B. Feiglova: Sinus maxillaris. Z. Morph. Anthrop. 59 (1967) 185–197

Hall, S. S., H. V. Thomas: Spontaneous hemorrhage into maxillary sinus. Arch. Otolaryng. 28 (1938) 371–375

Halle, M.: Externe oder interne Operation der Nebenhöhleneiterungen. Berlin. Klin. Wschr. 43 (1906) 1369–1404

von Haller, A.: Elementa Physiologiae Corporis Humanis. Bonsquet, Lausanne 1743

Hamberger, C. A., G. Hammer, G. Norlen et al.: Transantrosphenoidal hypophysectomy. Arch. Otolaryng. 74 (1961) 2–8

Hammer, G., C. Radberg: Sphenoidal sinus: an anatomical and roentgenological study with reference to transsphenoid hypophysectomy. Acta Radiol. (Stockh.) 56 (1961) 401–422

Hardy, J.: Transsphenoidal hypophysectomy. J. Neurosurg. 34 (1971) 582–594

Harrison, D. F. N.: Oro-antral fistulae. Brit. J. Clin. Pract. 15 (1961) 169–174

Hartz, H. J.: The lymphatics of the nose and nasopharynx, with consideration of the general lymphatic system. Trans. Amer. Acad. Ophthal. 16 (1911) 119–139

Hassmann, H.: Form, Maße und Verläufe der Schädelkanäle: des Canalis infraorbitalis, Canalis incisivus, Canalis palatinus major, Foramen spinosum und Meatus acusticus internus. Diss., Würzburg 1975

Hajek, M.: Pathologie und Therapie der entzündlichen Erkrankungen der Nebenhöhlen der Nase. Deuticke, Leipzig 1909

Hedewig, R.: Vergleichende anatomische Untersuchungen an den Jacobsonschen Organen. II. Teil: Galago crassicaudatus. Gegenbaurs Morph. Jb. 126 (1980)

de Heide, A. (1683): cited by H. Erhard 1910

Heineke, W.: Die chirurgischen Krankheiten des Kopfes. Enke, Stuttgart 1882

Heiss, R.: Der Atmungsapparat, I. Nasenhöhle, In: Möllendorf's Handbuch des Menschen, Bd. V/3. Springer, Berlin 1936 (S. 709–728)

Helms, J.: Die Bedeutung der Erstversorgung von Nasenverletzungen für die spätere Funktion. HNO 21 (1973) 77–78

Herberhold, C.: Störungen des Riechsinnes. Dtsch. Ärztebl. 75 (1978)

Heymann (1900): Heymanns Handbuch, Bd. III, 1. Hälfte (cited by P. J. Mink 1915)

Heymann and Ritter: Z. Laryng. Rhinol. 1 (1908) 1 (cited by L. Grünwald 1925)

Highmore, N. (1651): cited by M. C. Myerson 1932

Hilding, A. C.: The physiology of drainage of nasal mucus, IV: drainage of the accessory sinuses in man. Ann. Otol. (St. Louis) 53 (1944) 35–41

Hildmann, H., F. Lammert, A. Meertens, W. D. Scheerer: Über Zusammenhänge zwischen Nasenrachen, Tubaabstand und Oberkieferform. Laryng. Rhinol. Otol. 61 (1982) 573–576

Hirschfeld: cited after L. K. Rosenvold 1944

Hirschmann, A.: Über Endoskopie der Nase und deren Nebenhöhlen. Eine neue Untersuchungsmethode. Arch. Laryng. Rhinol. (Berl.) 14 (1903) 195 (cited after W. Draf 1978)

His: Anatomie menschlicher Embryonen, Bd. III. Leipzig 1885 (S. 46)

van der Hoeven, J.: Über Form-Abweichungen und Varianten der Nasenbeine. Z. Wiss. Zool. 11 (1860) 138–141

Holl, M.: Über die Fossa prenasales der menschlichen Schädel. Wien. Med. Wschr. 25 (1882) 753–756

Holzmann: cited after Schicketanz, H.-W., W. Schicketanz 1961

Hooper, R. S.: Orbital complications of head injury. Brit. J. Surg. 39 (1952) 126–138

Hopmann, W.: Anomalien der Choanen und des Nasenrachenraumes. Arch. Laryng. Rhin. (Berl.) 3 (1895) 48–67

Horsley, V.: On the technique of operations on the central nervous system. Brit. Med. J. 1906/II, 411–423

Houzè: Untersuchungen betreffend den Nasalindex im allgemeinen und den der Flamländer und Wallonen im besonderen. Arch. Anthrop. 20 (1891) (cited after Martin, R., K. Saller 1957)

Hovorka, O.: Die äußere Nase. Hölder, Wien 1893

Howarth, W. G.: Mucocele and pyocele of the nasal accessory sinuses. Lancet 1921/II, 744–746

Hoyer, H.: Beitrag zur Anthropologie der Nase. Morph. Arb. (Dr. G. Schwalbe) 4 (1895) 151–177

Hoyt, T. E., F. M. Turnbull, J. A. Kusske: Transantral transsphenoidal approach to the pituitary: technical note. J. Neurosurg. 59 (1983) 1102–1104

Hyrtl, J.: Handbuch der topographischen Anatomie, Bd. I. Braumüller, Wien 1853 (S. 192)

Hyrtl, J.: Lehrbuch der Anatomie des Menschen mit Rücksicht auf physiologische Anwendung, 18th ed., Bd. I, Braumüller Wien 1885

Ilberg, A.: Über die funktionelle Architektur der Nasenknorpel und ihre knöcherne Umgebung. Folia Oto-Laryng. 26 (1935) 239–257

Ingraham, F. D., D. D. Matson: Spina bifida and cranium bifidum, IV: an unusual nasopharyngeal encephalocele. New Engl. J. Med. 228 (1943) 815–820

Ishii, T.: In vorderster Abwehrfront: die Nase. Cholinerg und adrenerg gezügelt. Selecta 6 (1980) 460–461

Ishii, T., M. Toriyama: Acetylcholinesterase activity in the vasomotor and secretory fibers of the nose. Arch. Oto-Rhino-Laryng. 201 (1972) 1–10

Issing, P.: Wissenschaftliche Arbeit am Anatomischen Institut der Universität Würzburg, 1985

Jansen, A.: Zur Eröffnung der Nebenhöhlen der Nase bei chronischer Eiterung. Arch. Laryng. Rhin. (Berl.) 1 (1894) 135–157

Jennes, M. L.: Corrective nasal surgery in children. Eye, Ear, Nose Thr. Monthly 33 (1954) 583–591

Jeppesen, F., I. Windfeld: Dislocation of the nasal septal cartilage in the newborn. Acta Obstet. Gynec. Scand. 51 (1972) 5–15

Johnson, E. D.: Acute frontal sinusitis. Arch. Otolaryng. 47 (1948) 165–176

Johnston, J. B.: The nervus terminalis in man and mammals. Anat. Rec. 8 (1914) 185–198

Joseph, G.: Preliminary discussion on the thick septum problem. Rev. Laryng. 5 (1967) 111–115

Joseph, J.: Nasenplastik und sonstige Gesichtsplastik. Kabitzsch, Leipzig 1931

Joshinaga, T.: Anatomische Untersuchungen der Kieferhöhle bei Japanern. Int. Zbl. Laryng. 23 (1909) 11

Jost, G., B. Meresse, F. Torosian: Study of the junction between the lateral cartilage of the nose. Ann. Chir. Plast. 18 (1973) 175–182

Jovanovic, S.: Supernumerary frontal sinuses on the roof of the orbit: their clinical significance. Acta Anat. (Basel) 45 (1961) 133–142

Jung, H.: Gesichtspunkte der operativen Therapie der Choanalatresie. Laryng. Rhinol. Otol. 56 (1977) 425–431

Jüngken (1832): cited by A. Onodi 1915

Kageyama, I.: Wissenschaftliche Arbeit am Anatomischen Institut der Universität Würzburg, 1987

Kageyama, N., A. Kuwayama, T. Takahasi, M. Negoro, K. Ichihara: Diagnosis, treatment and postoperative results of Cushing's disease. Neurosurg. Rev. 8 (1985) 177–183

Kallius, E.: Geruchsorgan (Organon olfactus). In: Bardelebens Handbuch des Menschen, Bd. V Fischer, Jena 1905

Karmody, C. S., J. C. Gallagher: Nasoalveolar cysts. Ann. Otol. (St. Louis) 81 (1972) 278–283

Kasper, K. A.: Nasofrontal connections. Arch. Otolaryng. 23 (1936) 322–343

Kastenbauer, E. R.: Die Operation an Siebbein und Keilbeinhöhle kritisch betrachtet. Laryng. Rhinol. Otol. 54 (1975) 808–819

Kastenbauer, E.: Zur Pathogenese der Badesinusitis. HNO 16 (1968) Heft 10 (cited after C. P. Waggershauser 1980)

Keibel, F., F. P. Mall: Handbuch der Entwicklungsgeschichte des Menschen, Bd. II. Hirzel, Leipzig 1911

Keiter, F.: Über die Formentwicklung des kindlichen Kopfes und Gesichtes. Z. Menschl. Vererb. u. Konstit.-Lehre 17 (1933) 345–383

Keros, P.: Über die praktische Bedeutung der Niveauunterschiede der Lamina cribrosa des Ethmoids. Laryng. Rhinol. 11 (1962) 808

Key, A., G. Retzius: Studien in der Anatomie des Nervensystems und des Bindegewebes, Bd. I. Samson & Wallin, Stockholm 1875

Killian, G.: Zur Anatomie der Nase menschlicher Embryonen. Arch. Laryng. Rhin. (Berl.) 3 (1895) 17–47

Killian, G.: Die Nebenhöhlen der Nase in ihren Lagebeziehungen zu den Nachbarorganen. Fischer, Jena 1903

Killian, G.: Die Krankheiten der Kieferhöhle, Handb. d. Laryng. Rhin., Bd. III. 1898 (S. 50) (cited by Myerson 1932)

Kiesselbach, W.: Über spontane Nasenblutungen. Berl. klin. Wschr. 21 (1884) 375–377

Kiesselbach, W.: Über Nasenbluten. Wien. Med. Zg. (1885) 501

Klaff, D. D.: The surgical anatomy of the antero-caudal portion of the nasal septum: a study of the area of the premaxilla. Laryngoscope 66 (1956) 995–1020

Klaff, D. D.: Anatomy of the septum. Rhinology 8 (1970) 145–148

Klestadt, W.: cited by F. Montreuil 1949

Kley, W.: Die Unfallchirurgie der Schädelbasis und der pneumatischen Räume, Arch. Klin. Exp. Ohr.-, Nas.- u. Kehlk.-Heilk. 191, Kongreßbericht (1968) 1–216

Klinkosch, M.: Programma, quod visionem herniarum novumque herniae ventralis speciem proponit. In: Dissertationes medicae selectiores Pragenis, Vol. I. Walther, Prag 1764 (pp. 179–198)

Knox (1853): cited after J. Krmpotić-Nemanić 1977

Koch, J.: Kritisches Übersichtsreferat über die normale und pathologische Pneumatisation der Nebenhöhlen der Nase. Arch. Ohr.-, Nas.- u. Kehlk.-Heilk. 125 (1930) 174–218

von Koelliker, A.: Entwicklungsgeschichte des Menschen. Engelmann, Leipzig, 1879 (pp. 452, 765)

von Koelliker, A.: Der Lobus olfactorius und die Nervi olfactorii bei jungen menschlichen Embryonen. S.-B. Phys.-Med. Ges. Würzb. (1882) 68–72

von Koelliker, A.: Entwicklung des Auges und Geruchsorganes menschlicher Embryonen. Verh. Phys.-Med. Ges. Würzb. 17 (1883) Nr. 8

von Koelliker, A.: Handbuch der Gewebelehre des Menschen. Engelmann, Leipzig 1893/96

Kolmer, W.: Geruchsorgan. 1. Lage und Abgrenzung der Riechregion. In: Handbuch der mikroskopischen Anatomie des Menschen, Bd. III/1. Springer, Berlin 1927

Körner, O.: Die Vererbung anatomischer Variationen der Nase, ihrer Nebenhöhlen und des Gehörgangs. Die Ohrenheilkunde der Gegenwart und ihre Grenzgebiete 12 (1938) 1–6; 25–26; 45–47; 73–74; 85–99

Kortekangas, A. E.: Funktion und Funktionsprüfung der Nase und der Nasennebenhöhlen. In Berendes, J., R. Link, F. Zöllner: Hals-Nasen-Ohren-Heilkunde in Praxis und Klinik, Bd. I: Obere und untere Luftwege I. Thieme, Stuttgart 1977

Kowatscheff, L.: Besonderheiten der kindlichen Nase und ihre klinische Bedeutung. Z. Hals-, Nas.- u. Ohrenheilk. 48 (1943) 345–374

Kozielec, T., H. Jòzwa: Variation of the course of the facial artery in the prenatal period in man. Folia Morph. (Warszawa) 36 (1977), 55–61

Krauss, J.: Messungen zur cranio-cerebralen Topographie. Diss., Würzburg 1987

Kressner, A.: Die Indikation zur Median- und Kontralateraldrainage der Stirnhöhle und deren Durchführung. Arch. Ohr.-, Nas.- u. Kehlk.-Heilk. 157 (1951) 28–40

Krmpotić-Nemanić, J.: Entwicklungsgeschichte und Anatomie der Nase und der Nasennebenhöhlen. In Berendes, J., R. Link, F. Zöllner: Hals-Nasen-Ohren-Heilkunde in Praxis und Klinik, Bd. I: Obere und untere Luftwege I. Thieme, Stuttgart 1977

Krmpotić-Nemanić, J.: Anatomie, Variationen und Mißbildungen der Gefäße im Kopf-Hals-Bereich. Arch. Oto-Rhino-Laryng. 219 (1978) 1–91

Krmpotić-Nemanić, J., W. Draf, J. Helms: Chirurgische Anatomie des Kopf-Hals-Bereiches. Springer, Berlin 1985

Krmpotić-Nemanić, J., I. Kostović, P. Rudan, G. Nemanić: Morphological and histological changes responsible for the droop of the nasal tip in advanced age. Acta Oto-Laryng. (Stockh.) 71 (1971) 278–281

Kümmel: Tödliche Meningitis durch Duraverletzung bei einer intranasalen Abtragung der mittleren Muschel (Verhandlungen des Vereins Deutscher Laryngologen). Kabitsch, Würzburg 1913 (S. 174–179)

Kuhnt: cited after A. Onodi 1915

Lang, J.: Angioarchitektonik der terminalen Strombahn. In Meessen, H.: Handbuch der allgemeinen Pathologie, Bd. III/7. Mikrozirkulation. Springer, Berlin 1977

Lang, J.: Hypophysial region – anatomy of the operative approaches. Neurosurg. Rev. 8 (1985) 93–124

Lang, J.: Fossa cranialis anterior, mediale Bodenregion. Roundtable-Konferenz: Das frontobasale Trauma – Diagnostik und Behandlungsablauf. In Schuchardt, K., N. Schwenzer: Fortschritte der Kiefer- und Gesichts-Chirurgie, Bd. XXXII: Bildgebende Untersuchungsverfahren in der Mund-, Kiefer- und Gesichts-Chirurgie. Thieme, Stuttgart 1987 (S. 210–218)

Lang, J.: Über die Cellulae ethmoidales posteriores und ihre Beziehungen zum Canalis opticus. HNO 36 (1988) 49–53

Lang, J.: Klinische Anatomie der Nase, Nasenhöhle und Nebenhöhlen: Grundlagen für Diagnostik u. Operation. Akt. Oto-Rhino-Laryngol. Bd. 11. Thieme, Stuttgart 1988

Lang, J., C. Bachmann, S. Raabe: Über das postnatale Wachstum der Außennase. Gegenbaurs Morphol. Jb. 133 (1987) 5–32

Lang, J., R. Baumeister: Über das postnatale Wachstum der Nasenhöhle. Gegenbaurs Morph. Jb. 128 (1982) 354–393

Lang, J., S. Bressel: Über den Hiatus semilunaris, das Infundibulum und das Ostium des Sinus maxillaris, die vordere Ansatzzone der Concha nasalis media und deren Abstände zu Landmarken an der Außen- und Innennase. Gegenbaurs morphol. Jb. 134 (1988) 637–646

Lang, J., B. Brückner: Über dicke und dünne Zonen des Neurocranium, Impressionses gyrorum und Foramina parietalia bei Kindern und Erwachsenen. Anat. Anz. 149 (1981) 11–50

Lang, J., A. Haas: Über die Sagittalausdehnung des Sinus frontalis, dessen Wanddicke, Abstände zur Lamina cribrosa, die Tiefe der sogenannten Olfactorius-Rinne und die Canales ethmoidales. Gegenbaurs morphol. Jb. 134 (1988) 459–469

Lang, J., R. Haas: Neue Befunde zur Bodenregion der Fossa cranialis anterior. Verh. Anat. Ges. (Jena) 73 (1979) 77–86

Lang, J., P. Issing: Über Messungen am Clivus, den Foramina an der Basis cranii externa und den oberen drei Halswirbeln. Anat. Anz. 169 (1989) 7–34

Lang, J., H. Keller: Über die hintere Pfortenregion der Fossa pterygopalatina und das Ganglion pterygopalatinum. Gegenbaurs Morph. Jb. 124 (1978) 207–214

Lang, J., W. Kley: Über die Agnesie und Hypoplasie der Conchae nasales und des Septum nasi. HNO 29 (1981) 200–207

Lang, J., I. Mundorff-Vetter: Über die Knorpel der Außennase. Gegenbaurs Morph. Jb. 132 (1986), 861–874

Lang, J., G. Oehmann: Formentwicklung des Canalis opticus, seine Maße und Einstellung zu den Schädelebenen. Verh. Anat. Ges. (Jena) 70 (1976) 567–574

Lang, J., J. Pahnke: Wissenschaftliche Arbeit am Anatomischen Institut der Universität Würzburg (in preparation)

Lang, J., J. Papke: Über anatomische Grundlagen der blow-out-fractures der Orbita. 2. Arbeitstagung der Anatomischen Gesellschaft Würzburg, 8.–10. Oktober 1980

Lang, J., J. Papke: Über die klinische Anatomie des Paries inferior orbitae und dessen Nachbarstrukturen. Gegenbaurs Morphol. Jb. 130 (1984) 1–47

Lang, J., U. Reiter: Über die intrazisternale Länge von Hirnbahn- und Nervenstrecken (Nn. I–IV). Neurochirurgia (Stuttg.) 27 (1984) 125–128

Lang, J., W. Reiter: Über praktisch-ärztliche wichtige Maße des N. opticus, des Chiasma opticum und des Tractus opticus. Gegenbaurs Morph. Jb. 131 (1985), 777–795

Lang, J., C. Roth: Über die Fläche des Bodens der vorderen Schädelgrube und des Augenhöhlendaches sowie einige Winkel und Maße der Orbita. Anat. Anz. 156 (1984) 1–19

Lang, J., E. Sakals: Über die Höhe der Cavitas nasi, die Länge ihres Bodens und Maße sowie Anordnung der Conchae nasales und der Apertura sinus sphenoidalis. Anat. Anz. 149 (1981) 297–318

Lang, J., E. Sakals: Über den Recessus spheno-ethmoidalis, die Apertura nasalis des Ductus nasolacrimalis und den Hiatus semilunaris. Anat. Anz. 152 (1982) 393–412

Lang, J., K. Schäfer: Arteriae ethmoidales: Ursprung, Verlauf, Versorgungsgebiete und Anastomosen. Acta Anat. (Basel) 104 (1979) 183–197

Lang, J., F. Schlehahn: Foramina ethmoidalia and Canales ethmoidales. Verh. Anat. Ges. (Jena) 72 (1978) 433–435

Lang, J., F. Schulz: Über die Variabilität der Nasenarterien. Gegenbaurs Morph. Jb. 131 (1985) 551–566

Lang, J., H. Väth: Über die Abstände zwischen dem Ductus nasolacrimalis und dem Canalis palatinus major an der seitlichen Nasenwand sowie Distanzen zwischen Ostium pharyngeum tubae auditivae und Canalis palatinus major sowie Oberseite des Palatum molle. Anat. Anz. 168 (1989) 315–320

Lang, J., F. Schlehahn, H. P. Jensen, J. Lemke, J. Klinge, U. Muhtaroglu: Cranio-cerebral topography as a basis for interpreting computed tomograms. In: Lanksch, W., E. Kazner: Cranial Computerized Tomography. Springer, Berlin 1976

Lang, J., F. Schlehahn, K. Schäfer: Über den Inhalt der Canales ethmoidales. Verh. Anat. Ges. (Jena) 73 (1979a) 87–94

Lang, J., K.-A. Bushe, W. Buschmann, D. Linnert: Gehirn- und Augenschädel. In: Lang, J., (T. von Lanz), W. Wachsmuth: Praktische Anatomie, Bd. I/1B. Springer, Berlin 1979b

Lang, J., H.-P. Jensen, F. Schröder: Übergeordnete Systeme. In Lang, J., (T. von Lanz), W. Wachsmuth: Praktische Anatomie, Bd. I/1A. Springer, Berlin 1985

Lang, J., S. Bressel, J. Pahnke: Sinus sphenoidalis, klinische Anatomie des Zugansw.es zur Hypophysenregion. Gegenbaurs morphol. Jb. 134 (1988) 291–307

Lang, J., S. Bressel, A. Haas: Über den Ductus nasofrontalis bzw. das Ostium des Sinus frontalis und die vorderen Siebbeinzellen (in preparation)

Lang, W.: Injuries and diseases of the orbit. 1: traumatic enophthalmos with retention of perfect acuity of vision. Trans. Ophthalmol. Soc. U. K. 9 (1889) 41–45

Lange, F.: Die Sprache des menschlichen Antlitzes. Lehmann, München 1937

Langnickel, R.: Temporäre Erblindung nach endonasaler Siebbeinoperation. HNO 26 (1978) 172–173

Larsell, O.: The nervus terminalis. Ann. Otol. (St. Louis) 59 (1950) 414–438

Larsell, O., R. A. Fenton: Sympathic innervation of the nose: research report. Arch. Otolaryng. 24 (1936) 687–695

Lassau: cited by J. Krmpotić-Nemanić 1978

Lazarus, J.: Über Reflexe von der Nasenschleimhaut auf die Bronchiallumina. Arch. Anat. Physiol. (1891) 19–38

Lederer, F. L., R. Dinolt: Influence of avulsion of trigeminal nerve on human nose. Arch. Otolaryngol. 37 (1943) 768–784

Legler, U.: Beitrag zur Morphologie, Physiologie und Klinik des Vestibulum nasi vermittels eines neuzeitlichen Abdruckverfahrens. Z. Laryng. Rhinol. 46 (1967) 482

Legler, U.: Zur Morphologie und Nomenklatur des Vestibulum nasi anhand des Abdruckverfahrens. Z. Laryng. Rhinol. 47 (1968) 640

Legler, U.: Mißbildungen der Nase (mit Ausnahme der Gaumenspalten) Fremdkörper, Nasenbluten. In: Berendes, J., R. Link, F. Zöllner: Hals-Nasen-Ohren-Heilkunde in Praxis und Klinik, Bd. I: Obere und untere Luftwege I. Thieme, Stuttgart 1977

Leicher, H.: Die Vererbung anatomischer Variationen der Nase, ihrer Nebenhöhlen und des Gehörorgans. In: Die Ohrenheilkunde der Gegenwart und ihre Grenzgebiete, Bd. XII. 1928

Lembeck, F.: Zur Frage der zentralen Übertragung afferenter Impulse, III. Mitteilung. Das Vorkommen und die Bedeutung der Substanz P in der dorsalen Wurzel des Rückenmarks. Naunyn-Schmiedeberg's. Arch. Exp. Path. Pharmak. 219 (1953) 197–213

Lenz, H., W. Theelen, J. Eichler: Untersuchungen zum Nasenzyklus mit Hilfe rhinoanometrischer Messungen. HNO 33 (1985) 58–61

Lieutaud: Abcès des sinus frontaux sphénoidaux et maxillaires; mort. Mém. Acad. Roy. Sci. (1735) 18 (cited by R. W. Teed 1938)

Luc, H.: Une nouvelle méthode opérative pour la cuire radicale et rapide de l'empyème chronique du sinus maxillaire. Arch. Int. Laryng. 10 (1897) 273–282

Lundblad, L., J. Lundberg, E. Brodin et al.: Origin and distribution of capsaicin-sensitive substance P-immunoreactive nerves in the nasal mucosa. Acta Oto-Laryng. (Stockh.) 96 (1983a) 485–493

Lundblad, L., A. Saria, J. Lundberg et al.: Increased vascular permeability in rat nasal mucosa induced by substance P and stimulation of capsaicin-sensitive trigeminal neurons. Acta Oto-Laryng. (Stockh.) (1983b) 479–484

Lundgren, A., T. Olin: Muco-pyocele of sphenoidal sinus or posterior ethmoidal cells with special reference to the apex orbitae syndrome. Acta Oto-Laryng. (Stockh.) 53 (1961) 61–79

von Luschka, H.: Die Anatomie des menschlichen Kopfes. Laupp, Tübingen 1867

Macbeth, R.: Malignant disease of the paranasal sinuses. J. Laryng. 2 (1965) 592–612

McClatchey, K. D., R. V. Lloyd, J. D. Schaldenbrand: Metastatic carcinoma to the sphenoid sinus: case report and review of the literature. Arch. Oto-Rhino-Laryng. 241 (1985) 219–224

McCoy, J. R.: A plea for conservative methods in orthodontic treatment. Amer. J. Orthodont. 49 (1963) 161–182

McKenzie: cited by Thomson S. C., V. E. Negus 1948

McLaughlin C. R.: Absence of the septal cartilage with retarded nasal development. Brit. J. Plast. Surg. (1949) 61–64

Maier, H. N.: Über den feineren Bau der Wimpernapparate der Infusorien. A. f. P. K. 2 (1903)

Maisel, R. H., M. El Deeb, R. C. Bone: Sphenoid sinus mucoceles. Laryngoscope 83 (1973) 930–938

Malcolmson, K. G.: The vasomotor activities of the nasal mucous membrane. J. Laryng. 73 (1959) 73–98

Maltz, M.: New instrument: the sinuscope. Laryngoscope (St. Louis) 35 (1925) 805

Manelfe, C., A. Bonafé, P. Fabre, J.-J. Pessey: Computed tomography in olfactory neuroblastoma: one case of esthesioneuroepithelioma and four cases of esthesioneuroblastoma. J. Comput. Assist. Tomogr. 2 (1978) 412–420

Mann, W.: Die Lymphdrainage der Kieferhöhle. Laryng. Rhinol. Otol. 59 (1980) 782–785

Marcus, G.: Über einige Fälle von Pneumatisation des Orbitaldaches (Recessus supra-orbitalis). Anat. Anz. 76 (1933) 33–45

Martin, R., K. Saller: Lehrbuch der Anthropologie, Bd. I. Fischer, Stuttgart 1957

Masing, H.: Klinisch-anatomische Bemerkungen zur Cartilago septi nasi. Z. Laryng. Rhinol. 43 (1964) 604–612

Mayer: Beschreibung eines Sinus pterygoideus und jugalis beim Menschen. Schmidts Jb. Ges. Med. 31 (1841) 12–21

Menger, W., V. Kocoglu: Paranasale Sinusitiden im Säuglings- und Kindesalter und ihre Beziehung zu den Bronchitiden. Med. Welt (Stuttg.) 31 (1969), 1686–1693

Merkel, F.: Handbuch der topographischen Anatomie: Kopf. Viehweg, Braunschweig 1890

Merkel, F.: Handbuch der Anatomie. I. Bd. Viehweg, Braunschweig 1885–1890 (S. 100)

Merkel, F.: Jacobsonsches Organ und Pallia palatina beim Menschen. Anat. H. 1 (1892) 217–232

Messerklinger, W.: Die Endoskopie der Nase. Mschr. Ohrenheilk. 104 (1970) 451–456

Messerklinger, W.: Technik und Möglichkeiten der Nasenendoskopie. HNO 20 (1972a) 133–135

Messerklinger, W.: Nasenendoskopie: Der mittlere Nasengang und seine unspezifischen Entzündungen. HNO 20 (1972b) 212–215

Messerklinger, W.: Zur endoskopischen Anatomie der menschlichen Siebbeinzellen. Acta Oto-Laryng. (Stockh.) 75 (1973) 243–248

Messerklinger, W.: III Endoskopie der Nase und der Nebenhöhlen. In: Berendes, J., R. Link, F. Zöllner: Hals-Nasen-Ohren-Heilkunde in Praxis und Klinik, Bd. I: Obere und untere Luftwege I. Thieme, Stuttgart 1977

Messerklinger, W.: Schwierigkeiten bei der Kieferhöhlenspülung. Laryng. Rhinol. Otol. 59 (1980) 22–29

Messerklinger, W.: Über den Recessus frontalis und seine Klinik. Laryng. Rhinol. Otol. 61 (1982) 217–223

Metzenbaum, M.: Dislocation of the lower end of the nasal septal cartilage. Arch. Otolaryng. 24 (1936) 78–88

von Meyer, E.: Über eine basale Hirnhernie in der Gegend der Lamina cribrosa. Virchows Arch. path. Anat. 120 (1890) 309–320

Meyer, W.: Beiträge zur Kenntnis der Anatomie und Histologie der lateralen Nasendrüsen. Anat. Anz. 24 (1904) 369–381

von Mihalkovics, V.: Bau und Entwicklung der pneumatischen Gesichtshöhlen. Verh. Anat. Ges. (Jena) 10 (1896) 44–63

von Mihalkovics, V.: Handbuch der Laryngologie. Hölder, Wien 1896

Mikulics, J.: Zur operativen Behandlung des Empyems der Highmore-Höhle. Prag. Z. Ohrenheilk. 7 (1886) 257

Millard, D. R.: The triad of columella deformities. Plast. Reconstr. Surg. 31 (1963) 370–384

Milosslawski, M.: Die Sinus frontales. Diss., Moskau 1903 (cited after Jber. Anat. [Jena] 1905)

Mink, P. J.: Zur Pathologie und Therapie des Recessus sphenoethmoidalis. Arch. Laryng. Rhin. (Berl.) 29 (1915) 165–178

Mink, P. J.: Die Rolle des kavernösen Gewebes in der Nase. Arch. Laryng. Rhin. (Berl.) 30 (1916) 47–65

Montreuil, F.: Cysts of the nasal vestibule. Ann. Otol. (St. Louis) 58 (1949) 212–219

Morgagni, G. B.: Adversaria anatomica, 1706/19

Morrison, L. E.: Some relationships between embryology and surgery of the nose. Int. Rhinol. 8 (1970) 185–194

Mosher, H. P.: The anatomy of the sphenoid sinus and the method of approaching it from the antrum. Laryngoscope (St. Louis) 13 (1903) 177–215

Mosher, H. P.: The premaxillary wings and deviations of the septum. Laryngoscope 17 (1907) 840–867

Moss, M. L.: The role of the nasal septal cartilage in midfacial growth. In McNamara, J. A., Jr.: Factors Affecting the Growth of the Midface. Center for Human Growth and Development, Ann Arbor, MI, 1976

Most, A.: Über den Lymphgefäßapparat von Nase und Rachen. Arch. Anat. Physiol. (1901) 75–94

Mündich: cited by S. Salinger 1939

Müsebeck, K., H. Rosenberg: Temperaturmessung im Sinus maxillaris. Laryng. Rhinol. Otol. 59 (1980) 34–39

Myerson, M. C.: The natural orifice of the maxillary sinus. Arch. Otolaryng. 15 (1932)

Natvig, P., L. A. Sether, R. P. Gingrass, W. D. Gardner: Anatomical details of the osseous-cartilaginous framework of the nose. Plast. Reconstr. Surg. 48 (1971) 528–532

Naumann, H. H.: Rhinologische Grundlagen und Indikationen für korrigierende plastische Eingriffe im Nasenbereich. In: Gohrbrandt, E., J. Gabka, A. Berndorfer: Handbuch der plastischen Chirurgie, Bd. II. De Gruyter, Berlin 1966 (S. 1–44)

Naumann, H. H.: personal communication, 1987

Naumann, H. H., W. H. Naumann: Kurze Pathophysiologie der Nase und ihrer Nebenhöhlen (unter Ausschluß des Riechorgans): In: Berendes, J., R. Link, F. Zöllner: Hals-Nasen-Ohren-Heilkunde in Praxis und Klinik, Bd. I: Obere und untere Luftwege I. Thieme, Stuttgart 1977

Navarro, J. A. C., J. L. T. Filho, N. L. Zorzetto: Anatomy of the maxillary artery into the pterygomaxillopalatine fossa. Anat. Anz. 152 (1982) 413–433

Nikolić, V., A. Jo: Öffnungen und Dehiszenzen an der Vertikalplatte des Gaumenbeins: Anat. Anz. 121 (1967) 272–282

Noback, C. R.: The development anatomy of the human osseous skeleton during the embryonic, fetal and circumnatal periods. Anat. Rec. 88 (1944) 91–125

Nomina Anatomica, 5th ed. (approved by Eleventh International Congress of Anatomists at Mexico City, 1980). Williams & Wilkins, Baltimore 1983

Nowak, R., G. Mehls: Die Aplasien der Sinus maxillares und frontales unter besonderer Berücksichtigung der Pneumatisation bei Spaltträgern. Anat. Anz. 142 (1977) 441–450

Nowak, R., G. Mehls: Analytische Auswertung von Röntgennebenhöhlenaufnahmen bei Spaltträgern (im Vergleich mit einer gesunden Probandengruppe). Anat. Anz. 142 (1977) 451–470

Nowakowski, H.: Ergebn. inn. Med. Kinderheilk. (N. F.) 12 (1959) 219–301 (cited after R. Pfalz 1967)

Ohnishi, T.: Bony defects and dehiscences of the roof of the ethmoid cells. Rhinology 19 (1981) 195–202

Onodi, A.: Die Nasenhöhle und ihre Nebenhöhlen. Nach anatomischen Durchschnitten in 12 Holzschnittafeln dargestellt. Hölder, Wien 1893

Onodi, A.: The Anatomy of the Nasal Cavity and Its Accessory Sinuses: an Atlas for Students and Practitioners (translated from 2nd ed. by St. Clair Thompson) Lewis, London 1895

Onodi, A.: Das Verhältnis der Kieferhöhle zur Keilbeinhöhle und zu den vorderen Siebbeinzellen. Arch. Laryngol. Rhin. (Berl.) 11 (1901) 391–395

Onodi, A.: Die Dehiszenzen der Nebenhöhlen der Nase. Arch. Laryng. Rhin. (Berl.) 15 (1903) 62–71

Onodi, A.: Die Eröffnung der Kieferhöhle im mittleren Nasengange. Arch. Laryng. Rhin. (Berl.) 14 (1906) 154–160

Onodi, A.: Die Nebenhöhle der Nase beim Kinde. Kabitzsch, Würzburg 1911

Onodi, A.: Über die Lehre von den Augenleiden nasalen Ursprungs. Arch. Laryng. Rhin. (Berl.) 29 (1915) 430–436

Onodi: cited by K. Peter 1938

Onodi: cited by H. Richter 1932

O'Rahilly, R., D. Meyer: Roentgenographic investigation of the human skeleton during early fetal life. Amer. J. Roentgenol. 76 (1956) 455–468

Otto, H.-D., C. Opitz: Ein neues Konzept zur normalen und pathologischen Entwicklung des primären Gaumens. Teil 1. Das normale Schicksal der Hochstetterschen Epithelmauer. Anat. Anz. 163 (1987) 213–223

Pahnke, J.: Wissenschaftliche Arbeit am Anatomischen Institut der Universität Würzburg, 1986

Parker, L. S.: Mucocele of the right maxillary sinus with proptosis of the right eye. J. Laryng. 75 (1961) 507–509

Parkes, M. L., R. Kanodia: Avulsion of the upper lateral cartilage: etiology, diagnosis, surgical anatomy and management. Laryngoscope 91 (1981) 758–764

Patrzek: Über Verbiegungen der Nasenscheidewand bei Neugeborenen. Int. Klin. Rdsch. 4 (1890) 575

Paulsen: Experimentelle Untersuchung über die Strömung der Luft in der Nasenhöhle. S.-B. Akad. Wiss. Wien (1882) (cited by E. Zuckerkandl 1893)

Pearson, A.: The development of the nervus terminalis in man. J. Comp. Neurol. 75 (1941) 39–66

Pearson, A.: The development on the olfactory nerve in man. J. Comp. Neurol. 75 (1941) 100–217

Pedziwiatr, Z. F.: Das Siebbeinlabyrinth. I. Systematische Konzeption der Siebbeinmuscheln der Säugetiere. Anat. Anz. 131 (1972a) 367–377

Pedziwiatr, Z. F.: Das Siebbeinlabyrinth. II. Differenzierung und Systematik der Hauptmuschel bei einigen Gattungen der Säugetiere. Anat. Anz. 131 (1972b) 378–390

Pedziwiatr, Z. F.: Das Siebbeinlabyrinth. III. Das Siebbeinlabyrinth von 4–10 Monate alten menschlichen Feten. Anat Anz. 132 (1972c) 440–453

Peele, J. C.: Unusual anatomical variations of the sphenoid sinuses. Laryngoscope (St. Louis) 67 (1957) 208–237

Pellnitz, D.: Die Bedeutung von Ohrmuschel- und Nasenwachstum für die Indikationsstellung kosmetischer Operationen. Arch. Ohr.-, Nas.- u. Kehlk.-Heilk. 180 (1962) 387–392

Perna, G.: Die Nasenbeine. Eine embryologische und vergleichend-anatomische Untersuchung. Arch. Anat. Physiol., Anat. Abtl. (1906) 119–145

Perović, D.: Über eine eigenartige normal vorkommende Bildung an der unteren Nasenmuschel des Menschen. Z. Anat. Entwickl.-Gesch. 110 (1940) 597–633

Perović, D.: Beiträge zur Kenntnis der Entwicklung und des Baues des menschlichen Oberkiefers sowie des Sinus maxillaris. Bull. Int. Acad. Yougosl. Sci. Beaux-Arts 11 (1954)

Perović, D.: Über eine bisher unbeachtete Formation am Vomer sowie über wahre Begrenzung der Choanen. Z. Anat. Entwickl.-Gesch. 121 (1959) 1–8

Perović, D.: Was bedeuten die rätselhaften Gebilde, die auf der Crista choanalis vomeris auftreten? Z. Anat. Entwickl.-Gesch. 121 (1960) 417–430

Perwitzchky, R.: Die Temperatur und Feuchtigkeitsverhältnisse der Atemluft in den Luftwegen. Arch. Ohr.-, Nas.- u. Kehlk.-Heilk. 117 (1927) 1–36

Peter, F., H. Sicher: Anatomie und Technik der Wurzelspitzenresektion. Öst. Z. Stomat. 18 (1920) 223–238

Peter, K.: Das Centrum für die Flimmer- und Geißelbewegung. Anat. Anz. 15 (1899) 271–284

Peter, K.: Atlas der Entwicklung der Nase und des Gaumens beim Menschen mit Einschluß der Entwicklungsstörungen. Fischer, Jena 1913

Peter, K.: Vergleichende Anatomie und Entwicklungsgeschichte der Nase und ihrer Nebenhöhlen. In Denker, A., O. Kahler: Handbuch der Hals-Nasen-Ohren-Heilkunde, Bd. I. Springer, Berlin, Bergmann, München 1925

Peter, K.: Die Nase des Kindes. In: Handbuch der Anatomie des Kindes, Bd. II. Bergmann, München 1938

Petersen, R. J.: Canine fossa puncture. Laryngoscope (St. Louis) 83 (1973) 369–371

Petersen, J. M., S. C. Baldone, T. Srethadatta: Paranasal sinus aspergillosis: a report of two cases and review of the literature. JAOA (Apr. 81) 8 (1982) 549–553

Pfalz, R.: Veränderungen an Hals, Nase und Ohr durch endokrine Erkrankungen. HNO 15 (1967) 88–91

Pfeifer, G.: Die relativen Maßverhältnisse des wachsenden Gesichtes im Hinblick auf die zeitliche Indikation zu operativen Eingriffen. In Schuchardt, K.: Fortschritte der Kiefer- und Gesichtschirurgie Bd. IV. Thieme, Stuttgart 1958 (S. 67–81)

Pfeifer, G.: Angeborene Fehlbildungen des Gesichtes, der Kiefer- und der Mundhöhle. In Opitz, H., F. Schmid: Handbuch der Kinderheilkunde, Bd. IX. Springer, Berlin 1968

Pfeifer, G.: Die Craniogenese aus teratologischer Sicht. Nova Acta Leopoldina (N. F.) 58 262 (1986) 343–363

Pia, H. W., E. Grote, G. Hildebrandt: Giant pituitary adenomas. Neurosurg. Rev. 8 (1985) 207–220

Piersol, G. A.: Human Anatomy, 9th ed. Lippincott, Philadelphia 1930 (p. 1603)

Pirsig, W.: Die Regeneration des kindlichen Septumknorpels nach Septumplastiken. Acta Oto-Laryng. (Stockh.) 79 (1975) 451–459

Pirsig, W.: Operative Eingriffe an der kindlichen Nase. In: Berendes, J., R. Link, F. Zöllner: Hals-Nasen-Ohren-Heilkunde in Praxis und Klinik, Bd. II. Thieme, Stuttgart 1977a

Pirsig, W.: Septal plasty in children: influence on nasal growth. Rhinology 15 (1977b) 193–204

Plate, S., S. Asboe: Blindness as a complication of rhinosurgery. J. Laryng. 95 (1981) 317–322

Pollock, J. A., T. H. Newton: Encephalocele and cranium bifidum. In: Newton, T. H., D. G. Potts: Radiology of the Skull and Brain. Mosby, St. Louis 1971 (pp. 634–647)

Pollock, J. A., T. H. Newton, W. F. Hoyt: Transsphenoidal and transethmoidal encephaloceles: a review of clinical and roentgen features in eight cases. Radiology 90 (1968) 442–453

Port: Dtsch. Zahnärztl. Wschr. (1908) (cited after Schicketanz, H.-W., W. Schicketanz 1961)

Portmann (1926): cited by W. Draf 1978

Powell, N., B. Humphreys: Proportions of the Aesthetic Face: Thieme, Stuttgart 1984

Probst, C.: Hirnnervenläsionen bei Nasennebenhöhlenentzündungen, ein Fall von Sinus-cavernosus-Syndrom ohne Sinus-cavernosus-Thrombose. Arch. Klin. Exp. Ohr.-, Nas.- u. Kehlk.-Heilk. 204 (1973) 183–190

Proctor, B., G. T. Nager: The facial canal: normal anatomy variations and anomalies. Trans. Amer. Otol. Soc. 70 (1982) 49–77

Prott, W.: Zweifache Ausführungsgänge der Stirnhöhlen – eine anatomische Variante. Z. Laryng. Rhinol. 50 (1971) 821–822

Prott, W.: Röntgenologische Befunde zu normalen und atypischen Ausführungsgängen der Nasennebenhöhlen. Z. Laryng. Rhinol. 52 (1973) 96–109

Prott, W.: Liquorrhoe in die Kieferhöhle bei Arachnoidalzyste des Ethmoids – ein Beitrag zur klinischen Bedeutung des Canalis ethmoideomaxillaris (Canalis ethmoidalis). Laryng. Rhinol. Otol. 54 (1975) 689–691

Quiring, D. P., J. H. Warfel: cited after Krmpotić-Nemanić, J., W. Draf, J. Helms 1985

Radoievič, S., S. Jovanović, N. Lotrić: La fente orbitaire supérieure: morphologie et rapports avec les sinus paranasaux. Ass. Anat. 44 (1958) 647

Reidy, J. P.: The nasal septum. Ann. Roy. Coll. Surg. Engl. 43 (1968) 141

Reisman: cited by T. Ishii 1980

Reisman, R. E.: In vorderster Abwehrfront: die Nase. Die sekretorische Immunabwehr ist eigenständig. Selecta 6 (1980) 458

Rethi, L.: Experimentelle Untersuchungen über die Luftströmung in der normalen Nase, sowie bei pathologischen Veränderungen derselben und des Nasen-Rachen-Raumes. S.-B. Akad. Wiss. (Wien) 109 (1900) 17–36

Ricbourg, B., P. Cernea, J. P. Lassau, E. A. Cabanis, M. T. Iba Zizen: Vaskularisation der Mundöffnung. Rev. Stomat. (Paris) 77 (1976) 195–204

Richter, G. A.: Zur Pneumatisation des Stirnbeins unter besonderer Berücksichtigung atypischer Stirnhöhlendurchbrüche. Arch. Ohr.-, Nas.- u. Kehlk.-Heilk. 171 (1958) 330–334

Richter, H.: Die normale Entwicklung der menschlichen Nase, in Sonderheit der Siebbeinzellen. Arch. Ohr.-, Nas.- u. Kehlk.-Heilk. 131 (1932) 265–304

Richter, H.: Über eine Meningoencephalocele innerhalb der Stirnhöhle. Z. Laryng. Rhinol. 30 (1951) 41–43

Robinson, A. E., B. M. Meares, J. A. Goree: Traumatic sphenoid sinus effusion. Amer. J. Roentgenol. 101 (1967) 795–801

Roederer (1755): cited by H. Jung 1977

Rosenberger, H. C.: Growth and development of the naso-respiratory area in childhood. Ann. Otol. Rhinol. Laryngol. 43 (1934) 495–512

Rosenberger, J. P.: Nasal vestibular cysts. Arch. Otolaryng. 40 (1944) 288 (cited after F. Montreuil 1949)

Rosenfeld, M. G., J.-J. Mermod, S. G. Amara et al.: Production of a novel neuropeptid encoded by the calcitonin gene via tissue specific RNA processing. Nature 304 (1983) 129–135

Rosenmüller, J. C.: De simulari et nativa oss. varietate. Diss. Lips, 1804

Rosenvold, L. K.: Intracranial suppuration secondary to disease of the nasal septum. Arch. Otolaryng. 40 (1944) 1–15

Rowe, N. L.: Fractures of the orbit. Acta Stomat. Belg. 72 (1975) 681–685

Rowe, R. J., T. W. Daseler, A. M. Kinkella, W. Marshfield: Amer. Med. Ass. 201 (1967) 117 (cited by Plate, S., S. Asboe 1981)

Rudbek (1659): cited after H. J. Hartz 1911

Rudez, V.: Practical importance of the lateral displacement of the medial wall of the maxillary sinus. Acta Fac. Med. Zagreb. 14 (1966) Fasc. 1

Runge, H.: Die Beziehungen der Zahnkeime und Zahnwurzeln zur Oberkieferhöhle während des Kindesalters. Z. Anat. Entwickl.-Gesch. 85 (1928) 734–761

Salinger, S.: Endresults of external operations on the maxillary sinus. Arch. Otolaryng. 30 (1939a) 721–735

Salinger, S.: The paranasal sinuses. Arch. Otolaryng. 30 (1939b) 442–479

Salinger, S.: Paranasal sinuses: summaries of bibliographic material available in field of otolaryngology, Arch. Otolaryngol. 48 (1948) 430–462

Salinger, S.: The paranasal sinuses: summary of the listings in the Index Medicus. Laryngoscope 75 (1965) 1761–1799

Santorini, D.: Septemdecim Tabulae. Girardi, Parma 1775 (cited by E. Zuckerkandl 1892)

Sarnat, B. G., M. R. Wexler: Growth of the face and jaws after resection of the septal cartilage in the rabbit. J. Anat. 118 (1966) 755–768

Sasaki, C. T., D. G. Mann: Dilator naris function: a useful test of facial nerve integrity. Arch. Otolaryng. 102 (1976) 365–367

Schaeffer, J. P.: The sinus maxillaris and its relations in the embryo, child and adult man. Amer. J. Anat. 10 (1910) 313–368

Schaeffer, J. P.: Types of ostia nasolacrimalia in man and their genetic significance. Amer. J. Anat. 13 (1912) 183–192

Schaeffer, J. P.: The genesis, development and adult anatomy of the nasofrontal region in man. Amer. J. Anat. 20 (1916) 125–146

Schaeffer, J. P.: The Nose, Paranasal Sinuses, Nasolacrimal Passageways, and Olfactory Organ in Man. Blakiston, Philadelphia 1920 (pp. 125–129)

Scheff, G.: Der Weg des Luftstromes durch die Nase; auf Grund experimenteller und anatomischer Untersuchungen. Klin. Zeit- u. Streitfr. (Wien) 19 (1895) 37–63

Schicketanz, H.-W., W. Schicketanz: Mittelbare und unmittelbare Zahnschädigungen nach Kieferhöhleneingriffen. HNO 9 (1961) 169–175

Schloffer, H.: Erfolgreiche Operation eines Hypophysentumors auf nasalem Wege. Wien. Klin. Wschr. 20, Nr. 21 (1907) 621–624

Schlosshauer, B., K. H. Vosteen: Zur Diagnostik und Therapie der Carotisblutung nach Keilbeinhöhlenfrakturen. Arch. Ohr.-, Nas.- u. Kehlk.-Heilk. 165 (1954) 270–277

Schmid, F., U. Du Bala, R. Ewald: Die Entwicklung der Keilbeinhöhle. Mschr. Kinderheilk. 114 (1966) 309–311

Schmidt, H.-M.: Über Größe, Form und Lage von Bulbus und Tractus olfactorius des Menschen. Gegenbaurs Morphol. Jb. 119 (1973) 227–237

Schmidt, H.-M.: Über Maße und Niveaudifferenzen der Medianstrukturen der vorderen Schädelgrube des Menschen. Gegenbaurs Morph. Jb. 120 (1974) 538–559

Schmidt, H.-M.: Über die postnatale Entwicklung der Vertikalabstände zwischen der Lamina cribrosa und kraniometrischen Meßpunkten und Schädelebenen. Verh. Anat. Ges. (Jena) 69 (1975) 799–803

Schmitt, K. P.: Grenzbestimmung zwischen Vestibulum und Cavum nasi an Lebenden mittels Lastic-Abdruckverfahren sowie Größenvergleich zwischen innerem und äußerem Nasenloch. Med. Diss. Heidelberg 1968

Schroeder, U., H. Salzmann: Sehnervenschädigungen nach Eingriffen im Nasennebenhöhlenbereich. Arch. Klin. Exp. Ohr.,- Nas.- u. Kehlk.-Heilk. 205 (1973) 285–288.

Schubert, J., K. Seeliger: Die funktionelle Charakteristik der Mundspalte. In: Oral-Anatomie. 5. Interdisziplinäres Symposium der Oral-Anatomie mit internationaler Beteiligung vom 22. bis 25. November 1987 in Rostock. Wilhelm-Pieck-Universität, Rostock 1988 (S. 44–45)

Schultz-Coulon, H.-J., L. Eckermeier: Zum postnatalen Wachstum der Nasenscheidewand. Acta Oto-Laryng. (Stockh.) 82 (1976) 131–142

Scott, J. H.: The cartilage of the nasal septum. Brit. Dent. J. 95 (1953) 37–44

Scott, J. H.: Growth at facial sutures. Amer. J. Orthodont. 42 (1956) 381–387

Scott, J. H.: Studies in facial growth. Dent. Practit. Dent. Rec. 7 (1957) 344–345

Scott, J. H.: The growth of the human skull. J. Dent. Ass. S. Afr. 13 (1958) 133–142

Scott, J. H.: Further studies on the growth of the human face. Proc. Roy. Soc. Med. 52 (1959) 263–268

Scott, J. H.: The analysis of the facial growth from fetal life to adulthood. Angle Orthodont. 33 (1963) 110–113

Seifert, M.: Verbindungen der Nasenknorpel untereinander und zum knöchernen Skelett. Diss., Würzburg 1969

Seifert, K.: Die Ultrastruktur des Riechepithels beim Makrosmatiker. In: Bargmann, W., W. Doerr: Normale und pathologische Anatomie. Monographien in zwangloser Folge, Heft 21. Thieme, Stuttgart 1970 (S. 1–99)

Šercer, A.: Plastische Operationen an der Nase. In: Šercer, A., K. Mündnich: Plastische Operationen an der Nase und an der Ohrmuschel. Thieme, Stuttgart 1962

Sewall, E. C.: External operation on the ethmosphenoid frontal group of sinuses under local anesthesia: technic for removal of part of optic foramen wall for the relief of pressure on the optic nerve. Arch. Otolaryng. 4 (1926) 377

Seydel, O.: Über die Nasenhöhle der höheren Säugetiere und des Menschen. Gegenbaurs Morph. Jb. 17 (1891) 44–99

Shaheen, O. H.: Arterial epitaxis. J. Laryng. 89 (1975) Heft 1

Shaheen, O. H.: Nose and throat. In: Rob, C., R. Smith: Operative Surgery, 3rd ed. Butterworth, London 1976 (p. 632)

Sieglbauer, F.: Lehrbuch der normalen Anatomie des Menschen, 9th ed. Urban and Schwarzenberg, Wien 1963

Sieur-Jacob: Recherches anatomiques cliniques et opératoirs sur les fosses nasales et leurs sinus. Rueff, Paris 1901

Silberstein: Berl. Klin. Wschr. 43 (1906) 606 (cited by Plate S., s. Asboe 1981)

Simon, E.: Anatomy of the opening of the maxillary sinus. Arch. Otolarnyg. 29 (1939) 640–649

Skillern, R. H.: The catarrhal and suppurative diseases of the accessory sinuses of the nose. Lippincott, Philadelphia 1913 (p. 107)

Skillern, S. R.: Obliterative frontal sinusitis. Arch. Otolaryng. 23 (1936) 268–284

Sluder, G.: The role of the sphenopalatina (or Meckel's) ganglion in nasal headaches. Int. Rec. Med. 23 (1908) 989–990

Sluder, G.: The anatomical and clinical relations of the sphenopalatine (Meckel's) ganglion to the nose and its accessory sinuses. N. Y. Med. J. 90 (1909) 293–298

Smith, B., W. F. Regan, Jr.: Blow-out: fracture of the orbit: mechanism and correction of internal orbital fracture. Amer. J. Ophthal. 44 (1957) 733–739

Smith, C. G.: Incidence of atrophy of the olfactory nerves in man. Arch. Otolaryng. 34 (1941) 533–539

Soeprapto, M., A. Surjono: Bilateral choanal atresia. Paediat. Indones. 17 (1977) 255–260

von Spee, F.: Kopf. In: Bardelebens Handbuch der Anatomie des Menschen, Bd. I/2. Fischer, Jena 1896–1909

Spielberg, W.: Diagnosis of subacute and chronic inflammatory lesions of the mucosa lining the maxillary antrum of Highmore. N. Y. Med. J./Med. Rec. (N. Y.) 116 (1922a) 571

Spielberg, W.: Antroscopy of the maxillary sinus. Laryngoscope 32 (1922b) 441

Stenger, P.: Zur Technik der endonasalen Siebbeinoperation (einschließlich Keilbein und Stirnhöhle). Z. Ohrenheilk. (1912) 46–55

Stern, L.: Röntgenologische Betrachtung der Entwicklung und Ausdehnung der Nasennebenhöhlen. Hals-, Nas.- u. Ohrenarzt, 1. Teil 30 (1939) 169–199

Sternberg, M.: Ein bisher nicht beschriebener Kanal im Keilbein des Menschen und mancher Säugetiere. Ein Beitrag zur Morphologie der Sphenoidalregion. Arch. Anat. Physiol., Anat. Abt., Heft 5/6 (1890) 304–331

Stier, F.: Untersuchungen über die Verbiegungen der Nasenscheidewand. Diss., Rostock 1895

Stocksted, P.: The physiologic cycle of the nose under normal and pathologic conditions. Acta Oto-Laryng. (Stockh.) 42 (1952) 175

Straatman, N. J. A., C. T. Buiter: Endoscopic surgery of the nasal fontanel. Arch. Otolaryng. 107 (1981) 290–293

Straatsma, B. R., C. R. Straatsma: The anatomical relationship of the lateral nasal cartilage to the lateral nasal bone and the cartilaginous nasal septum. Plast. Reconstr. Surg. 8 (1951) 443–455

Straub, W.: Verletzungen der Orbita. Dtsch. Ärztebl. 21 (1972) 1347–1351

Streit, H.: Beitrag zur medianen Nasenfistel. Arch. Laryng. Rhin. (Berl.) 24 (1911) 454–458

Stubbe, C.: Variationsstatistische Untersuchungen an den Nerven- und Gefäßpforten des Gesichtsschädels. Diss., Würzburg 1976

Stupka, W.: Die Mißbildungen und Anomalien der Nase und des Nasenrachenraumes. Springer, Wien 1938

Suchannek, E.: Ein Fall von Persistenz des Hypophysenganges. Anat. Anz. 2 (1887) 520–525

Sunderlund, S., E. S. R. Hughes: The pupillo-constrictor pathway and the nerves to the ocular muscles in man. Brain 69 (1946) 301–309

Szilvássy, J.: Zur Entwicklung der Stirnhöhlen. Anthropol. Anz. 39 (1981) 138–149

Takagi, Y.: Human postnatal growth of vomer in relation to base of cranium. Ann. Otol. (St. Louis) 73 (1964) 238–247

Takagi, Y., J. F. Waters, J. F. Bosma: Anatomical studies of the epipharyngeal wall in relation to the base of the cranium. Ann. Otol. (St. Louis) 71 (1962) 366

Takahashi, R.: Surgery of the pterygopalatine fossa. A. N. L. 3 (1976) 1–29

Takahashi, R., M. Tsutsumi: Vidian neurectomy. O R L (Tokyo) 13 (1970) 719 (cited by R. Takahashi 1976)

Tanaka, T.: Ganglion sphenopalatinum des Menschen. Arb. 3. Abt. Anat. Inst. Kyoto 3 (1932) 91–115

Teed, R. W.: Meningitis from the sphenoid sinus. Arch. Otolaryng. 28 (1938) 589–619

Temesrekasi, D.: Mikroskopischer Bau und Funktion des Schwellgewebes der Nasenmuschel des Menschen. Z. Mikr.-Anat. Forsch. 80 (1969) 219–229

Terrahe, K.: Die hyperreflektorische Rhinopathie. HNO 33 (1985) 51–57

Terrahe, K., K. Mündnich: Gefahren und Komplikationen bei der transmaxillären Siebbein-Keilbeinhöhlenausräumung. Arch. Klin. Exp. Ohr.- Nas.- u. Kehlk.-Heilk. 205 (1973) 284–285

Terrahe, K., K. Mündnich: Gefahren und Komplikationen bei der transmaxillären Siebbein-Keilbeinhöhlen-Operation. Laryng. Rhinol. Otol. 53 (1974) 311–320

Theile, F. W.: Die Asymmetrien der Nase und des Nasenskelettes. Z. Rat. Med. (II. Folge) 6 (1855) 242

Thompson, J. N., M. W. Nicole, E. Wong, V. Passy, R. I. Kohut: Blindness following frontal sinus irrigation. Arch. Otolaryng. 106 (1980) 358–360

Thomson, S. C., V. E. Negus: Diseases of the Nose and Throat. Cassel, London 1948

Toldt, C.: Osteologische Mitteilungen. 1. Die Entstehung und Ausbildung der Conchae und der Sinus sphenoidales beim Menschen. Lotos, Jb. Naturwiss. (N. F.) 3/4 (1882) 1–20

Toldt, C.: Osteologische Mittheilungen. Zr. Heilk. (1883) (cited after E. D. Congdon 1920)

Tonndorf, W.: Zur Anatomie der Lamina cribrosa und der Crista olfactoria. Beitr. Anat. etc., Ohr. 23 (1926) 654–667

Topinard, P.: Anthropologie (Paris 1888), translated into German by R. Neuhauss, 2nd ed. Baldamus, Leipzig 1888

Tos, M., C. Mogensen: Density of mucous glands in the normal adult nasal septum. Arch. Oto-Rhino-Laryng. 214 (1976) 125–133

Tovi, F., J. Goldstein, J. Sidi: An unusual complication of maxillary sinusitis. J. Laryng. 97 (1983) 275–278

Tremble, G. E.: Distribution and comparison of nasal cilia. Arch. Otolaryng. 53 (1951) 481–491

Tunis, J. P.: Sphenoidal sinusitis in relation to optic neuritis. Laryngoscope (St. Louis) 22 (1912) 1157–1164

Turner, A. L.: The Accessory Sinuses of the Nose. Longmans, Green, New York 1902 (p. 43)

Turner, A. L., Porter, W. G.: The structural type of the mastoid process, based upon the skiagraphic examination of one thousand crania of various races of mankind. J. Laryng. 37 (1921) 115–121

Uddman, R., F. Sundler: Innervation of the upper airways. Clin. Chest Med. 7 (1986) 201–209

Valentin, A.: Die cytoskopische Untersuchung des Nasenrachens oder Salpingoskopie. Arch. Laryng. Rhin. (Berl.) 13 (1903) 401

Valentin, G.: Flimmerbewegung. In: Wagner, R.: Handbuch der Physiologie, Bd. I. Viehweg, Braunschweig 1842

van Alyea, O. E.: The ostium maxillare: anatomic study of its surgical accessibility. Arch. Otolaryng. 24 (1936) 553–569

van Alyea, O. E.: Ethmoid labyrinth. Arch. Otolaryng. 29 (1939) 881–902

van Alyea, O. E.: Sphenoid sinus anatomic study with consideration of the clinical significance of the structural characteristics of the sphenoid sinus. Arch. Otolaryng. 34 (1941) 225–253

van Alyea, O. E.: Frontal sinus drainage. Ann. Otol. (St. Louis) 55 (1946) 267–277

van der Hoeve, J.: Mucocèle der Keilbeinhöhle und hinteren Siebbeinzellen mit Atrophie des Sehnerven. Z. Augenheilk. 43 (1920) 223–242

van Gilse, P. H. G.: Zur Pneumatisation der Keilbeinhöhle. Z. Hals-, Nas.- u. Ohrenheilk. 3 (1922) (393) (cited by P. H. G. van Gilse 1926)

van Gilse, P. H. G.: Über die Bildung des Ostium sphenoidale anläßlich eines Präparates mit scheinbar fehlender Keilbeinhöhle. Acta Oto-Laryng. (Stockh.) 7 (1924/25) 192–198

van Gilse, P. H. G.: Über die Entwicklung der Keilbeinhöhle des Menschen. Beitrag zur Kenntnis der Pneumatisierung des Schädels von der Nase aus. Z. Hals-, Nas.- u. Ohrenheilk. 16 (1926) 202–298

Vetter, U., W. Pirsig, E. Heinze: Growth activity in human septal cartilage: age-dependent incorporation of labeled sulfate in different anatomic locations. Plast. Reconstr. Surg. 71 (1983) 167–179

Vetter, U., W. Pirsig, E. Heinze: Postnatal growth of the human septal cartilage. Acta Oto-Laryng. (Stockh.) 97 (1984) 131–136

Vidić, B.: The morphogenesis of the lateral nasal wall in the early prenatal life of man. Amer. J. Anat. 130 (1971) 121–140

Vidić, B., S. Radoievič: Note sur le prolongement du sinus sphénoidal dans la lame quadrilatère et l'apophyse clinoide postérieure. Acta anat. (Basel) 54 (1963) 368

Virchow, H.: Die anthropologische Untersuchung der Nase. Z. Ethnol. 44 (1912) 289–337

Virchow, R.: Cellular Pathology. Lippincott, Philadelphia 1863 (pp. 315–320)

Virchow, R.: Die krankhaften Geschwülste, Bd. III. Hirschwald, Berlin 1863–1867 (S. 456–463)

Vogt, K., F. Schrade: Anatomische Varianten des Ausführungsgangsystems der Stirnhöhle. Laryng. Rhinol. Otol. 58 (1979) 783–794

Waggershauser, C. P.: Badesinusitis am Bodensee und orbitale Komplikationen. Laryng. Rhinol. Otol. 59 (1980) 255–257

Waller: cited after W. Kley 1973

Watanabe, K., I. Watanabe: The ultrastructural characteristics of the capillary walls in human nasal mucosa. Rhinology 18 (1980) 183–195

Waterman, R. E., S. M. Meller: Alternations in the epithelial surface of human palatal shelves prior to and during fusion: a scanning electron microscope study. Anat. Rec. 180 (1974) 111–136

Weed, L. H.: Studies on the cerebro-spinal fluid. J. Med. Res. 31 (1914) 21–117

Wegener, U.: Meßvorgang und Normalwerte für ein neu entwickeltes Rhinomanometer. Diss., Würzburg 1983

Welcker, H.: Die Asymmetrien der Nase und des Nasenskelettes. Jubiläumsschrift, Geh. R. von Bischoff, Stuttgart 1882

Wertheim: cited after L. Grünwald 1925

Whitaker, S. R., P. M. Sprinkle, S. M. Chou: Nasal glioma. Arch. Otolaryng. 107 (1981) 550–554

Widdicombe, J. G.: The physiology of the nose. Clin. Chest Med. 7 (1986) 159–170

Wigand, M. E.: Transnasale, endoskopische Chirurgie der Nasennebenhöhlen bei chronischer Sinusitis. I. Ein bio-mechanisches Konzept der Schleimhautchirurgie. HNO 29 (1981) 215–221

Wigand, M. E.: personal communication, 1986

Wigand, M. E., W. Hosemann: Endoscopic ethmoidectomy for chronic sinu-bronchitis. In Meyers, E.: New Dimensions in Otolaryngology – Head and Neck Surgery, Vol. I. Elsevier, Amsterdam 1985 (pp. 549–552)

Wigand, M. E., W. Steiner: Endonasale Kieferhöhlenoperation mit endoskopischer Kontrolle. Laryng. Rhinol. Otol. 56 (1977) 421–425

Wigand, M. E., W. Steiner, M. P. Jaumann: Endonasal surgery with endoscopical control: from radical operation to rehabilitation of the mucosa. Endoscopy 10 (1978) 255–260

Wilson, J. W., J. A. Gehweiler: Teratoma of the face associated with a patent canal extending into the cranial cavity Rathke's pouch in a three-week-old child. J. Pediat. Surg., Vol. 5, Nr. 3 (1970) 349–359

Witt, E.: Ausbreitung der Stirnhöhlen und Siebbeinzellen über die Orbita. Med. Diss., Rostock 1908

Wolfensberger, M.: Zur Pathogenese des Pneumosinus maxillaris dilatans. HNO 32 (1984) 518–520

Woo, J. K.: Ossification and growth of the human maxilla, premaxilla and palate bone. Anat. Rec. 105 (1949) 737–761

Wood, J. F.: The anterior superior alveolar nerve and vessels. J. Anat. (London) 73 (1939) 583–591

Woollard, H. H.: Vital staining of the leptomeninges. J. Anat. (London) 58 (1924) 89–100

Wustrow, F.: Schwellkörper am Septum nasi. Z. Anat. Entwickl.-Gesch. 116 (1951) 139–142

Yoffey, J. M., C. K. Drinker: Some observations on the lymphatics of the nasal mucous membrane in the cat and monkey. J. Anat. 74 (1940) 45–52

Yoshinaga, T.: Anatomische Untersuchungen der Kieferhöhle bei Japanern. Internat. Zbl. Laryngol. 23 (1909) 11 (cited after Salinger, S. 1939)

Zahn, E.: Klin. Mbl. Augenheilk. 18 (1910) 338 (cited after Plate, S., S. Asboe 1981)

Zange, J.: Das Schwellgewebe der Nase, besonders in seiner Beziehung zu den Nebenhöhlen und ihre Ausführungsgänge. Arch. Ohr.-Nas.- u. Kehlk.-Heilk. 147 (1940) 103–113

Zange, J.: Operationen im Bereich der Nase und ihrer Nebenhöhlen. In: Thiel, R.: Handbuch der Ophthalmologie, Operationslehre. VEB Thieme, Leipzig 1950 S. 1091–1342

Zarniko (1940): cited by W. Draf 1978

Zehm, S.: Die Bedeutung des Nasenseptums für die traumatisch geschädigte Nase. In Schuchardt, K.: Fortschritte der Kiefer- und Gesichts-Chirurgie, Bd. XII. Thieme, Stuttgart 1967 (offprint)

Zehm, S.: Eosinophiles Granulom des Stirnbeines. HNO 13 (1965) 66–69

Ziegelmayer, G.: Äußere Nase. In Becker, P. E.: Humangenetik. Ein kurzes Handbuch in fünf Bänden, Bd. I/2. Thieme, Stuttgart 1969 (S. 56–81)

Zuckerkandl, E.: Normale und pathologische Anatomie der Nasenhöhle und ihrer pneumatischen Anhänge. Braumüller, Wien 1882 (S. 134–135)

Zuckerkandl, E.: Über den Zirkulationsapparat in der Nasenschleimhaut. Kaiserl.-Königl. Hof- und Staatsdruckerei, Wien 1884

Zuckerkandl, E.: Die Siebbeinmuscheln des Menschen. Anat. Anz. 7 (1892) 13–25

Zuckerkandl, E.: Normale und pathologische Anatomie der Nasenhöhle und ihrer pneumatischen Anhänge. Anatomie der Nasenscheidewand, Bd. II Braumüller, Wien 1892 (S. 6–9, 212–222 u. Tafeln)

Zuckerkandl, E.: Normale und pathologische Anatomie der Nasenhöhle und ihrer pneumatischen Anhänge. 2nd ed., Bd. I. Braumüller, Wien 1893 (S. 368–400)

Zuckerkandl, E.: Die Entwicklung des Siebbeins. Anat. Anz. 6 (1892) 261–264

Zuckerkandl, E.: Geruchsorgan. In Merkel, F., R. Bonnet: Ergebnisse der Anatomie und Entwicklungsgeschichte. Bergmann, Wiesbaden 1896

Index